C. R.
BSc.,
UNIT
KINGS
DERBY

CW00557043

Health Care and
Human Behaviour

Health Care and Human Behaviour

Edited by

ANDREW STEPTOE and
ANDREW MATHEWS

Department of Psychology
St. George's Hospital Medical School
University of London
England

1984

ACADEMIC PRESS

(Harcourt Brace Jovanovich, Publishers)

London   Orlando   San Diego   San Francisco   New York
Toronto   Montreal   Sydney   Tokyo   São Paulo

ACADEMIC PRESS INC. (LONDON) LTD.
24–28 Oval Road
London NW1 7DX

United States Edition Published by
ACADEMIC PRESS INC.
(Harcourt Brace Jovanovich Inc.)
Orlando, Florida 32887

British Library Cataloguing in Publication Data

Health care and human behaviour.
1. Medicine and psychology
I. Steptoe, A.   II. Mathews, A.
610   R726.5

ISBN 0–12–666460–9

LCCCN 83–73317

Typeset and printed in Great Britain at The Pitman Press, Bath

Contributors

H. Anisman Department of Psychology, Carleton University, Ottawa, Ontario K1S 5B6, Canada

S. Arndt Fachberich Erziehungswissenschaften der Universität Göttingen, 3400 Göttingen, Wilhelmsplatz 1, Federal Republic of Germany

M. H. Becker Department of Health Behavior and Health Education, School of Public Health, The University of Michigan, Ann Arbor, Michigan 48109, USA

G. W. Brown Department of Sociology, (Fraser Lodge), Bedford College, Regents Park, London NW1 4NS, England

T. K. J. Craig Department of Sociology, (Fraser Lodge), Bedford College, Regents Park, London NW1 4NS, England

R. L. Cromwell Department of Psychiatry, Division of Research, University of Rochester Medical Center, 300 Crittenden Boulevard, Rochester, New York 14642, USA

R. Grossarth-Maticek Interdiszplinares Forschungsprogramm Sozialwissenschaftliche Onkologie, Prospektive Epidemiologie und experimentelle Verhaltensmedizin, Hauptstrasse 27, 6900 Heidelberg, Federal Republic of Germany

D. W. Johnston Psychological Treatment Research Unit, The Warneford Hospital, Oxford OX3 7JX, England

S. V. Kasl Department of Epidemiology and Public Health, Yale University School of Medicine, 60 College Street, P. O. Box 3333, New Haven, Connecticut 06510, USA

W. Langosch Benedikt Kreuz Rehabilitationszentrum für Herz-und Kreislaufkranke, Fachbereich Psychologie/Psychotherapie, Südring 15, 7812 Bad Krozingen, Postfach 140, Federal Republic of Germany

J. C. Levenkron Department of Psychiatry, Division of Research, University of Rochester Medical Center, 300 Crittenden Boulevard, Rochester, New York 14642, USA

P. Maguire Department of Psychiatry, University Hospital of South Manchester, West Didsbury, Manchester M20 8LR, England

A. Mathews Department of Psychology, St. George's Hospital Medical School, University of London, Cranmer Terrace, Tooting, London SW17 0RE, England

V. Ridgeway Department of Psychology, St. George's Hospital Medical School, University of London, Cranmer Terrace, Tooting, London SW17 0RE, England

I. M. Rosenstock Department of Health and Health Education, School of Public Health, The University of Michigan, Ann Arbor, Michigan 48109, USA

P. Schmidt Fachbereich Gesellschaftswissenschaften der Universität Giessen, 6300 Giessen, Ludwigstrasse 23, Federal Republic of Germany

L. S. Sklar Department of Psychology, Carleton University, Ottawa, Ontario K1S 5B6, Canada

A. Steptoe Department of Psychology, St. George's Hospital Medical School, University of London, Cranmer Terrace, Tooting, London SW17 0RE, England

H. Vetter Interdiszplinares Forschungsprogramm Sozialwissenschaftliche Onkologie, Prospektive Epidemiologie und experimentelle Verhaltensmedizin, Hauptstrasse 27, 6900 Heidelberg, Federal Republic of Germany

Preface

Recent years have witnessed a rapid expansion in the applications of the behavioural sciences to medical problems outside the psychiatric domain. These range from analyses of the communications between doctors and patients to direct treatments with psychophysiological and behaviour modification programmes. Sophisticated psychosocial methodologies are also being used to identify the role of cognitive and emotional factors in the aetiology of medical disorders, and to alleviate the distress associated with modern clinical procedures.

Health Care and Human Behaviour outlines a number of significant developments in this area. It draws together leading authorities on different aspects of behavioural medicine and health care from Europe and North America. All have recently been involved in major research projects in their fields of expertise, and so write from a basis of practical as well as theoretical knowledge. A number of different research strategies is represented, each aimed at identifying the place of behaviour in medicine, and the ways in which it can be exploited in health care. We have divided the book into three major sections, each dealing with a different approach to the links between health and behaviour. These are prefaced by introductions that draw out some of the themes common to the chapters.

Part I of *Health Care and Human Behaviour* concerns the role of social and behavioural factors in the development of medical disorders. It is essential for the future of the discipline that advances in aetiological and intervention research progress in tandem. For, if treatments are not based on an understanding of causal aspects, therapeutic methods are at risk of being superficial and inappropriate. Parts II and III then describe a number of areas of practice and treatment to which behavioural scientists have made important contributions. Psychosocial interventions in non-psychiatric medicine can perhaps be seen as taking three forms. Firstly, there are a variety of procedures that facilitate medical and surgical treatments, improving the efficiency of their application and distribution. These behavioural adjuncts to treatment are discussed in the four chapters of Part II. Secondly, much research has been concerned with the psychosocial consequences of medical conditions, and the potential of behavioural techniques for the alleviation of distress. Finally, behavioural methods may be adopted as alternatives to conventional treatments. Examples of these two types of intervention are provided in Part III.

Inevitably, there are omissions from the coverage provided in this book. The selection of aetiological research is incomplete, while topics such as pain management, chronic illness behaviour and preventive behavioural procedures certainly deserve attention. These subjects must, however, be kept for more specialized volumes. Nevertheless, we hope that *Health Care and Human Behaviour* provides a useful overview of important trends in the application of behavioural sciences to medicine. The Editors are most grateful to all the contributors and other colleagues whose work and encouragement have led to the publication of *Health Care and Human Behaviour*. Special thanks are also due to Sue Wilson and Margaret Reuben for their secretarial support.

March, 1984   Andrew Steptoe
St. George's Hospital   Andrew Mathews

Contents

6. Compliance with Medical Advice   175
MARSHALL H. BECKER and IRWIN M. ROSENSTOCK

7. Psychological Care of Acute Coronary Patients   209
RUE L. CROMWELL and JEFFREY C. LEVENKRON

8. Psychological Preparation for Surgery   231
ANDREW MATHEWS and VALERIE RIDGEWAY

Part One

Psychosocial Factors in the Aetiology of Medical Disorders

Introduction

The contributions to Part I address the proposition that actions, emotions and the social environment influence the development of medical disorders. These factors may either have long-term effects on disease processes, or else trigger clinical symptoms in the predisposed, pathologically vulnerable individual. Research concerning the aetiological role of psychosocial factors derives from several disciplines. Firstly, the physiological and behavioural mechanisms that mediate between psychosocial experiences and organic pathology must be specified. Secondly, it is necessary to demonstrate that these mechanisms are sufficiently sensitive to behavioural and emotional challenges to account for clinical disorders; this problem is primarily studied in the experimental laboratory, where it is possible to determine whether functional modifications of an appropriate intensity and duration are elicited by environmental stimuli. Ultimately, however, the processes detailed experimentally must be confirmed in the clinical and epidemiological context. It is incumbent on the researcher into psychosocial aetiology to show that the patterns of the disease and adverse life experience are consistent with the putative mechanisms and hypothetical links. Moreover, the relevance of these processes to the individual patient needs to be documented.

The four chapters of Part I summarize much of the evidence in these different realms. The chapters are ordered to produce a progressive narrowing down in subject matter and research strategy, from broad statistical associations between illness and experience or incidents in the social environment, through personal life styles and actions, to the psychophysiological, endocrinological and immunological mechanisms mediating these effects within the organism. The first two contributions document the impact of acute events and chronic psychosocial stressors. Craig and Brown (Chapter 1) provide a detailed critique of questionnaire techniques for the evaluation of life events, underlining the methodological and empirical inadequacies of such procedures. The interview method they recommend takes account of the context in which life events occur, leading to a fuller understanding of the meaning of such events in the respondent's life. Although interview methods have been introduced comparatively recently, a sound data base linking life events with organic symptoms and some physical disorders is gradually being established.

Although self-administered paper and pencil methods appear to be of little value in the investigation of acute life events, questionnaire and other conventional survey instruments remain central to the studies of chronic life stress described by Kasl in Chapter 2. One of the major factors confusing research in this area is the vagueness of the elusive concept of stress, and Kasl offers a way forward through detailed analysis of the different elements contributing to personal experience in a specific environment. This is illustrated through research in occupational settings. Kasl's conclusions are optimistic, since the failure of many psychosocial disturbances to predict morbidity suggests that humans are remarkably adaptive and resilient when faced with adverse conditions. Craig and Brown also draw attention to the personal resources, coping abilities and social supports upon which people may draw when exposed to severe stresses.

The distinction between acute events and chronically stressful conditions is convenient but in no sense hard and fast. As Kasl points out, most acute adverse experiences have enduring consequences that may be of lasting significance in health and disease. Conversely, acute episodes may be superimposed on chronic harassment. The contrast between short and long term effects highlights a major issue in laboratory research concerning the mechanisms responsible for translating life experiences into organic pathology. Both Steptoe (Chapter 3) and Anisman and Sklar (Chapter 4) show that acute experimental paradigms have serious limitations when evaluating potentially pathological processes, since reaction patterns alter radically over time. Steptoe's chapter is primarily concerned with theories linking physiological and endocrine reactions to behavioural challenges on the one hand, and organic pathology on the other. He finds that much psychophysiological research is based on implicit models that lack strong empirical support. Progress depends on much closer definitions of experimental parameters at the expense of global descriptions of stressful stimuli. Nevertheless, for some disorders (particularly those of the cardiovascular system) cross-sectional data favouring psychophysiological mediation between behavioural stimulation and organic pathology has accumulated. The most pressing need at present is for long term prospective studies.

Anisman and Sklar detail the evidence for behavioural influences on immunological and neuroendocrine mechanisms in Chapter 4. Drawing on acute animal investigations, they find substantial evidence for the effects of behavioural stimulation on neurotransmitter pathways in several parts of the brain. Peripheral neuroendocrine and immunological parameters are also responsive, although effects are highly dependent on experimental parameters such as time course and duration of exposure and the availability of avoidance responses. The last part of Chapter 4 documents the manner in which behavioural factors may affect malignant tumour growth. These data provide the fundamental basis for discussions of psychological influences on cancer in humans. They are pertinent therefore to Chapter 11, where psychological interventions with cancer patients are described.

All four chapters in Part I draw attention to the diversity of potential mechanisms mediating the links between psychosocial environment and organic pathology. The possibilities are enumerated in most detail by Craig and Brown and by Steptoe, all of whom commend an attitude of scepticism concerning the pathological consequences of adverse experience. Although effects may emerge through direct influences on physiological stress responses and neuroendocrine processes, behavioural pathways must also be considered. Nor is this possibility absent in animal research. Anisman and Sklar point out how changes in behaviour, such as reduced eating or fighting, may modulate the effects of experimental stressors on immunological responses and tumour growth.

It will be evident to the reader that none of the contributors to Part I have glossed over the inconsistencies and inadequacies of much aetiological research. Kasl, for example, notes that data on environmental hazards such as noise, crowding and institutionalization are mixed and far from coherent. But this should not foster a pessimistic attitude; it is by confronting inconsistencies and teasing out discrepancies that further insight will be gained into intervening variables and adaptive mechanisms. These in turn give hope that aetiological research will have direct implications for the management and control of those psychosocial processes that affect health and well-being.

1

Life Events, Meaning and Physical Illness A Review

T. K. J. CRAIG and G. W. BROWN

Before asking whether physical manifestations of disease can arise from life events, it is necessary to look at methods of measuring the events themselves, and the troublesome methodological issues surrounding such aetiological studies.

MEASUREMENT OF LIFE EVENTS

The Schedule of Recent Experiences (SRE), developed by Holmes and Rahe (1967), has been much the most commonly used instrument and well illustrates what may be termed a *dictionary* approach to meaning. Rahe, in discussing its development, noted that interviews were used to assess the meaning of events, and, as expected, significance varied widely between individuals. However, one theme appeared common to most of the events: "The occurrence of each usually evoked, or was associated with, some adaptive or coping behaviour on the part of the involved individual". Thus, in the questionnaire, each item was "constructed to contain a life event whose advent is either indicative of, or requires a significant change in the ongoing life-pattern of the individual. The emphasis is on change from the existing steady state of adjustment and not on psychological meaning, emotional or social desirability" (Rahe, 1969, p. 98). Each broad type of event was given a simple definition and "weighted" in terms of its propensity to produce change and disruption, with the impli- cit assumption that events such as births of babies can be treated as

HEALTH CARE AND HUMAN BEHAVIOUR
ISBN 0–12–666460–9

comparable, in the sense that they are all likely to involve much the same amount of change and make broadly similar demands on adjustment. Assessment of the amount of disruption involved in each type of event was made by a body of judges (taken from the general population), on the basis of brief statements supplied by the investigators about each type of event. These judges were asked to allocate a score to each event in terms of an arbitrary score given to one event (usually loss of spouse). The amount of change involved in the event was then obtained by averaging the scores of the judges. Finally, it was assumed that the impact of different events is additive: the scores were summed with the implication that the greater the overall score, the greater the adverse effect.

Recent studies suggest that this time-consuming procedure may be unnecessary, in the sense that total scores of "life change" add nothing to those obtained by a simple count of events (Lorimer et al., 1979). Such a result is understandable in an instrument using a number of items which tend to be correlated (Lei and Skinner, 1980). The assumptions about comparability of apparently similar events (in terms of their demands on adjustment) have never, to our knowledge, been put to any direct test. Moreover, apparently similar levels of disruption can vary greatly in meaning. A birth may involve major changes for a woman (say a move to a new town and loss of job) but be seen as entirely welcome and positive, while to another woman it may bring about small changes in activity but be seen as unwelcome and disruptive. Totman has argued that meaning must be taken into account in the development of measures of change, but in practice he appears to have considered only net change in time spent on purposeful activity and the amount of net change in time spent on informal activity (Totman, 1979, p. 189). It is difficult to conceive of the issue being tackled effectively by dictionary-type instruments, which (as we have seen) ignore variability in context; and it remains uncertain how far scores on an instrument such as the Schedule of Recent Experiences reflect the impact of the disruptiveness of events, some aspects of meaning, or both.

We believe that the only effective way forward is to deal with individual variability in response and to measure both degree of disruptiveness and aspects of meaning, in order to sort out their respective aetiological contributions. Nonetheless, it is probably worth keeping two riders in mind. Even if meaning is important, it may not prove easy to deal with certain major changes in habit (say, a move from the country to a large city), the meaning of which may be beyond the comprehension of many caught up in them. Here, a straightforward description of the move may be the most effective way to proceed. There is also the possibility that for some events (for example, involvement in a particularly frightening road accident) meaning may differ so little between subjects that its exploration for the individual may be irrelevant.

Despite these qualifications, there is growing agreement that the meaning of "life events" needs to be taken into account. This has led to a number of interesting attempts with dictionary-type measures to reflect qualities of events other than amount of change in usual activity, such as in terms of their unpleasantness. In practice, this has meant dealing with characteristics of particular events rather than an overall score. But despite this concern with meaning, measurement is still in terms of classes of event; for instance, an investigator still has to make up his or her mind to characterize a birth as "pleasant" or "unpleasant". At best only *general meaning* is dealt with, and the variety of circumstances that might surround the birth of a child which would give it a different *specific meaning* for the individual are ignored.

A dictionary approach to life events almost always uses a respondent-based method to collect material. Before moving on to consider more intricate measures, it is perhaps worthwhile to summarize a few of its drawbacks. Typically, a standardized questionnaire is used and the subject asked whether or not a particular event, such as "illness of a relative" has occurred. It is respondent-based in the sense that it is the respondent who decides which relative and what illnesses to include. This vagueness is bound to lower the reliability and accuracy of the instrument and subject aetiological research to the threat of serious sources of bias (Brown and Harris, 1981). For example, it is possible that who is defined as a "relative", and what is serious enough to count as an "illness", may be influenced by a respondent's attempt to make sense of the fact that he or she has developed a particular disorder. The death of a distant uncle may only be mentioned because it happended to be closely juxtaposed in time with the onset of the respondent's own disorder. Prospective research would not necessarily rule out such threats to validity (Brown, 1981). It has been suggested, for example, that agreement on items of the SRE will be influenced by the subject's personality, attitudes or even mood at the time of its completion (Sarason *et al.*, 1975). Indeed, as Lauer (1973) has demonstrated, there are associations between high scores on the SRE and the Taylor Manifest Anxiety Scale. The Holmes–Rahe Schedule of Recent Experiences (SRE) has been criticized both in terms of such possible sources of invalidity and in terms of actual inaccuracy in reporting, irrespective of whether or not this is in any way linked to biased reporting of the kind just outlined (Brown, 1974, 1981; Jenkins *et al.*, 1979; Sarason *et al.*, 1975; Weshow and Reinhart, 1974). In a a recent enquiry, the average agreement between respondent and spouse about particular "events" during the previous two months was only about one third, and even when only potentially clear-cut incidents are included, agreement (using kappa) was only 0.42 (Yager *et al.*, 1981). This low level of agreement is almost certainly due to the vagueness of many of the questions of the SRE and its failure to question the respondent further about his or her replies. It is, therefore, possible that in certain circumstances respondent-based methods may, as a result of bias, exaggerate any association between life events and illness; and on other occasions, when to some degree such bias has been brought under control (say, in prospective research), their general inaccuracy and insensitivity may lead to a low association. Certainly, inconsistency in results has been the hallmark of research using respondent-based and dictionary approaches to meaning.

An alternative approach to measurement attempts to deal with meaning for the individual. We will refer to it as *contextual*, in recognition of the fact that *specific meaning* is dealt with by taking into account the circumstances surrounding a particular event. The Bedford College "Life Events and Difficulties Schedule" (LEDS), using a semi-structured interview, gathers as coherent and as full an account as possible of any incident which may be relevant to the research enquiry. First, the interviewer establishes the presence or otherwise of 40 types of possible event. Although the procedure differs markedly from that of the SRE, it is at this stage no more than a dictionary-type instrument. However, unlike other instruments, it covers the occurrence of ongoing difficulties as well as discrete life events (Brown and Harris, 1978, Chapter 8). Once the occurrence of an event or a difficulty has been established, a second level of interviewing allows the investigator to specify various aspects of meaning.

How far is it possible for this to be done and yet avoid potential bias? One way to avoid it would be to interview subjects before the development of any disorder. However, for most physical conditions it is probable that the time interval between event and onset is only a matter of weeks or even days; the number of interviews that would be necessary to pick up events before the disorder occurred would make such an approach quite impractical. Because of these logistic problems, some kind of retrospective design is likely to be necessary. It is essential that measurement of events can rule out the possibility that replies have been influenced by the kind of "effort after meaning" already outlined. With the LEDS, a set of previously developed rules and detailed questioning is used to decide whether or not an event is to be included. There is, therefore, no question of including the death of a distant uncle if this is not already covered by rules about what can and cannot be defined as an "event". Once the presence of an "event" is settled, its likely meaning is characterized by the use of ratings that take account of a person's biography and current circumstances. In assessing, say, the threat of having a third child in an overcrowded flat, raters make an estimate of what most persons in such circumstances would be likely to feel, by taking into account what is known of the person's plans and purposes, as these are reflected in his or her biographical circumstances. By ignoring self-reports about meaning, various potential sources of bias stemming from the respondent can be ruled out; and by using raters who are ignorant of such self-reports, potential bias stemming from the investigator is brought under control. It is important to note that the approach avoids altogether any judgement about the likely causal link between event and disorder; indeed, it is essential to keep from the raters who make the contextual ratings not only anything about what the subject said he or she felt, but also whether or not the event was followed by the onset of illness or disorder.

A crucial advantage of this approach is its ability to measure the "severity" of a given type of event. "Severity" in the LEDS is assessed in terms of the immediate or more protracted impact of stressful events, but can be utilized to measure other qualities, such as loss, danger and chances of resolution. The method has a high rate of inter-rater reliability for the occurrence, severity and dating of events (Brown and Harris, 1978, 1982). Evidence of "construct" validity is also provided by, for example, the association of severe "loss" events with onset of clinical depression, and severe "danger" with anxiety states, and events involving both "loss" and "danger" with the onset of mixed depressive and anxiety disorders (Finlay-Jones and Brown, 1981).

Returning to the measurement of events in general, there has been a fairly close correspondence between theoretical perspective and approach to measurement. Those emphasizing change and disruption have usually followed a respondent-based approach and utilized questionnaires, and those emphasizing the importance of specific meaning, an interview and investigator-based approach. However, some of the former group have amended the SRE to take account of general meaning, and have also tended to move towards a more flexible mode of interviewing. The life-event instrument and interview developed by Paykel and his colleagues, although dealing only with general meaning, was sufficient to establish an important aetiological link between life events and onset of depression (Paykel, 1974; Paykel et al., 1969). Research has now reached a point where it is essential to deal with specific meaning, if more effective theory is to be developed—for instance, in exploring the role of social support in buffering the impact of events. Nonetheless, the measurement of general meaning may be sufficient to make a case for causal links and much of the research we will review employs such an approach.

MEASUREMENT OF PHYSICAL SYMPTOMS

Any study of stress and physical symptoms must deal with the frequent association of somatic symptoms and affective disorders, particularly depression. For example, estimates of the prevalence of pain complaints among depressed in- and out-patients range between 60% and 100% (Von Knoring, 1965; Ward *et al.*, 1979), while recent reports of attenders at pain clinics have found that up to 87% of attenders met widely recognized criteria for major depressive disorder. Furthermore, there is evidence to suggest that some somatic symptoms are partially, or completely alleviated by treatment with anti–depressant drugs (Lindsay and Wykoff, 1981; Ward *et al.*, 1979). For the most part, studies of stress and physical illness gloss over these issues. There is usually no attempt made to separate symptoms due to "organic" pathology from those which simply reflect psychological states. This is surprising, given the evidence above, and the known prevalence of somatic symptoms of psychological origin among patients attending general practitioners and out-patient clinics (Culpin and Davies, 1960; Goldberg, 1970; Lipowski, 1967; Shepherd *et al.*, 1966).

Given current understanding, it is possible to classify somatic symptoms into three broad groups:

(i)   those whose basis can be shown to lie in structural damage to a specific organ or group of organs, with demonstrable morphological or physiological changes;

(ii) those whose origins are most clearly related to mental-state abnormalities, such as muscle-tension pains and the autonomic accompaniments of anxiety;

(iii) and a third group, which somewhat straddles these two, in so far as physical symptoms appear closely to mimic those of established organic disease, but where no structural or physiological basis can be demonstrated and which are not invariably associated with alterations of mental state. Such disorders include the "irritable colon syndrome" and "functional dyspepsia".

Of course, in practice, such separation may prove difficult, especially with those organic disorders which exhibit both morphological and psychiatric components (such as certain endocrine disorders, e.g. hypothyroidism). Nevertheless, we feel such attempts are imperative if progress is to be made towards demonstrating causal associations between stressful experience and physical ill-health.

Any such demonstration is complicated by evidence that a host of psychological and environmental factors directly influence attendance at health centres and helping agencies in general. As Mechanic points out, information used in the majority of life-event studies is bound to be influenced by individual differences in the propensity to perceive "illness" and to seek treatment: "Just as symptoms may be a cause of visiting the doctor, or taking time off work, they may also serve as an excuse to do so."

(Mechanic, 1974, p. 89). Mechanic showed that students who were "inclined to use the sick role" (as measured by a set of hypothetical questions) were also somewhat more frequent users of medical facilities when experiencing periods of stress (Mechanic and Volkart, 1961). To complicate the issues surrounding "illness behaviour" still further, there is evidence to suggest that after presenting particular symptoms to a family physician, whether or not a patient will be referred for specialist advice, and if so to what service, is influenced by cultural and socio-economic factors.

Finally, both illness onsets and events require precise dating before possible aetiological links can be established with any confidence. Neglect of this central issue is probably related to the widespread use of respondent-based instruments, which by their very nature rule out the kind of probing that is required.

STATISTICAL ISSUES

Most results in recent years have been presented in terms of the beguilingly straightforward notion of "variance explained" (r^2), based on squaring the correlation coefficient between "events" and "disorder". There must be some uncertainty about how far "variance explained" is a suitable notion to apply to data which is usually expressed in terms of simple dichotomized independent and dependent variables (e.g. event yes/no, disorder yes/no). However, the use of "dummy" variables in regression analysis has widespread acceptance and we believe "variance explained" to have more serious shortcoming as an index for aetiological research.

The amount of variance "explained" by life events is invariably low, usually no more than about 10%, and in studies using the SRE it it is commonly a good deal lower. Some reviewers have seen such results as indicating that life events are unlikely to have clinical or preventive importance (e.g. Andrews and Tennant, 1978). The likely error involved in this kind of interpretation can be readily illustrated by the fact that although most instances of lung cancer are associated with heavy smoking, much less than 1% of the variance is explained by this link. This apparently puzzling result is simple enough to explain: the index takes account of the fact not only that most with lung cancer are heavy smokers, but that most heavy smokers do not have lung cancer. Since the latter are far more common than the former, the fact that most with lung cancer are heavy smokers gets swamped in the "two-way" measure of association. This is much like the situation with depression. Although the majority developing depression experience an event before onset, usually involving a major loss or disappointment, most experiencing such events do not develop depression.

There has been extremely little discussion of the shortcomings of variance explained as a statistic, although warnings have occasionally been made (e.g. Rosenthal and Rubin, 1979). One of the confusions surrounding this issue is probably the notion of what is an "important" causal factor. "Variance explained" focuses on the sufficiency of a causal factor, but does not take account of its necessity, which is just as relevant in terms of causality. Thus, the presence of an invading bacterium, while a necessary condition of an infectious disorder, may contribute only a small amount to the "variance explained", since the symptoms depend crucially upon the state of host resistance or vulnerability, and a great many with the bacterium alone do not develop symptoms of the infection. Yet no-one could say that the tubercle bacillus was not important in the onset of tuberculosis.

It is, therefore, essential to consider alternatives. Paykel, in an excellent review, suggests three: attributable risk, relative risk and brought forward time (Paykel, 1978). "Attributable risk percent" is the proportion of disorder that can be attributed to the experience of risk factor. Although it is dependent on our knowledge of the frequency of cases of disorder under investigation in the general population, it can be estimated for case–control designs (e.g. Cole and MacMahon, 1971; Markush, 1977). The "x" index utilized by Brown and Harris (1978, pp. 117–121) is strictly comparable to "attributable risk percent".

"Relative risk" expresses the chance of developing a disorder as a ratio between the rate of the disorder among those exposed and those unexposed to the causal agent. The index can be used in most case–control designs, given that the number of people in the population affected by the disorder is relatively small compared with the number unaffected, as is the case for many psychiatric disorders and "specified" physical illnesses (MacMahon and Pugh, 1970).

"Brought forward time" is the average time by which a spontaneous onset can be considered to have been "brought forward" by the risk factor (Brown et al., 1973; Brown and Harris, 1978).

In the majority of studies of physical disorder these measures have not been used, probably because it is difficult to utilize them using the average scores employed in SRE studies. However, their utility can be demonstrated by examining work with psychiatric disorders using relative risk and attributable risk percent (Table I). Attributable risk percent, from an intuitive point of view, is a particularly satisfactory index of the importance of an aetiological effect, as it gives the proportion of cases associated with the putative causal risk factor, allowing for the fact that they will in some instances be associated by chance. It is most accurately estimated when there is knowledge of the rate of the putative causal agent in the general

TABLE I Illustrative findings concerning the impact of life events and other risk factors in terms of relative risk and attributable risk per cent

Condition	Risk factor	Method of life event measurement[c]	Relative risk	Attributable risk per cent[a]	Sources
A. Cases part of a random population survey					
Depression	Severe events	C–I	15.1	57	Brown and Harris, 1978
Streptococcal throat infection	Upsetting events	SR–D	12.6	29	Meyer and Haggerty, 1962
Death from cancer of lung	Smoking	–	6.6	83	Doll and Peto, 1976
B. Patients with a representative comparison sample from general population					
Schizophrenia	All life events	D–I	6.4	50	Brown and Birley, 1968
Depression	Severe events	C–I	5.6	49	Brown and Harris, 1978
Depression	Undesirable events	D–I	4.0	33	Paykel, 1974
Anxiety	Danger events	C–I	12.5	65	Finlay-Jones and Brown, 1981
Suicide	Undesirable events	D–I	5.8	49	Paykel et al., 1975
Organic illness general practice (women 18–50)	Severe events	C–I	3.6	27	Murphy and Brown, 1980
Appendicitis non-inflamed	Severe events	C–I	4.3	50	Creed, 1981
C. Patients and matched control series					
Myocardial infarction	All events 6 weeks before onset		3.6	20	Connolly, 1976[b]
Sudden death in women	Previous psychiatric history		12.0	49	Talbot et al. (1977)
Major physical illness	Psychiatric disorder		3.6	50	Eastwood and Trevelyan, 1972
Other physical illness			2.8	36	

[a]Estimated from published data for illustrative purposes. For calculation certain assumptions have had to be made (see Cole and MacMahon, 1971).
[b]Six-week event rates as reported in personal communication (Connolly, 1982).
[c]D = Dictionary; SR = Self report; C = Contextual; I = Interview.

population from which the cases are drawn. This cannot be obtained from a matched-comparison type of design, but it can often be estimated from published epidemiological data, or even from the sample under investigation when certain conditions are met (Cole and MacMahon, 1971).

While relative risk tends to be fairly closely correlated with attributable risk per cent, the two indices can differ in the sense that relative risk may be large, but because few of the total cases in the population are brought about by the causal agent, attributable risk is low. Table I shows that depression and cancer of the lung are both high on relative risk and attributable risk, despite a low variance explained. It is perhaps worth noting that it follows from the earlier discussion of variance explained that its size will be dependent on the rate of the disorder in the population studied. It is because cancer of the lung is such a rare condition compared to the frequency of smoking, that "variance explained" is so very low, despite its high attributable risk per cent. Variance explained can, therefore, be increased by not using representative samples, as in, say, a matched control design. Thus, in the study of 50 schizophrenic patients reviewed in Table I, the variance explained is 8%, but the comparison series of 325 persons is far too small to be a true reflection of the appropriate ratio of schizophrenic patients in the general population. If this were done, the variance explained would be well under 1%. In so far as a comparison series underestimates the correct ratio of those with and without the disorder in the general population, the value of variance explained will be "inflated", although it will usually still tend to be low.

Although we have emphasized the shortcomings of "variance explained", it is worth noting that "predictive power" gained from the knowledge of a risk factor can often be enhanced by taking into account further factors which interact with it, for example, the amount of social support experienced at the time of an event. A low amount of "variance explained" can, therefore, be a useful reminder that, even when there is a high attributable risk percent, a great deal more may still be needed to specify the conditions under which the putative causal agent will have an effect. However, the same point can be made by noting the proportion of persons with an appropriate causal agent who do not develop the disorder. It is, therefore, desirable to take account of a number of indices to understand the aetiological implications of a particular set of results. We merely argue that, when considered alone, attributable risk percent and relative risk are likely to be less misleading than "variance explained"; nevertheless, their limitations must also be borne in mind.

STRESS AND LIFE EVENTS

Anticipating somewhat the results of this review, it is possible to construct a number of simple models to explain the apparent causal relationship between stressful life events and physical symptoms (see Fig.1). These provide basic elements around which the review will be assembled.

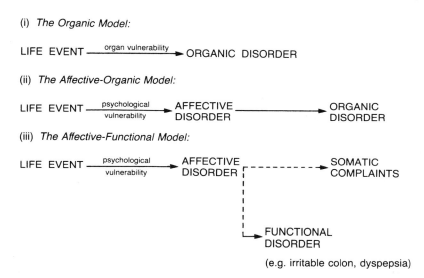

Fig. 1 Simple causal models relating life events and physical symptoms.

The organic model assumes direct causal association to exist between stress and organic disease, the particular organ system affected depending on some "organic vulnerability" (age, sex, genetic, previous physical disease and so forth).

The affective-organic model assumes that stressful events are only important in so far as they lead to an affective disorder, which in itself is the main risk factor for subsequent organic disorder. Appropriate vulnerabilities (psychological and organic) are important.

The affective-functional model seeks to explain physical symptoms either as somatic accompaniments of disturbed affect (muscle tension and palpitations in anxiety), or as "representations" of an affective disorder in which mood disturbance is minimal or denied by the patient.

A useful starting point for any review of stress and physical disorders is the work of Hinkle and his colleagues, which indicates that illness is distributed far from evenly in apparently fairly homogenous populations. Although Hinkle takes an extreme homeostatic view of the role of stress, emphasizing that stress can be a part of our most minor activities, the research itself dealt with what would appear to be far from trivial happenings. His findings are of particular interest as long time-periods are considered.

An early study used the health records of telephone company employees, as kept by the company's health centre. A reasonably good case was made that these were accurate for illness involving loss of time at work, although such a design has no way of ruling out a contribution from illness behaviour. Over a period as long as five to ten years, 10% of employees experienced one-third of the total number of episodes of illness (Hinkle *et al.*, 1956). It is noteworthy, given the potential bias introduced by illness behaviour, that findings persisted when only apparently major or potentially life-threatening illnesses were considered (e.g. heart disease, duodenal ulcer). The range of illnesses experienced by a person was directly related to the number of episodes, and usually a wide number of organ systems were involved. Illnesses appeared to occur in discrete time "clusters", at times when, with hindsight, the employees reported that their lives had been unsatisfying (Hinkle *et al.*, 1957, 1960).

In a number of subsequent prospective studies these general observations have been upheld. The first of these examined factors affecting the occurrence of acute episodes of relatively minor illness. A group of employees who worked in close physical proximity and came from broadly similar social and cultural backgrounds, were examined weekly for the development of symptoms of infection with common-cold viruses known to be prevalent in the community at the time. Given their close physical proximity, and the fact that most shared public transport facilities, it was presumed that their exposure to potential infection would be roughly comparable. Weekly observation over the six months of winter was supplemented by a personal diary of symptoms and activities. Development of respiratory illness was greatest in those women who had reported the majority of illnesses in the past, and in most cases, the infection appeared to be preceded by periods of physical strain or emotional arousal (Hinkle, 1974).

A further prospective study, again by Hinkle and his colleagues, failed to show associations (Hinkle *et al.*, 1974). There was no difference in occupational mobility between telephone company employees who died of coronary heart disease and those who died from other causes, or from those who remained alive. Furthermore, the rates of coronary heart disease in the most upwardly mobile group (those who had risen from shop-floor to managerial positions) were not statistically significantly different from those who had remained as workmen or foremen.

While these studies are of considerable interest, it is difficult to evaluate the likely overall impact of stressful experiences. Their measurement was crude, and Hinkle has argued that the effect of a social or interpersonal change on the health of individuals relates more to the previous health record and psychological characteristics of the individual than to any quality of the change itself. Furthermore, the noxious propensity of such changes were mediated by alterations in food intake, general activity, and exposure to potential sources of infection or physical trauma (Hinkle, 1974).

Another classic study reached rather more positive conclusions about the aetiological role of events. Meyer and Haggerty examined children at three-weekly intervals for streptococcal throat infections over the course of one year, during which time their parents were asked to keep a diary of events. There was an association between a family's experience of upsetting life events or chronic tension and the acquisition of infection, with or without symptoms (Meyer and Haggerty, 1962) (see Table I for results concerning frank illness). Although the study was not able to demonstrate just how far stress operated to influence the development of symptoms, it is of particular interest because of the suggestion that for some physical conditions at least, onset will follow emotional upset within a matter of a week or so. It is now fairly clear that this is the situation with the onset of florid symptoms of schizophrenia (Brown and Birley, 1968; Brown and Harris, 1978, pp. 124–126; Jacobs, Paykel and Prusoff, 1974; Leff and Vaughan, 1980) (see Table I).

About the time that these early studies were carried out, the bulk of research on life events and illness began to employ the SRE, developed by Holmes and Rahe. The initial work included studies of specific disorders, such as tuberculosis and inquinal hernia, as well as relatively minor health changes, and was based to a large extent on the use of health records and retrospective reporting of events (Holmes et al., 1957; Rahe, 1969; Rahe and Holmes, 1965). All appeared to demonstrate significant clustering of "changes" in the six months before onset of physical symptoms. However, as already noted, the SRE is incapable of finely dating life events and onset, and the studies may have reached quite erroneous conclusions about the time-period of relevance. It will be recalled that for streptococcal infections of the throat the two weeks before onset appeared to be critical. This discrepancy underlines a major unresolved issue—for physical illness, do events conform to what may be characterized as a depression model, in which impact may take as long as a year (although in practice most onsets occur within a few months), or a schizophrenia model, in which onset, if it is to occur, does so within a week or so of the event? It is probably also worth bearing in mind the third, as yet undocumented possibility, that for certain conditions, such as coronary heart disease, the impact of events may take several years before it has a visible effect in terms of illness.

Prospective research with naval personnel by Rahe and his colleagues broadly confirmed the earlier results, although the correlation between life-change scores and illness (either number of reported illnesses or those recorded on naval records) are very low: average correlations on one set of studies was 0.13 or 2% of variance (Rahe, 1974). The majority of illnesses in these naval studies were similar to the streptococcal infections studies by Meyer and Haggerty, in which the relevant time-period was two weeks, and yet no attempt was made to collect events for the six to eight months in which the men were at sea and during which time the record of illness utilized in the study was collected. Given this, it is possible that what predictive power life events had in these naval studies has little or nothing to do with events as such, but with the fact that the SRE is quite highly correlated with measures of personality and psychiatric dysfunction. Indeed, the fact that the best predictors of illness in the follow-up period were general psychosocial measures, such as being low paid, having an unskilled occupation and experiencing low job satisfaction, suggests that relevant life events were not recorded and that a verdict of "non-proven" seems the best scientific judgement to make about these otherwise apparently scientifically impressive prospective studies.

Of other prospective studies using the SRE which appear clearly to substantiate earlier cross-sectional work, in the sense of reporting a reasonably large association between life-changes and illness, one further study is worthy of special mention. In this study, 134 officer cadets completed the SRE for the preceding 18 months and subsequently a Health Checklist on each day of the initial two weeks' training period, and then again at intervals of four and eight months (Cline and Chosey, 1972). There was a significant positive correlation between the life-change scores after the 18 months preceding training and reported health-changes at two weeks four months, and eight months (Pearson's 'r' of 0.21, 0.34 and 0.30 respectively). It is possible that the inclusion of rather minor and vague complaints in the measure of illness ensured that an association due to response-set emerged. That is, someone tending to confirm the occurrence of vaguely formulated questions about life events might well, when seen at a later session, tend to report the occurrence of trivial and vague complaints.

A further prospective investigation by Theorell and his colleagues (1975) of a large number of Swedish middle-aged building workers, was unable to demonstrate a relationship between life-change scores and deaths or serious physical illness in the follow-up period. There was, however, a correlation between life-change and neurosis defined as suicide or psychiatric disorder associated with sick-leave for more than 30 days in the year. Similarly, Goldberg and Comstock (1976) in the United States were unable to demonstrate associations between experience of life-change and death or hospitalization for a major illness. It is of interest that, in the Swedish study, a crude measure of dissatisfaction did show some relationship with the development of myocardial infarction and death from all causes, and that one "life-change" (increased responsibility at work) preceded 19% of the infarcts and 9% of the total sample. Although these latter measures rely entirely on the reported feelings on the subject, the results are enough to remind us not to rule out the possibility of important psychosocial influences in the aetiology of coronary heart disease. The relationship of the crude measure of dissatisfaction both with myocardial infarction and the overall rate of death, possibly indicates that more general features of a person's life may play an aetiological role. The results also underline the point that very few life-event instruments have taken systematic account of ongoing long-term difficulties. Again, it would appear prudent not to place too much weight at present on these essentially negative findings.

SPECIFIC ILLNESS CONDITIONS

Theorell and Rahe (1971) report raised life-change scores prior to myocardial infarction in a retrospective study of an in-patient sample, and subsequently replicated these findings in an out-patient study (Rahe and Paasikivi, 1971). In the latter, the greatest "changes" occurred among coronary patients who died suddenly, before they could be admitted to hospital. This tendency for events to cluster before sudden death or an abrupt change in severity of pre-existing pathology has been demonstrated in other studies. That the more immediate impact of events may be important in "triggering" exacerbations of existing pathology is supported by a study of coronary heart disease using the earliest version of the LEDS. This was based only on the "dictionary" version, and assumed that all events defined as suitable for inclusion had a high likelihood of arousing significant emotion. For instance, hospital admissions of close relatives were only included if the condition was serious or the admission lasted at least one week. On average, a person in London experienced about three such events per year, although there was a wide distribution ranging from nil to over twenty. Connolly (1976) demonstrated that more patients than comparison subjects reported "independent" events (i.e. those which were on logical grounds unlikely to be directly related to the condition under study) in the few weeks prior to infarct. It should be noted that it was the occurrence of particular events, not number of events or a "life-change score", that was implicated. The result is, in fact, somewhat comparable to that obtained for schizophrenic patients and streptococcal infections of the throat (see Table I).

There have been relatively few studies of infectious conditions and dictionary-type measures. Amongst the more interesting is one exploring the effects of recent life stress on the development of experimentally induced common colds in 52 volunteer subjects (Totman et al., 1980). Life stress, measured by an instrument consisting of elements of the SRE and the LEDS, was related to the objective magnitude of infection (measured by assessing the amount of virus in nasal washings). The stress measure was designed to reflect changes in subjects' general levels of activity, although, as already noted, such an instrument is unable to determine whether it is the meaning of the change that is critical.

There has been little to suggest that raised life-change scores, using the SRE, bear any relation to neoplastic conditions. Studies of cervical cancer (Graham et al., 1971), breast cancer (Muslin et al., 1966) and lung cancer (Grissom et al., 1975) have all been negative. A positive result is reported by Lehrer (1980), though the conditions examined (gastric and the other bowel neoplasms) have notoriously insidious onsets which cannot be dated precisely and, as a respondent-based approach was utilized to cover the two years preceding first symptoms, the possibility that active disease was already present cannot be ruled out. Other research approaches to this question are discussed by Anisman and Sklar in Chapter 4.

The lack of association between events and peptic ulcer disease reported by Piper and his colleagues is interesting, given the widespread belief that these conditions are related to stress (Piper et al., 1981; Thomas et al., 1980). The frequency of life events for the two years preceding an exacerbation of duodenal ulcer was compared with the frequency of events in a matched comparison general population sample. Both groups had experienced similar numbers of events and life-change scores were similar in each. The only significant difference appeared to be that patients had more frequently changed residence in the two years preceding exacerbation.

SPECIFIC TYPES OF EVENTS

An alternative approach is based on the notion that is is the meaning of particular events that is critical, over and above their propensity to induce the need for change and readjustment in the objective sense. There have been three approaches to the measurement of meaning; two of these (general and specific meaning) we have already discussed, but before examining the literature on these in detail, one further notion, that of *individual* meaning, requires some elaboration.

Individual meaning deals with the subject's own perception and recall of the degree and kind of emotion experienced as a result of a particular life event. Byrne and Whyte (1980), for example, compared two groups of patients admitted to a coronary-care unit with severe chest pains, whose symptoms were attributable to organic disease processes (myocardial infarction) and those in whom no such morphological change could be demonstrated. The infarct patients did not report experiencing more events or more severe events in the "objective" sense, but they were more likely to describe negative reactions to the events they did experience. Similar conclusions have been drawn by others (e.g. Theorell, 1974; Vinokur and Selzer, 1975). Such an approach to the measurement of meaning is open to the very real criticism that subjects aware of the fact that they have suffered an infarct or other morphological change, may in an "effort after meaning" tend to perceive events as having been more unpleasant than they would have done were they questioned before symptoms of illness appeared (Brown, 1974; Paykel and Uhlenhuth, 1972). It is because of such potential bias that for the most part research has moved towards definitions of meaning beyond that of the self-report of already ill subjects, and we will not review further research carried out in this tradition.

As we discussed earlier, most studies of general meaning rely on a "dictionary-based" approach, in which the severity of an unpleasanat experience such as loss is held to be uniform across all examples of the particular loss in question. Bereavement has long been thought to play an important role in the genesis of a host of physical and mental health changes. Cross-sectional studies have demonstrated higher than average consultation rates, physical symptoms and mortality rates among the recently bereaved than among married persons of the same sex and similar age and social-class background (e.g. Maddison and Viola, 1968). Further, there are indications that cardiovascular disease rates are particularly elevated (Parkes *et al.*, 1969; Rees and Lutkins, 1967). More recent prospective studies have somewhat dampened the enthusiasm of these early reports. For example, through replicating observations of increased con-sulting rates following bereavement, it is clear that at least some of this can be explained as changes in help-seeking behaviour. This may reflect subjective assessments of health-changes brought about through alterations in mood, particularly feelings of irritation and anger (Parkes, 1970). Objective changes of physical health and increased rates of hospitalization appear to relate largely to populations with histories of pre-existing ill-health (Clayton, 1982). The results of research based on mortality data are only somewhat less equivocal. Increases in death rates from all causes following bereavement have been demonstrated in a number of studies (Cottington et al., 1980; Parkes et al., 1969; Rees and Lutkins, 1967; Talbott et al., 1977, 1981; Ward, 1976; Young et al, 1963), but largely negative results have been obtained from one research centre in well designed investigations (Clayton, 1974, 1979). To add to the confusion, most prospective studies have confirmed cross-sectional reports of increases in the use of known risk factors following bereavement, such as cigarette smoking and tranquilizer and hypnotic drug use, and these, rather than the more direct emotional impact of the bereavement, may well be the factor of direct aetiological significance.

But, as we have already indicated, the fact of a loss may well be a less important determinant of its emotional significance than the social and biographical context in which it occurs. This is suggested by some of the work of Parkes and of others, which indicates that facts such as the predictability of the death relate to outcome; sudden, unexpected deaths are usually felt as more stressful initially and carry greater risk of prolonged emotional disorder, often for up to three years after the bereavement, leading in some cases to pathological outcomes (Parkes, 1970, 1975). In a similar manner, prolonged illness involving much pain and physical mutilation prior to death and instances where the survivor has been intensively involved in caring for a sick relative appear to lead to less favourable outcomes, possibly because of promoting feelings of ambivalence and inadequacy in the caring relative (Maddison, 1968). In addition to these factors relating to the death itself, the social context in which it occurs (such as the presence of economic hardship, the availability of other close kin and emotional support) certainly influences the course of mourning and may well be crucially related to outcome (see Bowlby, 1980, for a detailed review of these factors). Certain puzzling inconsistencies in the research on bereavement may thus be due to a failure to go beyond bereavement in a dictionary-type sense.

There have been a large number of reports in which "losses" of various other kinds have been shown to precede the onset of physical symptoms; such "losses" often include relatively transient separations from family and home (Parens et al., 1966), changes in residence, more permanent separations such as divorce (Horne and Picard, 1979; Le Shan, 1959), and loss of employment (Kasl et al., 1975, see Chapter 2). While "loss" remains the most common quality of events to be examined utilizing a dictionary-based approach, other qualities (such as undesirability) have been assessed in a similar manner. For example, Fava and Pavan (1976) showed that patients with lower bowel disorders differed from those with acute appendicitis in having more "undesirable" and "exit" type events. But, however categorized, these investigations tend to remain limited by the use of *general meaning only*.

As we discussed in the introduction, one of the advantages of utilizing a contextual approach to meaning is the opportunity it provides to go beyond simple dictionary definitions of types of event to measure "severity" of experience following the same type of event. The approach has been used to study aetiological processes involved in depression (Brown and Harris, 1978), anxiety (Finlay-Jones and Brown, 1981) and physical illness in general (Murphy and Brown, 1980) (see Table I).

In the first test of this approach to physical illness, a group of 111 women, selected from a random sample of the general population, were studied because they reported on a screening questionnaire the recent development of new physical symptoms of moderate or severe intensity (Murphy and Brown, 1980). Every woman was interviewed about her psychiatric state during the past year, and about the presence of life events, using the LEDS. Thirty of the 111 women were excluded as having symptoms that could well be directly attributable to a psychiatric condition and were, therefore, likely to have no underlying "organic" basis. The remaining 81 women were compared with a group of 458 women, drawn from random samples of the general population, and matched for "life stage" and "social class", the two background variables known to relate to the frequency of life events. The proportion of women in the index group having a severe event (i.e. of the kind known to be capable of provoking a depressive disorder) was higher than in the comparison women. Events with less than severe threat showed no relationship to symptom onset. The association of severe events was confined to younger age-groups; women between 50 and 65 years of age showed instead a greater degree of pre-existing health difficulties which appeared to carry the bulk of predictive power. Furthermore, the relationship of severely threatening events to physical symptoms appeared to be mediated by an intervening psychiatric disorder of an affective nature; the mean length of time between the onset of the psychiatric disorder and onset of "organic" symptoms was seven weeks. By selecting a sample drawn from the general population, the risk of simply measuring consulting behaviour was much reduced, though not entirely eliminated, since the screening questionnaire was based on the self-report of the recent onset of physical symptoms.

Attributable risk per cent for those between 18 and 50 years is 27%, which is a good deal lower than the 57% obtained for severe events in relation to the onset of depression in the general population, but is similar to the 29% for streptococcal infections of the throat in children (See Table I—the later figure is only approximate, as certain assumptions had to be made about the data in the original report). The relative risk of 3.6

is also lower than for other conditions we have so far reviewed from Table I.

There must be some question about the diagnostic accuracy of the measure of physical illness in this study. While it proved possible to exclude "obvious" psychiatric syndromes presenting with somatic symptoms, the authors did not address the issue of "functional" disorders in detail, and such conditions may have been included in the "organic" group. A further study, however, using LEDS has recently been reported, which distinguishes "functional" and morphological groups. This will be discussed in some detail (Creed, 1981). The subjects were 119 patients aged 17 to 30 years, admitted for emergency appendectomy. At the time of interview and at the time of rating events, the investigator was unaware of the histologic appearance of the diseased organ. By studying patients only a few days post-operatively, there could be little doubt about the date of onset of acute pain. Subsequent histologic examinations enabled the patients to be classified as either belonging to those whose symptoms showed a definite inflammation of the appendix, and those in whom the appendix showed no, or only minimal, degree of inflammation. Both groups were compared to a comparison sample from the general population in terms of the presence of absence of events and psychiatric disorder.

Interestingly, although both diagnostic groups experienced more threatening events than the general population series, there were important differences in the severity of threat of the events occurring before onset. Those associated with an inflamed appendix tended to be upsetting in the short term (such as sitting examinations) and on the whole carried serious long-term implications far less often. By contrast, events for those patients found after the operation to have a non-inflamed appendix were severe in the sense of carrying serious long-term threatening implications, such as separation from a spouse. It is notable that these were the only type of event found in earlier research to be capable of bringing about the onset of either clinical depression or anxiety (Brown and Harris, 1978; Finlay-Jones and Brown, 1981).

Given this parallel with earlier research on depression, it is of interest that the non-inflamed group also experienced more symptoms of clinical depression in the month preceding the operation. Furthermore, the presence of such affective symptoms appeared to promote persistence of pain, lasting in many instances until the time of the follow-up interview one year later. Creed concluded that the abdominal pain in the non-inflamed group may be "caused" by the depression which precedes the onset of pain, and to this extent the findings are analogous to the earlier work by Murphy and Brown. However, for the majority of patients the relationship between severe events and pain appears to be a direct one. The presence of depressive symptoms, on the other hand, appeared to relate more closely to persistence of pain post-operatively, particularly in the non-inflamed group. (See note 1, p. 39.)

PSYCHIATRIC AND SOCIAL RISK FACTORS

The studies of Murphy and Brown (1980), and Creed (1981) raise the issue of affective disorder as intervening between life event stress and physical symptoms. Interpretation of most published studies on the role of depression is complicated by the multiplicity of measures of depression, and the apparent great variability in degree of severity taken to indicate a definite disorder. It is not unusual, for example, to find rather high rates of depressive disorder, suggesting that transient and perhaps trivial symptoms have been used as criteria of depression. However, these two recent studies have used clear-cut criteria and a high threshold of severity, and give definite support to the possibility that affective disorders may be more than simply prodromal manifestations of organic disease. If this is true, it should be possible to demonstrate increased prevalence of a variety of physical conditions in those suffering from chronic psychiatric disorders. There are, in fact, suggestions in studies of psychiatric patients of increases in mortality in the neuroses generally, and this mortality appears greatest in more severe neurotic disorders (Kerr *et al.*, 1969; Sims, 1973; Sims and Prior, 1978; Tsuang and Woolson, 1978). Whitlock and Siskind (1979) report on a follow-up study over a period of some four years of 129 patients aged 40 and over given a primary diagnosis of depression. During that time, nine male and nine female patients died, eight of these of cancer which had not been diagnosed at the time of psychiatric admission. For the men, cancer deaths were statistically significantly higher than expected. As the investigators are careful to point out, the possibility that the existence of cancer could have influenced the development of affective symptoms cannot be excluded and given the state of existing evidence, this may well be the safest provisional conclusion to draw. Nevertheless, positive findings are not solely confined to mortality studies in which the relative durations of the disease processes may be difficult to disentangle. In an impressive study, Eastwood and Trevelyan (1972) demonstrated an excess of major physical disease amongst a group of patients with psychiatric (largely affective) symptoms of a typically chronic nature. The study comprised 1471 randomly selected individuals, drawn from patients registered with a local general practice. Subjects were screened for the presence of psychiatric disorder and 124 "high scorers" were interviewed with a clinical psychiatric interview. A comparison series was made up of those patients giving negative responses to psychiatric items on the screening questionnaire and who matched the subjects on certain criteria. All those with psychiatric symptoms and all in the comparison series were examined physically and underwent physical screening tests covering a range of body systems. The psychiatric group as a whole had significantly more physical disease than the comparison group, those with at least one major physical condition comprising 32% of the psychiatric cases and 18% of the comparison series.

Finally, patients dying suddenly of myocardial infarction have been shown to have experienced a higher than expected prevalence of psychiatric disorder (Kuller and Perper, 1973; Talbott et al., 1977, 1981).

Not all studies have found such a definite association between physical morbidity and psychiatric disorder, but as Sims (1973) points out, morbidity and mortality figures for the neuroses in general may well have been under-estimated in such studies because of failure to use detailed tracing procedures. Of the more careful work with conflicting results, two deserve special mention. Robinson (1963) was unable to demonstrate an association between neuroticism and elevated blood pressure in a general population sample, while Goldberg and Comstock (1979) were unable to show any relationship between depression and subsequent physical illness. The latter described a matched case-control analysis in which 82 pairs of subjects were selected from a large-scale population study. Cases were those who were hospitalized or who died in the 12-month period following initial contact. However, it may be relevant that depression was established using rather sensitive standardized tests, suggesting that many with transient and mild affective disorders may have been included.

Given the possibility that chronic and relatively severe affective disorder might increase risk of physical morbidity, it is perhaps not unreasonable to explore further the extent to which milder, less chronic affective change may relate to the onset of physical morbidity. In an exhaustive review of early work on this subject, Le Shan (1959) commented on the frequency with which it had been reported that depressed mood or feelings of helplessness preceded the discovery of neoplastic disease. A well-known theoretical formulation, stemming from these early observations is the "giving-up/given-up" hypothesis of Engel and his co-workers (1967). In this view, stress may be linked to feelings of being overwhelmed expressed in the form of "It's all too much . . . I give up", and this associated with a sense of failure and loss of confidence in ability to function in an accustomed way. Perceptions of past failure are enhanced and expectations of the self are no longer seen as valid. The similarity of this state to mild depression is striking, though most investigators in this tradition have been careful to avoid equating the two.

Although there has been considerable support for this formulation, early observational studies may well have been subject to observer bias; for the most part investigators are aware of the presence and nature of physical illness when they were seeking evidence of feelings of "giving up". Of particular interest are studies in which raters have been "blind" to the diagnosis of physical conditions under investigation. For example, Schmale and Iker (1966) report that such attitudes (rated from the content of an open-ended interview conducted before the results of confirmatory diagnostic investigations were available), were present in 11 of 18 subjects whose final diagnoses were cervical cancer, and were able to replicate results in further studies (Schmale and Iker, 1971).

Given then these various indicators of the possible role of ongoing affective states and the suggestive evidence already reviewed that affective states, often as part of a reaction to severe events, may predispose a subject to physical illness, it is not unreasonable to ask how such emotional states could influence physical health. Perhaps the most popular explanation relates both the affective change and physical disorder to an underlying neurophysiologic and humoral mechanism common to both types of disorder (see Anisman and Sklar, Chapter 4; Steptoe, Chapter 3).

However, it is necessary to note that altered physiology consequent on stress following life events is not the only possible explanation of the apparent link between disorders of mood and physical illness. It is still necessary to take into account explanations involving changes in behaviour, such as cigarette consumption, which are well known to increase the risk of certain diseases directly, albeit over a relatively long period of use, and the effect of mood changes on "consulting" or "illness' behaviour, which are also well documented (Mechanic, 1974).

There is now a large body of evidence demonstrating that those in the lower social classes have higher mortality and morbidity rates than those in the middle or upper classes. Further, this elevated morbidity rate appears to involve a wide spectrum of diseases, suggesting a general rather than disease-specific explanation. The differential effect with class is to some extent explicable by higher levels of risk factors, such as smoking, obesity and exposure to a more dangerous physical environment. However, these factors only explain a relatively small part of the observed social-class gradient (usually in the order of 40%) (Marmot et al., 1978; Syme and Berkman, 1976), and so additional risk agents warrant further exploration. One of these, of central importance to this review, is the observation that lower-class persons report more severe life events of an unpleasant nature than those of the middle or upper classes (Brown and Harris, 1978; Meyers et al., 1974).

A further explanation lies in the observed differences in the quality of social relationships within different social groupings; for example, some studies based on industrial urban populations have shown that lower-class populations report fewer formal group affiliations and supportive intimate relationships (Brown and Harris, 1978; Berkman and Syme, 1979). The role of having warm intimate relationships as a protection against depression has already been mentioned, and similar claims have been made for physical illness symptoms (Cobb and Kasl, 1977; Gore, 1978). An interesting example of this latter observation is to be found in a study of the effects of social support available to a group of men recently made redundant, in which elevations in serum uric acid and cholesterol were significantly moderated by the presence of a supportive family network (Cobb, 1974). Finally, the presence of close emotional ties and support may well lie behind the lower morbidity rates of certain close-knit religious groups (Comstock et al., 1972), or, for that matter, help to explain the effects of urbanization on primitive rural cultures (Henry and Cassell, 1969; Scotch, 1963).

As the complex issues surrounding the relationship of chronic stress and physical health are reviewed elsewhere in this volume, we will note simply that chronic stress (measured as "major ongoing difficulties") showed no association with illness onset in either the study by Murphy and Brown (1980) or that by Creed (1981); a somewhat surprising finding, given the apparent relationship of such difficulties to the onset and course of depression (Brown and Harris, 1978).

CONCLUSIONS AND DISCUSSION

From the evidence provided in this review, we can safely conclude that there are at least three competing explanations to account for the development of physical *symptoms* following stressful life events (see Fig. 1). The least controversial of these relates to somatic symptoms which are clearly part of a definite affective disorder (probably depression), such as muscle-tension pains. It is established that the specific meaning of particular events can provoke an episode of clinical depression, and that the impact is formative in the sense that onset would not have occurred anywhere near the time that it did, or indeed, might not have occurred at all, without the occurrence of a particular event (Brown and Harris, 1978; Finlay-Jones and Brown, 1981). It follows that the same can be concluded about the role of events for any associated somatic symptoms.

The prevalence of depression or other symptoms of affective disorder in some functional disorders, together with their response to treatment with anti-depressant medication, point towards the conclusion that such disorders are best viewed as variants of affective illness. The evidence of one recent study of patients with appendicitis indicates that it is such a group of "functional" disorders amongst them that shows the clearest evidence for a formative effect of severe events with specific meaning. Indeed, findings for this group were almost identical to those obtained in earlier research for psychiatric patients suffering from depression (Creed, 1981). It is this observation, together with the well-documented effect of depression and stressful events on consulting behaviour, which leads many to conclude that the relationship between stress and physical illness is more apparent than real. Even after allowing for the effect of diagnostic misclassification and consulting behaviour, there remains some evidence for a third possibility, that of a relationship between life-event stress and *organic* disease. For the most part, this appears to be a "triggering" rather than "formative" effect; that is, the events provoked a disease which would probably have occurred before too long in any case. This is suggested by three observations.

(i) In many of the reports of stress and organic illness, there is evidence to suggest that there was pre-existing organic pathology to account for the new symptoms (e.g. atherosclerosis and myocardial infarction).

(ii) In so far as an event acts as a trigger, it seems likely that its immediate impact is in terms of general arousal. This has been repeatedly demonstrated to produce transient physiological changes in animals and human beings which lead to measurable decrements in the performance of already diseased or damaged organs; yet in healthy subjects, there is no convincing evidence that such circumscribed stress produces any enduring effect.

(iii) The events involved are often of only moderate severity and tend to occur within a few days or weeks of onset (Connolly, 1976; Creed, 1981; Meyer and Haggerty, 1962).

However, we only put this triggering perspective forward as the most likely possibility. We certainly do not wish to rule out altogether a directly "formative" effect on the basis of existing evidence. (See note 2, p. 39.)

There is, however, one additional complicating factor to be considered, concerning the role of events in organic disorder. This is the demonstration that psychiatric disorder, particularly when of an affective nature, may be a risk factor in its own right (Cottington *et al.*, 1980; Eastwood and Trevelyan, 1972; Murphy and Brown, 1980; Talbott *et al.*, 1981). Of course, if it is accepted that such affective disorders are brought about and perpetuated by severe events, it follows that for this reason alone there will be a link of a formative kind between events and physical illness; albeit one where there might be a delay of many months or years. With the introduction of this last possibility, we believe it is possible to construct a single scheme to reflect all four pathways we have discussed (Fig.2). In this

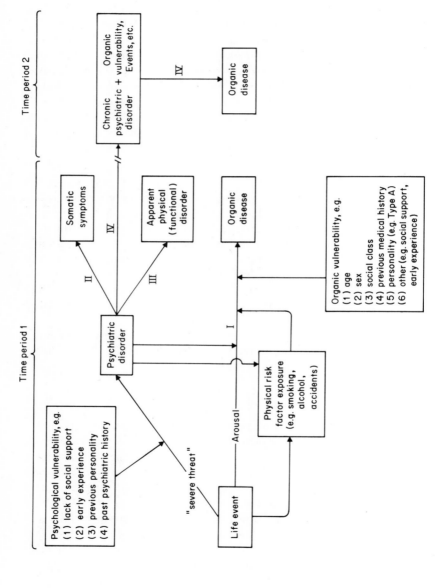

Fig. 2 Possible causal pathways relating life stress to physical disorder.

general model, we assume that the pathway taken will depend on the interaction of the event and the degree of specific psychological and organic vulnerability present at the time of the occurrence of the event. It suggests that general arousal consequent on the impact of an event will be sufficient to trigger organic symptoms in those subjects who are most at risk for a particular disease (pathway I) because of high loadings on one or more organic vulnerability factors (these would include such factors as age, existing physical conditions including the presence of infective agents in the body, and other risk agents such as smoking or alcohol consumption). In the absence of such factors there would be no immediate consequences arising from the arousal. In a similar way, events which are "severe" (i.e. in terms of their specific meaning) only increase the risk of developing an affective disorder in the presence of one or more psychological vulnerability factors. However, once such a disorder has formed, one of two possible routes may be followed. In the first (pathway II) symptoms are in reality those of an affective disorder with a somatic content, while in the second (pathway III) symptoms are predominantly somatic, with the affective content being masked or perhaps even denied by the subject.

In addition, the presence of such affective disorder may have further consequences. First, to increase consulting behaviour and thereby elevate apparent rates of physical illness in the short term. Secondly, over a much longer time-period, by enhancing "organic" vulnerability, pathway IV increases the risk of real rates of organic illness. Such organic illness may well be triggered by further life-event stress. Finally, both event stress and any subsequent affective disorder would lead to increased exposure to other risk agents, such as smoking and so further heighten organic vulnerability. However, this is best seen in terms of a longer time-period and pathway I.

To conclude, it will be clear that the role of life events and the aetiology of physical illness is far from resolved. The early reports of a link between stress and somatic symptoms have been confirmed, yet more recent research, handicapped by the use of dictionary-type measures of events and the use of questionnaires, has for the most part failed to deal with vital issues concerned with specificity: which illnesses are implicated, and how far different types of event relate to different illnesses and perhaps involve different time-periods. This cannot be done until research deals adequately with the complexity of both disease states and life events. A study reporting health-centre attendance or hospital admission as the "objective" measure of physical illness, will include individuals whose symptoms are based on particular organ-system dysfunction, as well as those whose symptoms are somatic manifestations of psychiatric disorder. Even though the possible selective biases arising from "illness behaviour" may have been dealt with, there can be no certainty about the homogeneity of the remaining subjects, as different physical disorders may well be more or less responsive to stress, and within particular disorders some will be more demonstrably related to "organic" change than others. Similar issues have been raised concerning the measures of life events in which different types of general, specific and individual meaning may play differing roles in aetiology. However, enough has been reasonably established to make us confident that further research, taking account of specificity of both psychiatric and organic conditions, will be productive; and, indeed, through its link with psychiatric disorder, stress stemming from life events may well prove to be a major factor in the aetiology of all forms of physical illness—somatic symptoms, functional disorders and organic disease.

REFERENCES

Andrews, G. and Tennant, C. (1978). Being upset and becoming ill: an appraisal of the relationship between life events and physical illness. *Med. J. Aust.* **I**, 324–327.

Berkman, L. F. and Syme, S. L. (1979). Social networks, host resistances and mortality: a follow-up study of Alameda County residents. *Am. J. Epidemiol.* **109**, 186–204.

Bowlby, J. (1980). "Attachment and Loss, Vol III: Loss, Sadness and Depression." Hogarth Press, London.

Brown, G. W. and Birley, J. L. T. (1968). Crises and life changes and the onset of schizophrenia. *J. Health Soc. Behav.* **9**, 203–214.

Brown, G. W., Sklair, F., Harris, T. and Birley, J. L. T. (1973). Life events and psychiatric disorder: 2. Some methodological issues. *Psychol. Med.* **3**, 74–87.

Brown, G. W. (1974). Meaning, measurement and stress. *In* "Stressfulness of Live Events: their Nature and Effects" (B. S. Dohrenwend and B. P. Dohrenwend, eds), pp. 217–243. Wiley, London.

Brown, G. W. and Harris, T. (1978). "The Social Origins of Depression: a Study of Psychiatric Disorder in Women." Tavistock Publications, London; Free Press, New York.

Brown, G. W. (1981). Life events, psychiatric disorder and physical illness. *J. Psychosom. Res.* **25** (5), 461–473.

Brown, G. W. and Harris, T. (1982). Fall-off in the reporting of life events. *Soc. Psychiat.* **17**, 23–28.

Clayton, P. J. (1973). Mortality and morbidity in the first year of widowhood. *Arch. Gen. Psychiat.* **30**, 747–750.

Clayton, P. J. (1979). The sequelae and non-sequelae of conjugal bereavement. *Am. J. Psychiat.* **136**, 1520–1534.

Clayton, P. J. (1982). Bereavement. *In* "Handbook of Affective Disorders (E. S. Paykel, ed.) pp. 403–415. Churchill Livingstone, London.

Cline, D. W. and Chosey, J. J. (1972). A prospective study of life changes and subsequent health changes. *Arch. Gen. Psychiat.* **27**, 51–53.

Cobb, S. (1974). Physiological changes in men whose jobs were abolished. *J. Psychosom. Res.* **18**, 245–258.

Cobb, S. and Kasl, S. V. (1977). "Termination: the Consequences of Job Loss." DHEW (NIOSH) Publication, Cincinatti.

Cole, P. and MacMahon, B. (1971). Attributable risk percent in case-control studies. *Br. J. Prev. Soc. Med.* **25**, 242–244.

Comstock, G. W. and Partridge, K. B. (1972). Church attendance and health. *J. Chron. Dis.* **25**, 665–672.

Connolly, J. (1976). Life events before myocardial infarction. *J. Hum. Stress* **2** (4), 3–17.

Cottington, E. M., Matthews, K. A., Talbott, E. and Kuller, L. H. (1980). Environmental events preceding sudden death in women. *Psychosom. Med.* **42**, 567–574.

Craig, T. K. J. and Brown, G. W. (1984). Goal frustration and life events in the aetiology of painful gastrointestinal disorder. In press.

Creed, F. (1981). Life events and appendicectomy. *Lancet* **i**, 1381–1385.

Culpan, R. and Davies, B. (1960). Psychiatric illness at a medical and a surgical out-patient clinic. *Comprehensive Psychiat.* **1**, 228–235.

Doll, R. and Peto, R. (1976). Mortality in relation to smoking: 20 years' observation of male British doctors. *Br. Med. J.* **2**, 1525–1536.

Eastwood, M. R. and Trevelyan, M. H. (1972). Relationship between physical and psychiatric disorder. *Psychol. Med.* **2**, 363–372.

Engel, G. L. (1967). A psychological setting of somatic disease: the giving up–given up complex. *Proc. Roy. Soc. Med.* **60**, 553–555.

Fava, G. A. and Pavan, L. (1976). Large bowel disorders, illness configuration and life events. *Psychother. Psychosom.* **27**, 93–99.

Finlay-Jones, R. and Brown, G. W. (1981). Types of stressful life event and the onset of anxiety and depressive disorders. *Psychol. Med.* **11**, 803–815.

Goldberg, D. (1970). A psychiatric study of patients with diseases of the small intestine. *Gut* **11**, 459–465.

Goldberg, E. L. and Comstock, G. W. (1976). Life events and subsequent illness. *Am. J. Epidemiol.* **104**, 146–158.

Goldberg, E. L., Comstock, G. W. and Hornstra, M. D. (1979). Depressed mood and subsequent physical illness. *Am. J. Psychiat.* **136**, 530–534.

Gore, S. (1978). The effect of social support in moderating the health consequences of unemployment. *J. Health, Soc. Behav.* **19**, 157–165.

Graham, S., Snell, L. N., Graham, J. B. and Ford, L. (1971). Social trauma in epidemiology of carcinoma of the cervix. *J. Chron. Dis.* **24**, 711–726.

Grissom, J. J., Weiner, B. J. and Weiner, E. A. (1975). Psychosocial correlates of cancer. *J. Consult. Clin. Psychol.* **43**, 113–114.

Henry, J. P. and Cassel, J. C. (1969). Psychosocial factors in essential hypertension: recent epidemiologic and animal experimental evidence. *Am. J. Epidemiol.* **90**, 171–200.

Hinkle, L. E. (1974). The effect of exposure to culture change, social change, and changes in interpersonal relationships on health. *In* "Stressful Life Events: their nature and effects" (B. S. Dohrenwend and B. P. Dohrenwend, eds), pp. 9–44. Wiley, New York.

Hinkle, L. E., Pinsky, R. H., Bross, I. D. and Plummer, N. (1956). The distribution of sickness and disability in a homogenous group of healthy adult men. *Am. J. Hygiene* **64**, 220–242.

Hinkle, L. E., Plummer, N., Metraux, R., Richter, R., Gittinger, J. W., Thetford, W. N., Ostfeld, A. M., Kane, F. D., Goldberger, L., Mitchell, W. E., Leichter, H., Pinsky, R., Goebel, D., Bross, I. D. and Wolff, H. G. (1957). Studies in human ecology, factors relevant to the occurrence of bodily illness and disturbances in mood, thought, and behavior in three homogenous population groups. *Am. J. Psychiat.* **114**, 212–20.

Hinkle, L. E., Redmont, R., Plummer, N. and Wolff, H. G. (1960). An examination of the relationship between symptoms, disability and serious illness in two homogenous groups of men and women. *Am. J. Pub. Health* **50**, 1327–1336.

Hinkle, L. E., Christenson, W. N., Benjamin, B., Kane, F. D., Plummer, N. and Wolff, H. G. (1974). The occurrence of illness among 24 'normal' women: evidences of differences in susceptibility to acute respiratory and gastrointestinal syndromes. Unpublished paper, presented before the American College of Physicians Annual Scientific Meeting, Miami Beach, May 1961.

Holmes, T. H. and Rahe, R. H. (1967). The social readjustment rating scale. *J. Psychosom. Res.* **11**, 213–218.

Holmes, T. H., Hawkins, N. G. and Davies, R. (1957). Evidence of psychosocial factors in the development of pulmonary tuberculosis. *Am. Rev. Tuberc. Pulm. Dis.* **75**(5), 768–772.

Horne, R. L. and Picard, R. S. (1979). Psychosocial risk factors for lung cancer. *Psychosom. Med.* **41**(7), 503–514.

Jacobs, S., Prusoff, B. A. and Paykel, E. S. (1974). Recent life events in schizophrenia and depression. *Psychol. Med.* **4**, 444–453.

Jenkins, C. D., Hurst, M. W. and Rose, R. N. (1979). Life changes: do people really remember? *Arch. Gen. Psychiat.* **36** (4), 379–384.

Kasl, S. U., Gore, S. and Cobb, S. (1975). The experience of losing a job: reported changes in health, symptoms, and illness behaviour. *Psychosom. Med.* **37**, 106–122.

Kerr, T. A., Schapira, K. and Roth, M. (1969). The relationship between premature death and affective disorder. *Br. J. Psychiat.* **115**, 1277–1282.

Kuller, L. H. and Perper, J. A. (1973). Myocardial infarction and sudden death in an urban community. *Bull. N.Y. Acad. Med.* **49**, 532–543.

Lauer, R. H. (1973). The social readjustment scale and anxiety: a cultural study. *J. Psychosom. Res.* **17**, 171–174.

Leff, J. and Vaughan, C. (1980). The interaction of life events and relatives' expressed emotion in the schizophrenia and depressive neurosis. *Br. J. Psychiat.* **136**, 146–153.

Lehrer, S. (1980). Life change and gastric cancer. *Psychosom. Med.* **42**(5), 499–502.

Lei, H. and Skinner, H. A. (1980). A psychometric study of life events and social adjustment. *J. Psychosom. Res.* **24**, 57–65.

LeShan, L. (1959). Psychological states as factors in the development of malignant disease: a critical review. *J. Nat. Cancer Inst.* **22**, 1–18.

Lindsay, P. G. and Wykoff, M. (1981). The depression pain syndrome and its response to antidepressants. *Psychosomatics* **22**, 571–577.

Lipowski, Z. J. (1967). Review of consultation and psychosomatic medicine, Part 2. *Psychosom. Med.* **29**, 201–224.

Lorimer, R. J., Justice, B., McBee, G. W. and Weinman, M. (1979). Weighting events in life event research. *J. Health Soc. Behav.* **20**, 306–307.

MacMahon, B. and Pugh, T. F. (1970). "Epidemiology: Principles and Methods." Little, Brown & Co., Boston.

Maddison, D. (1968). The relevance of conjugal bereavement to preventative psychiatry. *Br. J. Med. Psychol.* **41**, 223–233.

Maddison, D. and Viola, A. (1968). The health of widows in the year following bereavement. *J. Psychosom. Res.* **12**, 297–306.

Marmot, M., Rose, G., Shipley, M. and Hamilton, P. (1978). Employment grade and coronary heart disease in British civil servants. *J. Epidemiol. Community Health* **32**, 244–249.

Mechanic, D. (1974). Discussion of research programs and relations between stressful life events and episodes of physical illness. *In* "Stressful Life Events: their nature and effects" (B. S. Dohrenwend and B. P. Dohrenwend, eds), pp. 87–97. Wiley, New York.

Mechanic, D. and Volkart, E. H. (1961). Stress, illness behavior and the sick role. *Am. Soc. Rev.* **26**, 51–58.

Meyer, R. J. and Haggerty, R. J. (1962). Streptococcal infection in families: factors altering individual susceptibility. *Pediatrics* **29**, 539–549.

Meyers, J. K., Lindenthal, J. and Pepper, M. P. (1974). Social class, life events and psychiatric symptoms: a longitudinal study. *In* "Stressful Life Events: their nature and effects" (B. S. Dohrenwend and B. P. Dohrenwend, eds), pp. 191–205. Wiley, New York.

Murphy, E. and Brown, G. W. (1980). Life events, psychiatric disturbance and physical illness. *Br. J. Psychiat.* **136**, 326–338.

Muslin, H. L., Gyarfas, K. and Peiper, W. J. (1966). Separation experience and cancer of the breast. *Ann. N.Y. Acad. Sci.* **125**, 802–806.

Parkes, C. M. (1970). The first year of bereavement: a longitudinal study of the reaction of London widows to the deaths of their husbands. *Psychiatry* **33**, 444–467.

Parkes, C. M. (1975). Unexpected and untimely bereavement: a statistical study of young Boston widows and widowers. *In* "Bereavement: its psychological aspects" (B. Schoenberg, I, Gerber, A. Weiner, A. H. Kutschen, D. Peretz and A. C. Carr, eds). Columbia University Press, New York.

Parkes, C. M., Benjamin, B. and Fitzgerald, R. G. (1969). Broken heart: a statistical study of increased mortality among widowers. *Br. Med. J.* **1**, 740–743.

Paykel, E. S., Myers, J. K., Dienelt, M. N., Klerman, G. L., Lindenthal, J. J. and Pepper, M. P. (1969). Life events and depression: a controlled study. *Arch. Gen. Psychiat.* **21**, 753–760.

Paykel, E. S. (1974). Recent life events and clinical depression. *In* "Life Stress and Illness" (E, K. E. Gunderson and R. H. Rahe, eds), pp. 134–163. C. Thomas, Springfield.

Paykel, E. S. (1978). Contribution of life events to causation of psychiatric illness. *Psychol. Med.* **8**, 245–253.

Paykel, E. S. and Uhlenhuth, E. H. (1972). Rating the magnitude of life stress. *Can. Psychiat. Ass. J.* **17**, 5593–5600.

Paykel, E. S., Prussof, B. A. and Meyers, J. K. (1975). Suicide attempts and recent life events. *Arch. Gen. Psychiat.* **32**, 327–333.

Piper, D. W., McIntosh, J. H., Ariotti, D. E., Calogiuri, J. V., Brown, R. W. and Shy, C. M. (1981). Life events and chronic duodenal ulcer: a case control study. *Gut* **22**, 1011–1017.

Rahe, R. H. (1969). Life crisis and health changes. *In* "Psychotropic Drug Response: advances in prediction" (P. R. A. May and J. R. Wittenbourn, eds), pp. 92–125. C. C. Thomas, Springfield.

Rahe, R. H. (1974). The pathway between subjects' recent life changes and their near-future illness reports: representative results and methodological issues. *In* "Stressful Life Events: their nature and effects" (B. S. Dohrenwend and B. P. Dohrenwend, eds), pp. 73–86. Wiley, New York.

Rahe, R. H. and Holmes, T. H. (1965). Social, psychologic and psychophysiological aspects of inguinal hernia. *J. Psychosom. Res.* **8,** 35–44.

Rahe, R. H. and Paasikivi, J. (1971). Psychosocial factors and myocardial infarction II: out-patient study in Sweden. *J. Psychosom. Res.* **15,** 33–39.

Rees, W. D. and Lutkins, S. G. (1967). Mortality of bereavement. *Brit. Med. J.* **4,** 13–16.

Robinson, J. O. R. (1963). A study of neuroticism and casual arterial blood pressure. *Br. J. Soc. Clin. Psychol.* **2,** 56–64.

Rosenthal, R. and Rubin, D. (1979). A note on variance explained as a measure of the importance of events. *J. Appl. Soc. Psychol.* **9,** (5), 395–396.

Sarason, I. G., De Monchaux, C. and Hunt, T. (1975). Methodologic issues in the assessment of life stress. *In* "Parameters of Emotion" (L. Levi, ed.), pp. 499–509. Raven Press, New York.

Schmale, A. and Iker, H. (1966). The psychological setting of uterine cervical cancer. *Ann. N.Y. Acad. Sci.* **125,** 807–813.

Schmale, A. and Iker, H. (1971). Hopelessness as a predictor of cervical cancer. *Soc. Sci. Med.* **5,** 95–100.

Scotch, N. A. (1963). Sociocultural factors in the epidemiology of Zulu hypertension. *Am. J. Pub. Health* **53,** 1205–1213.

Shepherd, M., Cooper, B., Brown, A. C. and Kalton, G. W. (1966). "Psychiatric Illness in General Practice." Oxford University Press, London.

Sims, A. (1973). Mortality in neurosis. *Lancet,* **ii,** pp. 1072–1076.

Sims, A. and Prior, R. (1978). The pattern of mortality in severe neurosis. *Br. J. Psychiat.* **133,** 299–305.

Syme, S. L. and Berkman, L. F. (1976). Social class, susceptibility and sickness. *Am. J. Epidemiol.* **104** (1), 1–8.

Talbott, E., Kuller, L. H. and Detre, K. (1977). Biologic and psychosocial risk factors of sudden death from coronary disease in white women. *Am. J. Cardiol.* **39,** 858–864.

Talbott, E., Kuller, L. H., Perper, J. and Murphy, P. A. (1981). Sudden unexpected death in women: biologic and psychosocial origins. *Am. J. Epidemiol.* **114** (5), 671–682.

Theorell, T. (1974). Life events before and after onset of a premature myocardial infarction. *In* "Stressful Life Events: their nature and effects" (B. S. Dohrenwend and B. P. Dohrenwend, eds), pp. 101–117. Wiley, New York.

Theorell, T. and Rahe, R. H. (1971). Psychosocial factors and myocardial infarction I: an in-patient study in Sweden. *J. Psychosom. Res.* **15,** 25–31.

Theorell, T., Lind, E. and Floderus, G. (1975). The relationship of disturbing life changes and emotions to the early development of myocardial infarction and other serious illnesses. *Int. J. Epidemiol.* **4,** 281–293.

Thomas, J. H., Greig, M. and Piper, D. W. (1980). Chronic gastric ulcer and life events. *Gastroenterology* **78,** 905–911.

Totman, R. (1979). "Social Causes of Illness." Souvenir Press, London.

Totman, R., Kiff, J., Reed, S. E. and Craig, W. (1980). Predicting experimental colds in volunteers from different measures of recent life stress. *J. Psychosom. Res.* **24,** 155–163.

Tsuang, M. T. and Woolson, R. F. (1978). Excess mortality in schizophrenia and affective disorders. *Arch. Gen. Psychiat.* **35,** 1181–1185.

Vinokur, A. and Selzer, M. L. (1975). Desirable versus undesirable life events: their relationship to stress and mental distress. *J. Personality Soc. Psychol.* **32,** 329–337.

Von Knoring, L. (1965). The experience of pain in depressed patients. *Neuropsycho-biology* **1**, 155–165.

Ward, A. M. W. (1976). Mortality of bereavement. *Br. Med. J.* **1**, 700–702.

Ward, N. G., Bloom, V. L. and Friedel, R. O. (1979). The effectiveness of tricyclic antidepressants in the treatment of coexisting pain and depression. *Pain* **7**, 331–341.

Wershow, H. J. and Reinhart, G. (1974). Life change and hospitalization: a heretical view. *J. Psychosom. Res.* **18**, 393–401.

Whitlock, F. A. and Siskind, M. (1979). Depression and cancer. *Psychol. Med.* **9**, (4), 747–752.

Yager, J., Grant, I., Sweetwood, H. L. and Gerst, M. (1981). Life-event reports by psychiatric patients, non-patients, and their partners. *Arch. Gen. Psychiat.* **38**, 343–347.

Young, M., Benjamin, B. and Wallis, C. (1963). The mortality of widowers. *Lancet* **ii**, 454–456.

NOTES ADDED IN PROOF

1. One final study in this tradition is of relevance. Craig and Brown (1984), investigating the presence of severe events prior to the onset of gastrointestinal pain in 140 consecutive referrals to three gastrointestinal clinics and in a matched healthy comparison series, confirmed the findings of the appendicitis study. Severe life events involving loss and disappointment were much more often associated with the onset of functional disorders, defined as the absence of verifiable organic pathology on confirmatory investigative procedures such as endoscopy. A new measure of "goal frustration" was developed. In keeping with other qualitative dimensions of the LEDS it was a contextual measure, rated by independent assessors who were kept in ignorance as to whether the the respondent was a patient or a healthy comparison subject. Goal frustration was defined as the irreversible obstruction of the attainment of a goal or ambition which had been decided upon and worked toward by the subject well prior to the frustrating event. Patients with confirmed organic disease were a good deal more likely to have experienced at least one such goal frustrating event prior to first onset of symptoms than were patients with functional disorders or the healthy comparison subjects. Furthermore, such events were usually followed by the development of a mild affective disorder of the quality and severity reported in Murphy and Brown's earlier work with organic patients.

2. Indeed, it is likely that for certain disorders such formative effects may emerge with the exploration of new dimensions of meaning, as appears to be the case with gastrointestinal pain (Craig and Brown, 1984).

2
Chronic Life Stress and Health
STANISLAV V. KASL

INTRODUCTION

Recent volumes on stress (e.g. Elliott and Eisdorfer, 1982; Goldberger and Breznitz, 1982) confirm and reinforce a set of conclusions which are derivable from an examination of the last decade of stress research. Firstly, the concept of stress appears indispensable, but the reasons for this are far from apparent. It is, however, a quixotic enterprise to search for, and then insist on, a single set of conceptual and operational definitions of stress. Nevertheless, strong research design methodology, with interpretable measures of impact, strong causal inferences and study of underlying mechanisms and mediating processes, can propel the stress field forward, even if theoretical and conceptual confusion remains.

Perhaps the least satisfactory (and most easily remedied) aspect of the current state of stress research is the fact that the term "stress" continues to be used in fundamentally different ways: as an environmental condition, as the response to that condition, or as some relationship between environmental demands and the person's ability to meet these demands. However, it is possible to detect the beginnings of a terminological consensus (Elliott and Eisdorfer, 1982) which favours "stressor" as the environmental condition of interest and "stress reaction" as the relevant response. Beyond this, consensus is yet to be reached regarding the unique defining criteria for stressful stimuli and stress responses.

There are many reasons why the concept of stress remains troublesome and refractory to consensually endorsed modifications. Basically, it is not even clear if we wish to retain the term with its strong ties to the vernacular (and thus exploit its vagueness, its surplus meanings, and its high polemical value), or if we are trying to arrive at a useful scientific construct through increasing refinement and precision, and interplay with accumulating

HEALTH CARE AND HUMAN BEHAVIOUR
ISBN 0–12–666460–9

empirical evidence. If the latter, then should we adopt a strategy of working inductively ("upwards") from low level generalizations, or deductively ("downwards") from a full-blown theoretical formulation? Can we define the unique stimulus conditions of interest ("stressor") without any reference to outcomes? Can we designate a unique set of outcomes which will indicate the impact of a stressor? Should the concept of stress also encompass relational constructs (e.g. linking properties of the environmental condition to the characteristics of the organism) and intervening steps (e.g. appraisal processes, emotional reactions, coping strategies), or should these be variables which, though crucial to the research design, are exogenous to the concept?

Stress is one of the scientific concepts endowed with a built-in negative correlation between conceptual richness and subtlety on the one hand, and operational feasibility on the other. As the concept is improved along one dimension, the other one poses more problems. The balance of current stress research is tipped in favour of conceptual richness. The emphasis appears to be on a subjective ("Stress is, if you think it is stress") and idiographic ("one man's meat is another man's poison") approach to stress in the study of the health impact. McGrath's (1970) widely used definition is a good example: "A (perceived) substantial imbalance between demand and response capability under conditions where failure to meet demand has important (perceived) consequences". This definition has a pleasant aura of precision about it, but in fact the burden of defining the central concept is shifted onto several secondary concepts, and creates many methodological headaches. For example, it drives us away from the study of actual environmental conditions, and weakens our ability to reconstruct the causal chain from health outcomes back to some pathogenic aspect of the environment. Moreover, it seduces us into studying the easy but methodologically suspect association between perceived and self-reported responses or outcomes. Furthermore, it adds an open-ended indeterminancy to our research designs, since we are less certain that in any particular setting, we have assessed all the relevant and important mediating and modifying variables.

Many investigators have effectively finessed the issue of conceptualizing stress by proposing some list of concrete environmental conditions which are to be thought of as stressors. These may then be examined for their impact on human health. Such lists may be purely intuitive, or somewhat guided by theory, usually only an implicit one. Sometimes, the lists also reflect empirical evidence on adverse health consequences that has already been collected. The most useful lists appear to be those which are restricted to one particular social role or environmental setting (e.g. work environment), where there is also a good back-log of empirical evidence on adverse outcomes, and a rich theory which dimensionalizes that particular environmental setting. For example, Landy and Trumbo (1976) offer the following list of stressors: job insecurity, excessive competition, hazardous working conditions, task demands, and long or unusual working hours. Others have offered similarly useful lists of stressful work conditions (Gross, 1970; Holt, 1982; McGrath, 1976).

The stress and disease literature on humans reveals that two broad classes of stressors have been examined: environmental conditions (stimuli, events) and characteristics of the individual, such as personality traits. F. Cohen *et al.* (1982) propose 4 types of environmental stressors: (i) acute and time-limited; (ii) stressor sequences (series of events, resulting from an initiating event, such as divorce); (iii) chronic intermittent stressors (e.g. repeated conflicts with one's boss); and (iv) chronic stressors (e.g. long-lasting parental discord). While the boundaries of this time-oriented classification are obviously too imprecise to provide a firm definition of scope, the intent of this chapter is to deal with the last two types of events.

Stress research which focuses on a characteristic of the person as the stressor is somewhat more ambiguous. Frequently, it is not clear how that focal characteristic enters into the fundamental stress paradigm of stressor → biological and/or psychosocial reaction health consequence. There are several possibilities. The characteristic or trait many increase the chances of exposure to a stressor; persons exhibiting coronary prone behaviour patterns may self-select work situations where they are over-loaded or under deadline pressures. Alternatively, the characteristic may be a modifier which enhances the stressor → reaction connection; for example, response to certain social situations can be enhanced by extreme shyness (Zimbardo, 1982). Thirdly, the characteristic itself may be an endogenous source of distress (a sufficient cause) which initiates some biologic reaction leading to health consequences in the absence of environmental stimuli. The concept of endogenous depression is illustrative of this possibility. Finally, the characteristic may not be involved in aetiology, but is instead a consequence of health status changes. For example, the higher rate of anxiety and "neuroticism" observed in case-control studies of persons with and without myocardial infarction is clearly a consequence of the MI and not a risk factor of aetiological significance (Jenkins, 1976). For the purposes of defining the boundaries of this chapter, the primary interest is in the characteristics of persons which act in the manner suggested by the first two possibilities only.

Broadly-based reviews of stress factors in disease tend to cover rather similar ground to reviews of some other central concept, such as emotion (e.g. Henry, 1982), or even simply overviews of general psychosocial factors in disease (e.g. McQueen and Siegrist, 1982). Such ambiguity suggests that it may be more productive to try to clarify mechanisms and pathways involved, than to quibble over whether a stressor or a stress reaction are involved.

In summary, it is the intent of this review to examine the health consequences of certain enduring or chronically intermittent stressors. The term "stressor" is used atheoretically in its vernacular usage. It does not presume a full consensus on defining characteristics among the investigators. The role of personal characteristics in stressor exposure or in modification of stressor–reaction–disease linkages will also be considered. Direct effects of environmental conditions (such as asbestos and cancer) and simple effects of medical care variables (such as social class and accesss to quality medical care) will not be considered.

THE DISTINCTION BETWEEN LIFE EVENTS AND CHRONIC LIFE STRESSES

While this is a perfectly reasonable distinction intended to subdivide the task allocated to different reviewers, the reader who wishes to gain a more unified perspective of the stress field should approach it with some scepticism. This distinction implies that we have two seperable bodies of research literature: those dealing with acute changes where the stressors are the adaptive demands of the change itself, and those dealing with enduring situations where the adaptive demands persist because they inhere in the stable aspects of the situation.

Logical analysis will reveal just how difficult this distinction is. Consider the job of a foreman, which is associated with higher rates of peptic ulcer (Pflanz, 1971; Susser, 1967). A promotion from worker to foreman is both an acute change and the start of exposure to a different work environment which is associated with a different risk of disease. Higher rates of ulcer following promotion can be attributable either to the acute change or the new chronic environment. Higher rates which appear with some delay could mean the accumulation of effects from the chronic environment, or a delay in the clinical manifestations of the impact of the acute stressor. The tapering off of the increase in rates with years on the new job could signal an acute stressor effect, or it could mean that the chronic effects do not cummulate indefinitely, and that successful adaptations to the chronic stressor take a while to learn. In short, both differential rates as well as the temporal patterns of these rates, may be insufficient to distinguish the acute from the chronic stressor dynamics.

When two environments are associated with equal risk of disease, then elevated rates following change from one to the other have perhaps a simpler interpretation. However, in the vast majority of instances we are either studying environments which are unequal in disease risk or, more commonly, we do not even know what the risks are. The recent evidence from Helsing and Szklo (1981) that elevated mortality rates for males after bereavement (no elevations were found for widows) did not taper off with years since bereavement, prompted the inquiry of whether we are dealing with an acute stressful life event or a change to a situation chronically associated with higher risk (Susser, 1981). The usual mortality and morbidity analyses by marital status are, of course, quite ambiguous with this respect (e.g. Bloom *et al.*, 1978). Similarly, a recent overview of the literature on health consequences of migration reveals that most of the evidence is utterly ambiguous as to whether a study is documenting an impact of the experience *per se* or of the differential risks associated with the two environments (Kasl and Berkman, 1983).

PROBLEMS WITH THE CONCEPT OF CHRONICITY

From the beginnings of research on the stress concept, the temporal dimension, embodied in the notion of the General Adaptation Syndrome, has been a crucial aspect of the formulation. The time dimension is particularly salient for this chapter with its focus on chronic stressors and the more distal outcomes, changes in health status.

Let us start with a logical analysis of the stress paradigm: stressor → biological and/or psychosocial reaction → health status change. It would appear that disease outcomes will primarily result from enduring stressors that lead to enduring reactions (which represent enduring elevations of a relevant risk factor). These in turn will produce the structural changes that are associated with manifestations of overt clinical disease. When these requirements are not fulfilled, a disease outcome may still be expected when some other conditions hold. Notably, these would be either a disease process, such as that involving sudden cardiac death (Eliot and Buell, 1981) or perforated peptic ulcer (Wolf *et al.*, 1979), where acute but intense arousal can precipitate the condition, or else a situation where the stressor, though only acute, has initiated biological and/or psychosocial reactions which then endure.

The psychosomatic literature is replete with evidence linking acute stressors to acute biological changes. For example, a recent review of plasma lipid variability (Dimsdale and Herd, 1982) has shown that free fatty acids are almost always found elevated in the context of a stressful event. The evidence for serum cholesterol is weaker while that for triglycerides is quite inconsistent. Aside from the problem that the strongest evidence is for a biological marker which has an uncertain role in atherogenesis and as a risk factor for coronary heart disease, the main point is that we cannot extrapolate from this kind of evidence to the conclusion that exposure to similar but chronic stressors would lead to chronic elevations of such biological markers. Field studies of real-life, relatively enduring situations may paint a much more complicated picture. For example, Friedman *et al.* (1958) showed that cholesterol levels go up for a considerable period among tax accountants as the tax deadline approaches and workload goes up. However, Reynolds (1974) did not observe similar cholesterol changes in employees who were responsible for launching the space vehicle for moon landing and were working for a considerable period under severe deadline pressure. And cross-sectional associations between cholesterol and various indicators of stable job pressures consistently yield non-significant correlations for a large variety of occupational categories (Caplan *et al.*, 1975; French *et al.*, 1982).

The psychosomatic literature on blood pressure leads to much the same conclusions. In spite of the innumerable studies on acute changes in response to acute stressors, the consensus is that these do not add up to an endorsement of the aetiological role of enduring psychosocial stressors in the incidence of hypertension (e.g. Bunney *et al.*, 1982; Jenkins, 1981; Weiner, 1977). Field studies of enduring powerful social stressors, such as those in the inner city (Harburg *et al.*, 1973) or crowding in the residential environment (Kasl and Harburg, 1975) and the prison setting (D'Atri *et al.*, 1981), have yielded only very weak associations with blood pressure levels.

Another problem is how to view chronic-intermittent stressors (e.g. Burchfield, 1979), in contrast to either acute or uninterrupted chronic stressors. Do transitory, self-limiting, reversible elevations of a biological marker or risk factor represent an increased risk of a disease simply because of the repetitive nature of such elevations? The answer presumably depends on the mechanisms involved: changes in plasma lipids may be more benign than changes in blood coagulation time. And under some circumstances, such as industrial noise, which is both intermittent and unpredictable (S. Cohen *et al.*, 1982), the effect on blood pressure regulation may be worse than that of uninterrupted chronic noise.

The temporal dimension of stressors and their periodicity may create complex findings, such as in the case of the immune system. With many possible measures of immunity available, the general conclusion appears to be that stressors may decrease, as well as enhance, susceptibility to disease (see Anisman and Sklar, Chapter 4, for details of this evidence).

However, perhaps the most troublesome, and in some ways most neglected, aspect of the time dimension in stressor-outcome relationships is the situation in which the chronic stressor persists but the biological and/or psychosocial reaction does not. In a recent review of endocrine responses to stress, Rose (1980) cites many instances where the endocrine responses, though sensitive to acute stressors, undergo extinction when the individuals are re-exposed to those stressors, or are exposed to chronic stressors. For example, in a study of paramedics and firefighters, urinary corticoids for either group were substantially the same on days worked and days off (Dutton et al., 1978). Similarly, a study of helicopter medics found that urinary 17-OHCS levels were similar on days in which the medics flew and days when they remained in base (Bourne et al., 1967). Experienced pilots studied during strenuous flight failed to show elevations of growth hormone or prolactin (Pinter et al., 1979). Rose's general comment is worth quoting: "We have become impressed with the fact that individuals adapt or accommodate to most stressful stimuli upon being re-exposed to them and thus, the stimuli lose their stressful quality" (Rose, 1980, p. 255).

The phenomenon pointed out by Rose need not be confined to endocrine responses. In a study of male blue collar workers losing their jobs because of a permanent plant shutdown (Cobb and Kasl, 1977; Kasl, 1982; Kasl and Cobb, 1979 and 1980), the vast majority of the dependent variables (physiological, mental health, and work-role deprivation) showed a similar pattern of changes over time. In short term comparisons, involving the period of some 4–6 weeks before plant closing to some 4–6 weeks after shutdown, these variables were highly sensitive to whether or not the man was re-employed or unemployed on the second occasion, with elevated levels associated with unemployment. However, in longer term comparisons (4–6 weeks to 4–6 months after shutdown), men who continued to remain unemployed came down to "normal" levels, similar to those of men who were re-employed by that time.

These findings seem to create problems for the stressor–disease paradigm. A number of important questions are raised by such data. Does this phenomenon represent an active coping process, or does it involve some kind of a passive habituation (a process of extinction not involving higher cortical processes), or even perhaps a built-in biological time curve of reactivity? And can we identify these different processes? Are there identifiable characteristics of stressors which are reliably associated with the difference between chronic vs diminishing reactivity? What is the significance of the possible pattern of findings (noted by Rose, 1980) which suggest that some endocrine responses (e.g. catecholamines) may adapt to stressors more slowly than others (e.g. cortisol) and may in addition be maintained in elevated states by specific environmental demands, such as for attention and vigilance? Finally, are the reactions studied necessary links in the causal chain which eventually leads to disease outcomes? For example, are the endocrine responses necessary antecedents to changes in the immune system, or may changes in immune status emerge as "direct" results of exposure to chronic stressors? Does the extinction of the endocrine response make a difference in the linkage between changed immune status and risk of disease development? These last questions on linkages to disease outcomes are particularly important in view of the general observation that the whole research area on stress and human health contains precious few studies which encompass both the necessary proximate biological and/or psychosocial reactions, as well as the distal disease outcomes (Elliott and Eisdorfer, 1982).

TOWARDS A PARADIGM FOR CHRONIC-REACTIVITY: EXAMPLES FROM THE WORK SETTING

The above discussion and an earlier review of the literature (Kasl, 1977) makes it clear that, in addition to the chronicity of the stressor, we also need to be concerned with other stressor characteristics and specific person characteristics, in order to understand the circumstances which lead to chronic reactivity. What we want to understand is what makes adaptation and coping either easy, or difficult, or nearly impossible. Because the occupational stress research literature is the most extensive one, we shall draw on examples from it.

As a start, we may speculate that the pathogenic process whereby the work environmental conditions lead to chronic reactivity and, eventually, to disease outcomes, has the following characteristics (Kasl, 1981): the stressful work condition is enduring rather than acute; failure to meet the demands of the work setting has serious consequences (e.g. high level of responsibility for such outcomes as the lives of others, expensive equipment, or profits); habituation or adaptation to the chronic situation is difficult because of environmental constraints, as well as the need to maintain some form of involvement, vigilance or arousal; there is a "spill-over" of the effects of the work role on other areas of functioning (e.g. family, leisure), so that the daily impact of the demanding job situation becomes cumulative and health-threatening, rather than being daily defused or erased, when it would have little long-term impact.

In the above enumeration of characteristics, the first two are relatively straightforward, while the latter two remain rather vague and elusive. Let us turn to a selection of findings from diverse studies in order to see if collectively they suggest some inductive generalizations and if they can help clarify these vague parameters.

   (i)   Airline pilots show increased heart rate during and after take-off. This happens irrespective of the length of their flying experience. There is no apparent heart rate elevation in flight, but there may be some at approach and landing, depending upon weather conditions (Smith, 1967).

(ii)   Military pilots of high performance single engine jets show elevated blood pressure throughout flights, and particularly so at take-off and landing (Roman, 1963).

(iii) Pilots of jet fighter bombers landing on aircraft carriers have elevated levels of serum cortisol, while the radar intercept officers, not involved in piloting the plane but equally exposed to the danger, have normal levels (Rubin, 1974).

(iv)   In a study of 17-OHCS levels in a combat situation, on the day of the anticipated attack, the captain and the radio operator showed an increase in corticosteroid levels, while the enlisted men showed a decrease (Bourne et al., 1968).

(v)   Workers paid on a piecework basis (pay proportional to output) or being switched from salary to piecework show chronically higher or stably increased catecholamine levels (Levi, 1974; Timio and Gentili, 1976).

(vi)   Female clerks working overtime show elevated catecholamine levels at work (during regular hours and overtime hours) and even in the evening at home away from work (Frankenhaeuser, 1979; Rissler, 1977).

(vii) Difficult rush hour commuting to and from work is associated with higher catecholamine levels, higher blood pressure, and aggravation of pre-existing cardiovascular symptoms (Lundberg, 1976; Stokols and Novaco, 1981).

(viii) After a vacation period, more industrial workers are likely to show a rapid adrenaline decrease after exposure to stressors than at other times (Johansson, 1976). Conversely, the speed of unwinding from work is likely to influence the spillover effects of work stressors on leisure activities (Frankenhaeuser, 1977).

(ix)   Sawmill workers, who show the highest levels of catecholamines and who show no decreases toward the end of the day, have jobs with the following characteristics: work pace controlled by machine, highly repetitive yet involving skilled judgements made at very short intervals, and highly constraining with the need to maintain the same posture (Frankenhaeuser and Gardell, 1976; Gardell, 1976; Johansson et al., 1978).

(x)   Jobs which are characterized by the combination of relatively high job demands and relatively narrow latitude with respect to decision-making and other on-the-job behaviours appear to be associated with excess risk for coronary heart disease (Karasek et al., 1981 and 1982).

(xi)   Only a relatively small subset of air traffic controllers show repeated
       elevations of cortisol levels for occasions when the workload
       increases; these are men judged most competent by their peers and
       who show high investment in their work (Rose *et al.*, 1978).

While this listing of results may appear like a hodgepodge of diverse
findings, it is possible to discern certain themes which may define a little
more precisely the conditions of chronic reactivity. They include external
pacing of work demands, such as that created by machines or payment
mechanisms; tasks requiring a high level of continuous attention or
vigilance; relatively drastic consequences of inadequate task performance;
psychological and physical constraints on the way the tasks are performed;
exogenous influences (e.g. commuting, vacations, leisure activities) which
reduce ability to recover from elevated levels caused by enodgenous (at
work) demands; personal characteristics which may enhance the influence
of any of the above.

The job of the air traffic controller appears paradigmatic for the above
analysis and has received a good deal of attention recently (Crump, 1979).
In centres of high density traffic the demands are chronic, adaptation is
difficult, the need to maintain vigilance is unabated, and the level of
responsibility for lives and equipment is high. One relatively unexplored
aspect is the role of work team social supports in buffering the effects of the
work environment. Air traffic controllers have been found to have more
hypertension, diabetes and peptic ulcer than a comparison group of pilots
examined in a comparable manner (Cobb and Rose, 1973). In addition, air
traffic controllers acquire these diseases at a younger age than pilots and
those in centres of high traffic density are more affected than others. Higher
rates of mild-to-moderately severe illness, and problems with impulse
control after work have also been noted (Rose *et al.*, 1978). Cross-sectional
analyses of data at one point in time may not reveal higher blood pressure
levels compared to other occupations (Caplan *et al.*, 1975), but this appears
to be a function of the limitations of cross-sectional compared to prospective designs (Rose *et al.*, 1978a), rather than an inconsistency in the total
pattern of findings.

There may be other job categories with demands similar to those to
which air traffic controllers are exposed. For example, the role of train
dispatchers before the advent of electronic equipment bears some resem-
blance, and at least one author (McCord, 1948) has commented on their
curtailed longevity. The obervation of excess cardiac mortality among West
German sea pilots may also fit this picture (Zorn *et al.*, 1977).

It should be noted that, in the above sketch for a paradigm of chronic
reactivity, the work stressor conditions which have been analysed all

represent, broadly speaking, excessive demands or overload conditions. It is not clear to what extent we also need to be concerned with work conditions of underload: the inadequately challenging jobs, the lack of one's skills and abilities. As a broad generalization, it would appear that these conditions affect adversely mental health indicators, but have a lesser impact on physical health status (Kasl and Cobb, 1983). Thus their neglect here has some justification because of the emphasis on physical health. However, it certainly cannot be ruled out that certain health outcomes, such as coronary heart disease are sensitive to conditions of underload, such as monotony and insufficient job responsibility (Alfredsson et al., 1982; Theorell and Floderus-Myrhed, 1977).

HEALTH EFFECTS OF OCCUPATIONAL STRESS

The occupational stress research literature is extensive and well-reviewed (e.g. Cooper and Payne, 1980; Holt, 1982; Kahn et al., 1982; McLean, 1979). Volumes on job stress reduction and management are also beginning to appear in numbers (e.g. Beech et al., 1982; Cooper, 1981; McLean, 1981), perhaps prematurely. It is the intent of this section to provide an overview of this literature and to allow the interested reader to pursue selected themes in greater depth.

A detailed methodological evaluation of the research approaches has been provided elsewhere (Kasl, 1978). Suffice it to note here a number of problems. These include; the insufficient use of prospective epidemiologic designs, in which a cohort of subjects is picked up prior to incidence of disease and risk factor data are collected prospectively; the neglect of biological risk factors or markers in order to document the antecedent, additive, interactive, or mediating role of the stressors of interest; the inability to rule out diverse confounding variables, particularly those associated with self-selection into stressor exposure; the ambiguous role of the subjective variables (perceptions and evaluations of the stressors), which are supposed to be the crucial linkages between stressors and disease outcomes. These subjective parameters are usually only weakly related to the objective environmental conditions, their antecedents are unclear (but presumably involve, in part, stable personal characteristics), and they may be confounded with outcomes (either because the measurement processes for both are similar or because these subjective variables are influenced by the outcomes in the fashion of "reverse causation", involving cognitive reappraisal or attribution processes).

The best studies exploit research opportunities presented by "natural" experiments. Such settings sometimes offer the possibility of prospective longitudinal designs, with highly comparable naturally occurring control groups, and minimal problems of self-selection. A recent Belgian study of coronary heart disease (CHD) among male bank employees (Kittel *et al.*, 1980) is a good illustration of this strategy. Two cohorts of clerks and executives, initially free of CHD, were followed for 10 years. In one cohort, the subjects worked in a private bank with a typically commercial function; moreover, changes in management policy moved toward a more dynamic enterprise and linked promotion to greater competitiveness. In the second cohort, the subjects worked in a semi-public savings bank; they had fewer responsibilities, the struggle for promotion was minimal, and no major changes in management policy took place. Over the 10-year period, the first cohort experienced a 50 per cent higher rate of "hard" events (fatal or non-fatal myocardial infarction, sudden death) than the second cohort, after controlling for the major coronary risk factors in a multiple logistic function. The excess of new events in the first cohort was particularly striking among men in the higher quintiles of coronary risk factors. An earlier report of CHD prevalence among monks (Caffrey, 1969) also represented this strategy of pinpointed contrast. Within both the Benedictine and Trappist orders, which differ in diet and life-style, the priests who had more responsibilities had higher CHD rates than the brothers with few responsibilities. Both studies, however, lacked data on psychosocial and behavioural intervening processes, which would have helped clarify the linkage between stressors and disease outcomes.

Analyses of disease-specific mortality rates continue to be a popular way of attempting to identify possibly stressful occupations. Such analyses (e.g. Guralnick, 1963) have shown that certain occupational groups (such as college presidents, professors and teachers) die from atherosclerotic heart disease at a lower than expected rate, while other groups (such as lawyers and judges; physicians and surgeons; pharmacists; insurance agents and brokers; real estate agents and brokers) have higher than expected rates. Since these differences are reasonably large (about two to one), but involve groups rather comparable on social status, level of physical activity, physical hazards in the work environment, and so on, it is not unreasonable to ask whether differential job stressors might not be involved. The mortality differences between teachers and physicians have been observed in several countries (King, 1970). Moreover, it has also been noted that general practitioners have twice as high rates of incidence of myocardial infarction (and mortality from it) as do other types of physicians (Morris *et al.*, 1952).

Unfortunately, the interpretation of mortality differentials due to occupations is frequently speculative. For example, the high rates of coronary heart disease mortality among policemen, sheriffs, and marshals (Guralnick,

1963) could be completely a function of self-selection into those occupations: lower-middle class men who smoke, tend to be overweight and have higher levels of blood pressure and cholesterol. Furthermore, mortality statistics do not tell us at which point(s) of the disease development spectrum the suspect work stress variable may make its impact: on health habits, on level of biological risk factors, on incidence of new events (for a given level of risk factors), and on case fatality. For example, the recent analysis of CHD mortality in British civil servants included data on risk factors and life style habits and was thus able to show that the excess mortality for those in the lowest grades was insufficiently explained by their higher levels of risk factors (Marmot et al., 1978). The strategy of comparing mortality ratios of men in selected occupations to the mortality experience of their wives (e.g. Carruthers, 1980) is another strategy for attempting to gain more precision, but the technique still appears rather problematic.

Useful leads may also come from cross-sectional studies or morbidity prevalence differentials involving rather similar occupations or work settings. Thus Russek (1962) has reported that those specialities in medicine, dentistry and law which were rated by experts as more "stressful" (unspecified) had higher rates of CHD, as determined from mailed questionnaires. Even though a later report (Russek, 1965) revealed a positive association between stressfulness and cigarette smoking, and analyses within smoking categories showed a much more tenuous relationship between stressfulness and CHD rates, the original association between speciality and CHD risk is clarified rather than invalidated. Suggestive results were also noted in a study of NASA personnel (French and Caplan, 1970). Prevalence rates of CHD among managers were significantly higher than among scientists and engineers and, as a group, the managers also had higher levels of role conflict, subjective quantitative overload, and amount of responsibility.

A quite different research strategy for identifying stressful occupational groups is to select dangerous or demanding occupations (initially, an intuitive judgement) and then describe the comparative stresses on these jobs. Health outcomes are generally not included in such studies. Groups which have been studied in this fashion include coal miners (Althouse and Hurrell, 1977), fighter pilots (Aitken, 1969), policemen (Davidson and Veno, 1980; Kroes et al., 1974; Margolis, 1973) and air traffic controllers (Crump, 1979; Singer and Rutenfranz, 1971; Smith, 1973). The common finding from these efforts is that the dangerous or demanding aspects of jobs are seldom mentioned as sources of stress or dissatisfaction and one is left a bit puzzled about the initial intuition which led us to study these jobs. For example, the most common "stress" reported by policemen involves administrative issues and contacts with the court system. Does this reveal a weakness of the self-report methodology and its inability to penetrate defensiveness, or is it appropriate to take these results at face value? A cautious investigator must reserve judgement and not be swept by the immense publicity about the purported stressfulness of the policeman's job and the toll it exacts (Davidson and Veno, 1980). The high divorce rate among the police for example may reflect the changes in values, attitudes and life style which are precipitated by becoming a policeman, rather than being linked to stress *per se*.

Holt (1982) provides an excellent overview of the specific conditions at work which have been examined, as stressors, for their health impact. One often investigated dimension is *workload*, and there is an increasingly popular formulation which asserts that jobs or organizational roles which are associated with overload, excessive demands, and many responsibilities represent settings of high CHD risk (Kasl, 1978). Supporting evidence includes the findings that elevated risk is related to working excessive hours and/or holding down more than one full-time job (House, 1974) and being in a high level executive job but having a typically low level of education for that job category (Hinkle *et al.*, 1968). The precise nature of this evidence, however, suggests that grand formulations may be premature. One study may show excess risk associated with two jobs, but not overtime, another may show higher risk for overtime, but not for hours of work at home, and still another may show excess risk due to working many hours. In a prospective study of myocardial infarction (MI) among Swedish construction workers (Theorell and Floderus-Myrhed, 1977), a "workload" index which increased the risk for MI contained items which dealt with having *too little* responsibility or experiencing recent changes toward less responsibility. Possibly, the underlying risk factor is general job dissatisfaction, an interpretation supported by other reports (Jenkins, 1976; Sales and House, 1971). Finally, we must also remember that men in higher levels of management often have lower, not higher, rates of CHD than those in lower levels (Hinkle *et al.*, 1968; Marmot *et al.*, 1978; Pell and D'Alonzo, 1963). Since workload and responsibility tend to be positively associated with management level, additional factors must play a crucial role. They may include organizational resources available to the executive to deal with the workload, wide job decision latitude (Karasek *et al.*, 1981) which permits effective coping, company selection or self-selection processes which promote those who deal with the workload effectively, and so on.

The workload dimension also seems implicated (suggestively but not at all conclusively) in studies which assess, not the work environment itself, but some reaction to it. Specifically, several prospective and retrospective studies of MI (e.g. Paffenbarger *et al.*, 1966; Russek, 1965; Thomas and

Greenstreet, 1973; Wardwell *et al.*, 1968; see Jenkins, 1976 and 1981 for reviews of this evidence) have repeatedly identified one specific area of symptoms and complaints as a risk factor: reports of sleep disturbance, feeling tired on awakening, being exhausted at the end of day, unable to relax. However, these reports of fatigue and exhaustion have not been linked to environmental conditions, such as an objectively demanding job. Instead, the fact that these symptoms are related to father's occupational level, but not the subject's, and that they predict from the time before the subjects began their work careers, suggest that we are dealing with a pre-existing trait variable rather than a response to situational demands (or prodromal symptomatology).

Another aspect of the work environment frequently examined for health impact is *shiftwork* (e.g. Mott *et al.*, 1965; Rentos and Shepard, 1976; Tasto and Colligan, 1978; Winget *et al.*, 1978). There is little question that certain complaints (particularly sleep disturbances, fatigue, digestion and elimination problems) are associated with shiftwork. Workers whose shifts rotate once a week continually have their circadian rhythms and social life disrupted, and they are the ones who report most complaints. Continuous employment on the evening shift greatly interferes with many social interactions. In addition to the social disruption and the disorganization of time-oriented psysiology (eating, sleeping, body temperature, etc.), those working in the evenings or on rotating shifts may have an excess of rheumatoid arthritis and and possibly peptic ulcer (Mott *et al.*, 1965). In general, workers in fixed afternoon and rotating shifts also give evidence of poorer mental health on a variety of indices (Kasl, 1973).

The shiftwork studies also indicate a good deal of interaction among variables in producing the health impact. For example, complaints related to insomnia are particularly common when shiftwork involves an interaction of variables such as working a night shift and living in poor housing with inadequate sound insulation (Thiis-Evensen, 1958). Specific complaints, such as those regarding sleep, depend partly on individual differences in diurnal variations in levels of activity, such as preferring high levels of activity in the morning vs in the evening (Torsvall and Akerstedt, 1980). Psychosomatic complaints associated with night-work appear to be related to changes in serum gastrin levels as well as to a stable trait variable, neuroticism (Akerstedt and Theorell, 1976).

The findings from shiftwork studies are not always clearly interpretable, because of self selection issues: in many settings, voluntary choices and financial inducements are involved in working a particular shift and pre-existing differences among workers may appear as impact of the shift. It is also not clear to what extent the findings should be interpreted within a stress framework. For example, sleep disturbances as a result of trying to sleep during the day in a noisy environment may represent simple and direct cause-effect associations, with no need to involve elaborate stress formulations.

Various aspects of *organizational structure* have also been examined for their possible linkages to health outcomes (Holt, 1982; Kahn, 1981; Kahn *et al.*, 1982; Katz and Kahn, 1978). However, much of this work deals with mental health variables, job satisfaction, and absenteeism. For example, large organizations with a "flat" organizational structure (relatively few levels in the organization) are associated with higher levels of job dissatisfaction, absenteeism, and, frequently, accidents. Having a staff position (versus a position on the production line) is also related to higher job dissatisfaction. Jobs which are at "boundaries" of organizations often have elevated disease rates. For example, external salesmen are at excess risk for peptic ulcer (Ihre and Muller, 1943) and Benedictine priests working outside the monastery had 65% higher rate of myocardial infarction than Benedictine priests inside the monastery (Quinlan and Barrow, 1966). The concept of "boundariness" is admittedly difficult to operationalize and quantify. Nevertheless, the job of the foreman, so frequently at the interface between union and management, could also be considered a "boundary" job. As was noted already, foremen have an excess of peptic ulcer disease (Pflanz, 1971; Susser, 1967) and, in some industries, may have an excess of CHD as well (Pell and D'Alonzo, 1963).

Even though the focus of this chapter is on chronic conditions, it is worth noting briefly the literature on *change in the work role*, because of the relatively enduring changes involved. *Retirement* is a good example of a change which is both an acute event as well as the beginning of enduring exposure to a new set of environmental conditions. The research literature on retirement is in rather good agreement that, on the average, there is no adverse impact on mental and physical health associated with the transition from work to retirement (Kasl, 1980; Minkler, 1981). Furthermore, variations in post-retirement outcomes are most convincingly seen as reflecting continuities or pre-retirement status (particularly in physical health, social and leisure activities, general well-being and satisfaction), so that it is even difficult to argue that "no adverse impact on average" hides a mixture of beneficial and adverse outcomes of retirement, depending on various circumstances. Nevertheless, there probably is a minority of individuals whose attachment to the work role is so strong (and whose life cycle perspective on the work role views normal retirement age as inappropriate) that involuntary retirement can be followed by depression or other illnesses, although this has not been adequately documented.

Studies of *occupational mobility* and disease outcomes, particularly CHD, have revealed inconsistent and ambiguous findings (Berkanovic and

Krochalk, 1977; Jenkins, 1976, Kasl, 1978), often showing no impact (e.g. Lehman *et al.*, 1967). The basic problem is that such studies have been much too superficial and the measurement of mobility has been insensitive to the life cycle perspective (e.g. career goals and aspirations) and the underlying changes in "person-environment fit" (e.g. better or poorer fit between a person's skills and the new job demands) precipitated by the job mobility.

The research on the health effects of *unemployment* is currently in turmoil. Powerful effects of unemployment on mortality have been suggested by ecological (aggregate) analyses of business cycle fluctuations (e.g. Brenner, 1979; Brenner and Mooney, 1982; Bunn, 1979). However, this method has major weaknesses which gave gone unanswered (Kasl, 1979 and 1981) and there is a great need for assessment by different methodologies to see if the results will be confirmed. A modification of the macro-social approach to aggregated data, supplemented by longitudinal survey data, has yielded somewhat inconsistent results, pointing towards a modest adverse impact at best (Catalano and Dooley, 1977 and 1979; Dooley and Catalano, 1979; Dooley *et al.*, 1981). And the previous mentioned results of our own longitudinal survey (Cobb and Kasl, 1977; Kasl, 1982; Kasl and Cobb, 1979 and 1980) revealed acute effects but not chronic changes, thus suggesting very limited support for the unemployment mortality connection. Certainly, the current salience of this problem will lead to additional research efforts and findings which may offer a resolution to this disagreement.

It might be noted that the occupational stress and health literature has dealt predominantly with men and that research efforts on *women* are only now beginning to acquire momentum (Haw, 1982). Much of this work is at a fairly primitive stage, using cross-sectional data and depending on simplistic operationalizations (e.g. cross-classifications of subjects by marital status, work status, and presence of children) to get at complex constructs, such as conflict between roles or stresses of multiple roles. Many problematic or crucial variables remain unmeasured, such as the self-selection factors which relate to working status (career goals, family finances, etc.) and the protective or beneficial effects of the work role. The tentative conclusion thus far is that the adverse health effects of multiple roles on women have not been demonstrated.

The Framingham study has been the basis of some fine prospective analyses of work and CHD in women (Haynes and Feinleib, 1980; Haynes *et al.*, 1980). The results revealed only a slight (non-significant) excess of CHD among working women. This effect was strongest in the comparison of clerical workers with non-working women, particularly for clerical workers with significant family responsibilities. Decreased job mobility and an unsupportive boss were also found to be CHD risk factors among the clerical workers. Women's working status also was found to influence the role of other psychosocial risk factors: among working women, behaviour Type A and suppressed hostility proved to be stronger predictors of CHD, while among housewives, being easygoing and showing tension symptoms were the two scales which were the stronger predictors of CHD.

It is useful to conclude this section on occupational stress with Locke's (1976) characterization of desirable conditions at work (based more on evidence from job satisfaction and mental health measures, than physical outcomes): (i) work represents mental challenge (with which the worker can cope successfully) and leads to involvement and personal interest; (ii) work is not physically too tiring; (iii) rewards for performance are just, informative and in line with aspirations; (iv) working conditions are compatible with physical needs and they facilitate work goals; (v) work leads to high self-esteem; and (vi) agents in the work place help with the attainment of job values.

THE RESIDENTIAL ENVIRONMENT AND HEALTH

There is an extensive research literature on the physical and mental health impact of the residential environment. However, unlike the studies of the occupational environment, the residential literature seldom makes use of explicit stress–theoretical formulations. This seems appropriate, for many of the cause–effect relationships are of a simple, direct nature: poor environmental design and home accidents, presence of house dust and allergies, faulty heating and carbon monoxide poisoning, presence of lead–containing interior paint and lead poisoning (Spivey and Radford, 1979). To be sure, these environmental conditions are necessary but not sufficient for the adverse health outcome to take place. Psychosocial characteristics, including stress reactions, could be involved in the causal matrix. For example, family conflict could alter parental supervision of small children, which in turn changes the potential connection between lead paint and lead poisoning into an actuality. However, these are mere speculations which need to be documented.

Evaluating the impact of many residential settings is made difficult by problems of self-selection which confound the relationships. For example, the apparent impact of retirement residential communities on health and well-being of the elderly can be partly or completely a function of pre-existing goals, plans, and aspirations for a specific retirement setting, and the relation of these to the person's assessment of what he or she actually experiences in that setting (Kasl and Rosenfield, 1980). Institutional settings, such as long-term hospitals or nursing homes, appear to be powerful environmental influences on the health status of its elderly residents and the excess mortality associated with moves to such settings has been amply documented (e.g. Rowland, 1977). However, the self-selection bias in this instance is so powerful (individuals who are in a seriously debilitated or incapacitated conditions are admitted at the point when pre-existing adverse changes in health status have taken place) that such mortality data are quite useless. Lawton (1977) has expressed astonishment that "to date no complete longitudinal control group study allowing a critical test of the effects of institutionalization has been reported" (p. 293). What we do have, among the interpretable research designs, are studies of patient and environmental characteristics which relate to *differential* outcomes. Prominent among these is the work of Lieberman and his colleagues, which suggests that health-enhancing institutional environments are those which foster autonomy and more personalization of residents, are more integrated into the community, allow privacy and leave locus of control to a greater extent with the patients, and are not permissive regarding deviant behaviour (e.g. Lieberman, 1974; Tobin and Lieberman, 1976; Turner *et al.*, 1972). It can be readily seen that these are not parameters of the physical setting of these institutions, but rather its policies, its rules and regulations. This is typical of the whole social–ecological perspective on environmental influences on health status where the dominant emphasis is on psychosocial rather than physical parameters (e.g. Moos, 1979).

One of the aspects of the residential setting which has received a good deal of attention, and which is potentially quite compatible with a stressor and stress reaction theoretic framework, is the work on *crowding* and *density*. While fundamental issues regarding conceptualization and specification of underlying psychosocial processes remain to be worked out, some kind of a distinction between population density (e.g. in the neighbourhood) and crowding within the dwelling unit is now well accepted (Aiello and Baum, 1979; Baldassare, 1979; Epstein, 1981). A recent overview of this field would suggest that, with the exception of infectious diseases, the results of impact have been quite inconsistent; the need to control adequately for confounding variables remains a paramount issue (Cox *et al.*, 1982).

Much of the work represents ecological correlations between residential characteristics of census tracts or geographical areas and mortality or institutional contact rates (e.g. hospital admissions, crime statistics), aggregated for the same areas (e.g. Brennan and Lancashire, 1978; Galle *et al.*, 1972; Levy and Herzog, 1974; Manton and Myers, 1977. For overviews, see Hinkle and Loring, 1977; Kasl, 1976). While this work gives the general impression that, after adjusting for socio-demographic variables, some impact of crowding and density does remain (but not always in the expected direction; see Levy and Herzog, 1974), many technical problems of statistical adjustments (e.g. problems of partialling out effects of highly correlated variables in elaborate multivariate analyses) remain. One highly illuminating re-analysis was carried out by Ward (1975), who showed that, as one introduces more refined measures of social variables (class and ethnicity), the apparent contribution of population density to pathology is reduced.

Some of the recent work on residential crowding, carried out from an epidemiological or social survey perspective (i.e. non-ecological) has been done by two research teams who have recently engaged in a heated controversy over their findings (Booth et al., 1980; Gove and Hughes, 1980). The more useful aspect of the debate concerns the use of objective vs subjective ("experience of crowding") indices and the limitations of the persons/room index. However, the more telling but less illuminating aspect of the debate is over just how *small* the effects are. Even under extreme conditions of residential crowding the impact is small (e.g. Mitchell, 1971). Overall, studies which involve individuals (not aggregate data) and objective indices of crowding rarely explain more than 2–3% of the variance.

Unfortunately, a good deal of the density and crowding research is working with superficial or opaque variables. For example, the meaning of a specific value on an index of crowding is altered by the presence of young children or by single person households, variables which on their own can mask or confound the apparent impact of crowding. Similarly, an index of areal density may reflect luxurious high-rise apartments in one setting and crowded inner city slums in another.

The research literature on living in high-rise housing (e.g. Gillis, 1977; Kaminoff and Proshansky, 1982; Power, 1970; Stevenson et al., 1967) is consistent with the crowding research, and fails to suggest that such a residential setting is inherently stressful. Some problems appear fairly predictably, such as supervision of small children's outdoor play or lack of perceived control over the environment, especially its social aspects. Other problems, such as crime, may also be heightened by the high-rise setting. However, the health impact of such problems is yet to be demonstrated. In any case, the impact of the high-rise setting cannot be expected to be uniform. It may be affected by sex, stage of life cycle, housing goals, aspirations, expectations of future mobility and ability to establish friendship contacts and social supports.

In general, the residential environment appears to have limited impact on health, and leaves little room for explorations of stress–disease associations. Wilner's classical study of 20 years ago (Wilner et al., 1962) on health benefits of improved housing showed minimal effects, thereby setting the stage for overthrowing intuitive and "common sense" beliefs about the impact of housing (e.g. Schorr, 1963). General reviews of the literature (e.g.

Hinkle and Loring, 1977; Kasl and Rosenfield, 1980) have supported the following conclusions. Firstly, the link between residential parameters (objectively defined) and subjective perceptions and evaluations (such as housing satisfaction) is a strong one. The next link, from such perceptions and evaluations to desire to make a residential move, is also strong. The further links with certain outcomes, such as fairly superficial indicators of social interaction, are also reasonably well established. However, the links to distal disease outcomes are rare and seem to involve specific and "mechanistic" hazard-to-disease connections, which seldom require the help from a stress formulation.

OTHER ENVIRONMENTAL EXPOSURES

Research evidence has accumulated on the impact of exposure to a variety of environmental factors, such as noise, heat, air pollution, traffic congestion, and other more specialized conditions. Recent reviews are available for much of this work (Baum *et al.*, 1981; Bell, 1981; Cohen and Weinstein, 1981; Evans and Jacobs, 1981; Stokols and Novaco, 1981). Other factors, such as electric shock or cold pressor, have been only examined in laboratory setting and will not be considered.

The study of the processes involved in possible health impact of such environmental exposures is made difficult by the presence of several interrelated processes. Hazards which are perceptible to the senses, or when the person has been made aware of his or her exposure, are subject to a process of cognitive appraisal. This process is under the influence of many host characteristics, including the outcome variables we wish to study. Variations in the appraisal can have a major influence on behavioural effects. A relatively simple physical parameter has now become a complex psychophysical stimulus. The appraised hazard may lead to arousal (activation) and to efforts at coping and adaptation, which may have their own behavioural and biological effects, which may in turn strongly influence the outcomes of interest, and are affected by the nature of the appraisal and many host characteristics. Many of the behavioural and health outcomes that are studied are heavily influenced by prior years of learning and socialization and prior health history and by major social–environmental variables, such as the marriage and the family. Variables defining the environmental exposure are likely to account only for a small part of the variance in the behavioural outcomes. Biases in measurement and spurious effects may easily swamp this sought-for small effect.

Evaluation of the evidence is made difficult by its fragmentary nature. With respect to air pollution, for example, we have the documentation of the relationship to respiratory disease, but this does not include evidence on the role of psychosocial processes (Whittemore, 1981). On the other hand, we have studies which examine the influence of objectively determined levels of air pollution on awareness, perception of severity, complaining to authorities, and indicators of proximate impact, such as annoyance or being "bothered". The role of many modifying variables, such as perceived adaptability, coping strategies, habituation and desensitization processes and general neighbourhood satisfaction has also been examined, and complex dynamics have been clearly revealed (Creer et al., 1970; Evans and Jacobs, 1981; Hohm, 1976; Lindvall and Radford, 1973). This rich evidence, however, does not add up to a complete linkage with disease outcomes, and only indirectly implicates possible stress processes.

The evidence on the impact of *noise* is the most extensive, and illustrates some of the generic conceptual and methodological issues involved. General reviews have vacillated between two views. On the one hand, it is argued (Kryter, 1972) that harmful effects of noise as a physical stimulus have not been demonstrated, because it is likely that the harmful effects are due to the psychological meaning of the stimulus not its physical properties (e.g. noise on the job may mean threat of bodily harm from machinery and it is perhaps this threat which has long term consequences). On the other hand, it is suggested (Goldsmith and Jonsson, 1973) that long-term effects of noise have not yet been adequately studied, and that many possibly harmful effects (on symptoms, impairment of function, feelings, interference with activities) may be direct effects of the physical properties of the stimulus. Studies of specific relationships, such as airport noise and birth defects (Jones and Tauscher, 1978; Edmonds et al., 1979) or airport noise and mental hospital admissions (Abey-Wickrama et al., 1969; Jenkins et al., 1981), have yielded inconsistent findings. Data on children, however, seem more consistent and suggest long-term effects on blood pressure, auditory discrimination, distractability and, possibly, reading ability (S. Cohen et al., 1979, 1980 and 1982; Cohen and Weinstein, 1981).

There is ample evidence that the impact of environmental noise on psychological and behavioural outcome has many modifiers. For example, residents near a motorway are less disturbed by the noise coming from the motorway if they are heavy users of it (Hitchcock and Waterhouse, 1979). Residents near airports are more annoyed by the noise if they are afraid of crashes or if they have various negative attitudes towards the airport and the personnel (Cohen and Weinstein, 1981).

Most interesting are the results of a recent British study of mental health effects of aircraft noise (Jenkins et al., 1981; Tarnapolsky et al., 1980; Watkins et al., 1981), which illustrate a pattern of findings which is puzzling and troublesome, but not unusual in studies of environmental exposures.

Essentially, a substantial association (gamma = 0.50) was observed between objectively measured noise (The Noise and Number Index, NNI) and the level of being bothered and annoyed. Being bothered and annoyed was also associated with levels of various symptoms, with use of any drugs and with use of psychotropic drugs only. However, the objective indicator of noise, NNI, was *not* related to these same outcomes. Moreover, within each level of annoyance, higher symptom levels and higher use of drugs was observed in the *lower* NNI areas. The study examined many other variables, such as psychiatric hospital admissions and outpatient visits to general practitioners, but none showed a significant impact of the objective noise levels. The results of an earlier study of airport noise and community symptom levels obtained findings fully consistent with the British data (Graeven, 1974). Overall, one has the impression of dealing with an intervening variable which does not intervene: the subjective perception or appraisal of noise and bothersomeness is an intervening variable in a non-existent overall relationship between objective noise and indices of impact!

These findings point to the confusing and confounding role of the attribution process. It may be presumed to be the strongest when we are dealing with highly ambiguous environmental exposures, where the major source of impact, if there is any, comes from the psychological appraisal process. This would apply to the Three Mile Island accident (Houts and Goldhaber, 1981), to exposures to high voltage direct current transmission lines (Gatchel et al., 1981), and to incidents of industrial "mass psychogenic illness" (Smith et al., 1978). The TMI results are particularly illuminating: by October, 1980 (some 18 months after the accident), the level of symptoms among residents within 5 miles of the TMI nuclear plant was comparable to that for residents living 41–55 miles away. However, residents near TMI were still much more likely to attribute their symptoms to the accident than were residents from farther away. Similarly, a study of men after a natural disaster (flooding) showed "self-perceived influence of flood on health", even though no differences in the number and nature of illnesses between exposed and unexposed respondents were observed (Melick, 1978).

PERSONAL AND BEHAVIOURAL CHARACTERISTICS MODIFYING STRESSOR EFFECTS

The studies which fall into this category help us to identify characteristics or attributes of susceptible or vulnerable individuals, and to understand the processes mediating between stressors and disease outcomes. The research literature is very large and only a brief sketch, outlining the major themes, will be given here.

One type of study identifies a risk factor for a disease outcome, thereby improving our ability to predict incidence. For example, greater emotional and behavioural distance to parents, reported by medical students, is a predictor of cancer incidence (and suicide) in later years (Thomas et al., 1979). The association appears robust, and later analyses revealed the specific importance of the father–son relationship and showed that the association survived statistical controls for smoking, drinking, and radiation exposure (Shaffer et al., 1982). However, specific causal processes are not established using this strategy.

The recent evidence that a negative global self-assessment or one's health status is a risk factor for higher mortality above and beyond one's actual ("objective") health status is another fascinating finding in search of aetiological mechanisms (Kaplan and Camacho, 1983; Mossey and Shapiro, 1982). Persons with negative self-assessments of health do have fewer healthy life style habits and fewer social contacts, but these are separate predictors of mortality, not accounting for the predictive power of the self-assessments of health (Berkman and Syme, 1979; Wingard et al., 1982).

The work on the Type A or Coronary-Prone Behaviour Pattern has finally begun to move away from treating it as an isolated stable personality characteristic, towards studying it in interaction with other variables, primarily those relating to the work setting (e.g. Chesney et al., 1981; Davidson and Cooper, 1980). It is not yet clear what kind of a modifier variable it is, or how it interacts with relevant work environment variables, such as job demands and deadline pressures. The finding that, among air traffic controllers, those who were less hard driving were at greater risk of future hypertension, would seem to suggest that in certain demanding work settings, being a Type A reduces rather than increases CHD risk (Rose et al., 1978). However, since Type A's had higher illness rates, it would seem that we cannot really make a choice between two relevant formulations: either Type A people in Type A work settings experience high person–environment fit and, consequently, low stress; or Type A persons are particularly stimulated in Type A work settings (high stress) and thus their CHD risk is synergistically enhanced. Of course, it is possible that both formulations apply, depending on which aspect of the Type A construct we are considering. For example, with respect to competitiveness Type A's may thrive in such a work setting (high P–E fit), while with respect to low environmental control. Type A's may be aroused physiologically, thus enhancing their CHD risk. Additional complexity is introduced by our inability to separate out three relevant processes: Type A's self-selecting certain work setting; Type A's creating certain job conditions; Type A's responding to certain job conditions.

The richest and most complex work on modifiers of stressor effects concerns the work on coping and adaptation, and social supports and social networks. Coping and evaluation is an area of considerable theoretical development (Coelho *et al.*, 1974; Holroyd and Lazarus, 1982; Lazarus, 1966), but assessment procedures suitable for epidemiologic investigations of stressor–disease associations are a relatively recent development (e.g. Folkman and Lazarus, 1980; Ilfeld, 1982; Pearlin and Schooler, 1978). Consequently, the major contribution of this area thus far has been to our understanding of coping with illness (e.g. Cohen and Lazarus, 1979; Moos, 1977), and of processes influencing course of pre-existing disease (e.g. Kasl, 1983), but not yet toward understanding of incidence of new disease. The relevance of coping processes to surgery and recovery after myocardial infarction are discussed in more detail in Chapters 7 and 8.

Research on social support and social networks (or at least the use of these terms in titles) has become popular, but fundamental issues of conceptualization and measurement (as in the case of stress) remain to be resolved. The conceptualizations at the moment are varied (e.g. Cobb, 1976; Gore, 1981; Kaplan *et al.*, 1977; Lieberman, 1982; Lin *et al.*, 1979, Porritt, 1979) and conceptual overlap between different formulations is somewhat confusing. While many different concepts and processes have been proposed, the measurement methodology to implement these is lagging behind. The empirical evidence at the moment is quite sporadic; for areas where most systematic work has been done, such as stress at work, the results suggest surprisingly weak effects (e.g. LaRocco *et al.*, 1980; Winnbust *et al.*, 1982). For specific disease outcomes, such as angina pectoris, social support processes may play an important role in incidence (Medalie and Goldbourt, 1976). However, it appears possible that the role of support and network variables is more important for medical care behaviours and for processes relating to course of illness (Kasl, 1983) than to incidence of new disease.

CONCLUDING COMMENTS

Attempts to provide an overview of a large and complex area of research are bound to suffer to some extent from over-simplifications, distortions and the idiosyncratic biases of the reviewer. The primary bias of this chapter is one of methodological scepticism. This stance appears justified on two grounds. Firstly, the possible link between stress and disease has received a generous airing in the scientific and lay press, and a critical commentary is unlikely to stifle continued interest in this area. Secondly, the dominant popular and scientific bias, in the face of ambiguous evidence, is to see vulnerability in human organisms (stressors causing disease) and a critical commentary raises the alternative possibility of successful adaptability.

REFERENCES

Abey-Wickrama, I. Brook, M. E. A., Gattoni, F. E. G. and Herridge, C. F. (1969). Mental hospital admissions and aircraft noise. *Lancet* **ii,** 1275–1278.

Aiello, J. R. and Baum, A., eds (1979). "Residential Crowding and Design." Plenum Press, New York.

Aitken, R. C. B. (1969). Prevalence of worry in normal aircrew. *Br. J. Med. Psychol.* **42,** 283–286.

Akerstedt, T. and Theorell, T. (1976). Exposure to night work: serum gastrin reactions, psychosomatic complaints and personality variables. *J. Psychosom. Res.* **20,** 479–484.

Alfredsson, L., Karasek, R. and Theorell, T. (1982). Myocardial infarction risk and psychosocial work environment: An analysis of the male Swedish working force. *Soc. Sci. Med.* **16,** 463–467.

Althouse, R. and Hurrell, J. (1977). "An Analysis of Job Stress in Coal Mining." DHEW (NIOSH) Publication No. 77–217, U.S. Government Printing Office, Washington, D.C.

Baldassare, M. (1979). "Residential Crowding in Urban America." University of California Press, Berkeley.

Baum, A., Singer, J. E. and Baum, C. S. (1981). Stress and the environment. *J. Soc. Issues* **37**(1), 4–35.

Beech, H. R., Burns, L. E. and Sheffield, B. F. (1982). "A Behavioural Approach to the Management of Stress." Wiley, Chichester.

Bell, P. A. (1981). Physiological, comfort, performance, and social effects of heat stress. *J. Soc. Issues* **37** (1), 71–94.

Berkanovic, E. and Krochalk, P. C. (1977). Occupational mobility and health. *In* "Advances in Psychosomatic Medicine, Vol. 9: Epidemiologic Studies in Psychosomatic Medicine" (S. V. Kasl and F. Reichsman, eds), pp. 132–139. Karger, Basel.

Berkman, L. F. and Syme, S. L. (1979). Social networks, host resistance, and mortality: a nine-year follow-up study of Alameda Country residents. *Am. J. Epidemiol.* **108,** 186–204.

Bloom, B. L., Asher, S. J. and White, S. W. (1978). Marital disruption as a stressor: a review and analysis. *Psychol. Bull.* **85,** 867–894.

Booth, A., Johnson, D. R. and Edwards, J. N. (1980). In pursuit of pathology: The effects of human crowding. *Am. Sociol. Rev.* **45,** 873–878.

Bourne, P. G., Rose, R. M. and Mason, J. W. (1967). Urinary 17-OHCS levels. Data on seven helicopter ambulance medics in combat. *Arch. Gen. Psychiat.* **17,** 104–110.

Bourne, P. G., Rose, R. M. and Mason, J. W. (1968). 17-OHCS levels in combat. *Arch. Gen. Psychiat.* **19,** 135–140.

Brennan, M. E. and Lancashire, R. (1978). Association of childhood mortality with housing status and unemployment. *J. Epidemiol. Comm. Health* **32,** 28–33.

Brenner, M. H. (1979). Mortality and the national economy. A review and the experience of England and Wales, 1936–1976. *Lancet* **ii**, 568–573.

Brenner, M. H. and Mooney, A. (1982). Economic change and sex-specific cardiovascular mortality in Britain 1955–1976. *Soc. Sci. Med.* **16**, 431–442.

Bunn, A. R. (1979). Ischaemic heart disease mortality and the business cycle in Australia. *Am. J. Pub. Health* **69**, 772–781.

Bunney, W., Jr., Shapiro, A., Ader, R., Davis, J., Herd, A., Kopin, I. J., Jr., Krieger, D., Matthysse, S., Stunkard, A., Weissman, M. and Wyatt, R. J. (1982). Panel report on stress and illness. *In* "Stress and Human Health" (G. R. Elliott and C. Eisdorfer, eds), pp. 257–337. Springer-Verlag, New York.

Burchfield, S. R. (1979). The stress response: A new perspective. *Psychosom. Med.* **41**, 661–672.

Caffrey, B. (1969). Behavior patterns and personality characteristics related to prevalence rates of coronary heart disease in American monks. *J. Chron. Dis.* **22**, 93–103.

Caplan, R. D., Cobb, S., French, J. R. P., Jr., Harrison, R. V. and Pinneau, S. R., Jr. (1975). "Job Demands and Worker Health." HEW Publication No. (NIOSH) 75–160, Washington, D.C.

Carruthers, M. (1980). Hazardous occupations and the heart. *In* "Current Concerns in Occupational Stress." (C. L. Cooper and R. Payne, eds), pp. 3–22. Wiley, Chichester.

Catalano, R. and Dooley, D. (1977). Economic predictors of depressed mood and stressful life events in a metropolitan community. *J. Health Soc. Behav.* **18**, 292–307.

Catalano, R. and Dooley, D. (1979). The economy as a stressor: A sectoral analysis. *Rev. Social Economy* **37**, 175–188.

Chesney, M. A., Sevelius, G., Black, G. W., Ward, M. M., Swan, G. E. and Rosenman, R. H. (1981). Work environment, Type A behavior, and coronary heart disease risk factors. *J. Occup. Med.* **23**, 551–555.

Cobb, S. (1976). Social support as a moderator of life stress. *Psychosom. Med.* **38**, 300–314.

Cobb, S. and Kasl, S. V. (1977). "Termination: The Consequences of Job Loss." HEW Publication No. (NIOSH) 77–224, Cincinnati.

Cobb, S. and Rose, R. M. (1973). Hypertension, peptic ulcer, and diabetes in air traffic controllers. *J. Am. Med. Ass.* **224**, 489–492.

Coelho, G. V., Hamburg, D. A. and Adams, J. E., eds (1974). "Coping and Adaptation." Basic Books, New York.

Cohen, F. and Lazarus, R. S. (1979). Coping with stresses of illneess. *In* "Health Psychology—A Handbook" (G. C. Stone, F. Cohen and N. E. Adler, eds), pp. 217–254. Jossey-Bass, San Francisco.

Cohen, F., Horowtiz, M. J., Lazarus, R. S., Moos, R. H., Robins, L. N., Rose, R. M. and Rutter, M. (1982). Panel report on psychosocial assets and modifiers of stress. *In* "Stress and Human Health" (G. R. Elliott and C. Eisdorfer, eds), pp. 149–188. Springer-Verlag, New York.

Cohen, S. and Weinstein, N. (1981). Nonauditory effects of noise on behavior and health. *J. Soc. Issues* **37**,(1), 36–70.

Cohen, S., Glass, D. C. and Phillips, S. (1979). Environment and health. *In* "Handbook of Medical Sociology" (H. E. Freeman, S. Levine and L. G. Reeder, eds), pp. 134–149. Prentice-Hall, Englewood Cliffs, N.J.

Cohen, S., Evans, G. W., Krantz, D. S. and Stokols, D. (1980). Physiological, motivational, and cognitive effects of aircraft noise on children. *Am. Psychologist* **35**, 231–243.

Cohen, S., Krantz, D. S., Evans, G. W. and Stokols, D. (1982). Community noise, behavior, and health: The Los Angeles Noise Project. *In* "Advances in Environmental Psychology, Vol. 4: Environment and Health" (A. Baum and J. E. Singer, eds), pp. 295–317. Erlbaum, Hillsdale, N.J.

Cooper, C. L. (1981). "The Stress Check." Prentice-Hall, Englewood Cliffs, N.J.

Cooper, C. L. and Payne, R., eds (1980). "Current Concerns in Occupational Stress." Wiley, Chichester.

Cox, V. C., Paulus, P. B., McCain, G. and Karlovac, M. (1982). The relationship between crowding and health. *In* "Advances in Environmental Psychology, Vol. 4: Environment and Health" (A. Baum and J. E. Singer, eds), pp. 271–294. Erlbaum, Hillsdale, N.J.

Creer, R. N., Gray, R. M. and Treshow, M. (1970). Differential responses to air pollution as an environmental health problem. *J. Air Pollut. Control Ass.* **30**, 814–818.

Crump, J. H. (1979). Review of stress in air traffic control: Its measurement and effects. *Aviat., Space, and Envir. Med.* **50**, 243–248.

D'Atri, D. A., Fitzgerald, E. F., Kasl, S. V. and Ostfeld, A. M. (1981). Crowding in prison: The relationship between changes in housing mode and blood pressure. *Psychosom. Med.* **43**, 95–105.

Davidson, M. J. and Cooper, C. L. (1980). Type A coronary-prone behavior in the work environment. *J. Occup. Med.* **22**, 375–383.

Davidson, M. J. and Veno, A. (1980). Stress and the policeman. *In* "White Collar and Professional Stress" (C. L. Cooper and J. Marshall, eds), pp. 131–166. Wiley, Chichester.

Dooley, D. and Catalano, R. (1979). Economic, life and disorder changes: time-series analyses. *Am. J. Comm. Psychol.* **7**, 381–396.

Dooley, D., Catalano, R., Jackson, R. and Brownell, A. (1981). Economic, life, and symptom changes in a nonmetropolitan community. *J. Health Soc. Behav.* **22**, 144–154.

Dutton, L. M., Smolensky, M. H., Leach, C. S., Lorimer, R. and Hsi, B. P. (1978). Stress levels of ambulance paramedics and fire fighters. *J. Occup. Med.* **20**, 111–115.

Edmonds, L. D., Layde, P. M. and Erickson, J. D. (1979). Airport noise and teratogenesis. *Arch. Envir. Health* **34**, 243–247.

Eliot, R. S. and Buell, J. C. (1981). Environmental and behavioral influences in the major cardiovascular disorders. *In* "Perspectives on Behavioral Medicine" (S. M. Weiss, J. A. Herd and B. H. Fox, eds), pp. 25–39. Academic Press, Orlando, New York and London.

Elliott, G. R. and Eisdorfer, C., eds (1982). "Stress and Human Health." Springer-Verlag, New York.

Epstein, Y. M. (1981). Crowding stress and human behavior. *J. Soc. Issues* **37**(1), 126–144.

Evans, G. W. and Jacobs, S. V. (1981). Air pollution and human behavior. *J. Soc. Issues* **37**(1), 95–125.

Folkman, S. and Lazarus, R. S. (1980). An analysis of coping in a middle-aged community sample. *J. Health Soc. Behav.* **21**, 219–239.

Frankenhaeuser, M. (1977). Job demands, health, and wellbeing. *J. Psychosom. Res.* **2**, 313–321.

Frankenhaeuser, M. (1979). Psychoneuroendocrine approaches to the study of emotion as related to stress and coping. In "Nebraska Symposium on Motivation" (H. E. Howe and R. A Dienstbier, eds), pp. 123–161. University of Nebraska Press, Lincoln.

Frankenhaeuser, M. and Gardell, B. (1976). Underload and overload in working life: outline of a multidisciplinary approach. J. Hum. Stress 2, 35–46.

French, J. R. P., Jr. and Caplan, R. D. (1970). Psychosocial factors in coronary heart disease. Industr. Med. Surg. 39, 383–397.

French, J. R. P., Jr., Caplan, R. D. and Harrison, R. V. (1982). "The Mechanisms of Job Stress and Strain." Wiley, Chichester.

Friedman, M. D., Rosenman, R. D. and Carroll, V. (1958). Changes in serum cholesterol and blood clotting time in men subjected to cyclic variation of occupational stress. Circulation 17, 852–861.

Galle, O., Gove, W. and McPherson, J. M. (1972). Population density and pathology: what are the relations for man? Science 176, 23–30.

Gardell, B. (1976). "Job Content and Quality of Life." Prisma, Stockholm.

Gatchel, R. J., Baum, A. and Baum, C. S. (1981). "Stress and Symptom Reporting as Related to the CV Line." Human Design Group, Olney, Maryland.

Gillis, A. R. (1977). High-rise housing and psychological strain. J. Health Soc, Behav. 18, 418–431.

Goldberger, L. and Breznitz, S. eds (1982). "Handbook of Stress." Free Press, New York.

Goldsmith, J. R. and Jonsson, E. (1973). Health effects of community noise. Am. J. Pub. Health 63, 782–793.

Gore, S. (1981). Stress-buffering functions of social supports: An appraisal and clarification of research models. In "Stressful Life Events and Their Contexts." (B. S. Dohrenwend and B. P. Dohrenwend, eds). pp. 202–222. Prodist, New York.

Gove, W. R. and Hughes, M. (1980). The effects of crowding found in the Toronto study: Some methodological and empirical questions. Am. Sociol. Rev. 45, 864–870, 878–886.

Graeven, D. B. (1974). The effects of airplane noise on health: An examination of three hypotheses. J. Health Soc. Behav. 15, 336–343.

Gross, E. (1970). Work, organization, and stress. In "Social Stress" (S. Levine and N. A. Scotch, eds), pp. 54–110. Aldine, Chicago.

Guralnick, L. (1963). "Mortality by Occupation and Cause of Death." Vital Statistics—Special Reports, Vol. 53, Nos. 3, 4 and 5, Washington, D.C.

Harburg, E., Erfurt, J. C., Chape, C., Hauenstein, L. S., Schull, W. J. and Schork, M. A. (1973). Socio-ecological stressor and Black-White blood pressure: Detroit. J. Chron. Dis. 26, 596–611.

Haw, M. A. (1982). Women, work, and stress: A review and agenda for the future. J. Health Soc. Behav. 23, 132–144.

Haynes, S. G. and Feinleib, M. (1980). Women, work, and coronary heart disease: prospective findings from the Framingham Heart Study. Am. J. Pub. Health 70, 133–141.

Haynes, S. G., Feinleib, M. and Kannel, W. B. (1980). The relationship of psychosocial factors to coronary heart disease in the Framingham study. Part III. Eight-year incidence of coronary heart disease. Am. J. Epidemiol. 111, 37–58.

Helsing, K. J. and Szklo, M. (1981). Mortality after bereavement. Am. J. Epidemiol. 114, 41–52.

Henry, J. P. (1982). The relation of social to biological processes in disease. *Soc. Sci. Med.* **16**, 369–380.

Hinkle, L. E., Jr. and Loring, W. C., eds. (1977). "The effect of the Man-Made Environment on Health and Behavior." DHEW Publication No. (CDC) 77-8318, Washington, D.C.

Hinkle, L. E., Jr., Whitney, L. H., Lehman, E. W., Dunn, J., Benjamin, B., King, R., Plakun, A. and Fehinger, B. (1968). Occupation, education, and coronary heart disease. *Science* **161**, 238–246.

Hitchcok, J. and Waterhouse, A. (1979). Expressway noise and apartment tenant response. *Envir. Behavior* **11**, 251–267.

Hohm, C. (1976). A human ecological approach to the reality and perception of air pollution. *Pacif. Sociol. Rev.* **19**, 21–44.

Holroyd, K. A. and Lazarus, R. S. (1982). Stress, coping, and somatic adaptation. *In* "Handbook of Stress" (L. Goldberger and S. Breznitz, eds), pp. 21–35. Free Press, New York.

Holt, R. H. (1982). Occupational stress. *In* "Handbook of Stress" (L. Goldberger and S. Breznitz, eds), pp. 419–444. Free Press, New York.

House, J. S. (1974). Occupational stress and coronary heart disease: A review and theoretical integration. *J. Health Soc. Behav.* **15**, 12–27.

Houts, P. S. and Goldhaber, M. K. (1981). Psychological and social effects on the population surrounding Three Mile Island after the nuclear accident on March 28, 1979. *In* "Energy, Environment, and the Economy" (S. Majumdar, ed), pp. 151–164. Pennsylvania Academy of Sciences, Harrisburg.

Ihre, B. J. E. and Muller, R. (1943). Gastric and duodenal ulcer. *Acta Med. Scand.* **116**, 33–57.

Ilfeld, F. W., Jr. (1982). Marital stressors, coping styles, and symptoms of depression. *In* "Handbook of Stress" (L. Goldberger and S. Breznitz, eds), pp. 482–495. Free Press, New York.

Jenkins, C. D. (1976). Recent evidence supporting psychologic and social risk factors for coronary disease. *New Engl. J. Med.* **294**, 987–994, 1033–1038.

Jenkins, C. D. (1981). Behavioral factors in the etiology and pathogenesis of cardiovascular diseases: sudden death, hypertension, and myocardial infarction. *In* "Perspectives on Behavioral Medicine" (S. M. Weiss, J. A. Herd and B. H. Fox, eds), pp. 41–54. Academic Press, Orlando, New York and London.

Jenkins, L., Tarnapolsky, A. and Hand, D. (1981). Psychiatric admissions and aircraft noise from London airport: four-year, three-hospitals' study. *Psychol. Med.* **11**, 765–782.

Johansson, G. (1976). Subjective wellbeing and temporal patterns of sympathetic adrenal medullary activity. *Biol. Psychol.* **4**, 157–172.

Johansson, G., Aronsson, G. and Lindstrom, B. P. (1978). Social psychological and neuroendocrine stress reactions in highly mechanized work. *Ergonomics* **21**, 583–599.

Jones, F. N. and Tauscher, J. (1978). Residence under an airport landing pattern as a factor in teratism. *Arch. Envir. Health* **33**, 10–12.

Kahn, R. L. (1981). "Work and Health." Wiley Interscience, New York.

Kahn, R. L., Hein, K., House, J., Kasl, S. V. and McLean, A. (1982). Report on stress in organizational settings. *In* "Stress and Human Health" (G. R. Elliott and C. Eisdorfer, eds), pp. 81–117. Springer-Verlag, New York.

Kaminoff, R. D. and Proshansky, H. M. (1982). Stress as a consequence of the urban physical environment. *In* "Handbook of Stress" (L. Goldberger and S. Breznitz, eds), pp. 380–409. Free Press, New York.

Kaplan, B. H., Cassel, J. and Gore, S. (1977). Social support and health. *Med. Care* **15**(Suppl. 1–5), 47–58.

Kaplan, G. A. and Camacho, T. (1983). Perceived health and mortality: A nine-year follow-up of the Human Population Laboratory cohort. *Am. J. Epidemiol.* **117**, 291–304.

Karasek, R., Baker, D., Marxer, F., Ahlbom, A. and Theorell, T. (1981). Job decision latitude, job demands, and cardiovascular disease: A prospective study of Swedish men. *Am. J. Pub. Health* **71**, 694–705.

Karasek, R. A., Theorell, T. G. T., Schwartz, J., Pieper, C. and Alfredsson, L. (1982). Job, psychological factors, and coronary heart disease. *Adv. Cardiol.* **29**, 62–27.

Kasl, S. V. (1973). Mental health and the work environment: an examination of the evidence. *J. Occup. Med.* **15**, 509–518.

Kasl, S. V. (1976). Effects of housing on mental and physical health. In "Housing in the Seventies, Working Papers 1." pp. 286–304. U.S. Department of Housing and Urban Development, Washington, D.C.

Kasl, S. V. (1977). Contributions of social epidemiology to studies in psychosomatic medicine. In 'Advances in Psychosomatic Medicine, Vol. 9: Epidemiologic Studies in Psychosomatic Medicine" (S. V. Kasl and F. Reichsman, eds), pp. 160–223. Karger, Basel.

Kasl, S. V. (1978). Epidemiological contributions to the study of work stress. In "Stress at Work" (C. L. Cooper and R. Payne, eds), pp. 3–48. Wiley, Chichester.

Kasl, S. V. (1979). Mortality and the business cycle: some questions about research strategies when utilizing macro-social and ecological data. *Am. J. Pub. Health* **69**, 784–788.

Kasl, S. V. (1980). The impact of retirement. In "Current Concerns in Occupational Stress" (C. L. Cooper and R. Payne, eds), pp. 137–186. Wiley, Chichester.

Kasl, S. V. (1981). The challenge of studying the disease effects of stressful work conditions. *Am. J. Pub. Health* **71**, 682–684.

Kasl, S. V. (1982). Strategies of research on economic instability and health. *Psychol. Med.* **12**, 637–649.

Kasl, S. V. (1983). Social and psychological factors affecting the course of disease: An epidemiological perspective. In "Handbook of Health, Health Care, and the Health Professions" (D. Mechanic, ed.), Free Press, New York.

Kasl, S. V. and Berkman, L. (1983). Health consequences of the experience of migration. *A Rev. Pub. Health* **4**, 67–88.

Kasl, S. V. and Cobb, S. (1979). Some mental health consequences of plant closing and job loss. In "Mental Health and the Economy" (L.A. Ferman and J. P. Gordus, eds), pp. 255–299. Upjohn Institute for Employment Research, Kalamazoo.

Kasl, S. V. and Cobb, S. (1980). The experience of losing a job: some effects on cardiovascular functioning. *Psychother. Psychosom.* **34**, 88–109.

Kasl, S. V. and Cobb, S. (1983). Psychological and social stresses in the work place. In "Occupational Health: Recognizing and Preventing Work-Related Disease" (B. S. Levy and D. H. Wegman, eds), pp. 251–263. Little, Brown & Co., Boston.

Kasl, S. V. and Harburg, E. (1975). Mental health and the urban environment: Some doubts and second thoughts. *J. Health Soc. Behav.* **16**, 268–282.

Kasl, S. V. and Rosenfield, S. (1980). The residential environment and its impact on the mental health of the aged. In "Handbook of Mental Health and Aging" (J. E. Birren and R. B. Sloane, eds), pp. 468–498. Prentice Hall, Englewood Cliffs, N.J.

Katz, D. and Kahn, R. L. (1978). "The Social Psychology of Organizations" 2nd edn. Wiley, New York.

King, H. (1970). Health in the medical and other learned professions. *J. Chron. Dis.* **23,** 257–281.

Kittel, F., Kornitzer, M. and Dramaix, M. (1980). Coronary heart disease and job stress in two coohorts of bank clerks. *Psychother. Psychosom.* **34,** 110–123.

Kroes, W. H., Margolis, B. L. Nad Hurrell, J. J. (1974). Job stress in policemen. *J. Police Sci. Admin.* **2,** 145–155.

Kryter, K. D. (1972). Non-auditory effects of environmental noise. *Am. J. Pub. Health* **62,** 389–398.

Landy, F. J. and Trumbo, D. A. (1976). "Psychology of Work Behavior." Dorsey Press, Homewood, Ill.

LaRocco, J. M., House, J. S. and French, J. R. P., Jr. (1980). Social support, occupational stress and health. *J. Health Soc. Behav.* **21,** 202–218.

Lawton, M. P. (1977). The impact of the environment on aging and behavior. *In* "Handbook of the Psychology of Aging" (J. E. Birren and K. W. Schaie, eds), pp. 276–301. Reinhold, New York.

Lazarus, R. S. (1966). "Psychological Stress and Coping Process." McGraw-Hill, New York.

Lehman, E. W., Schulman, J. and Hinkle, L. E., Jr. (1967). Coronary deaths and organizational mobility. *Arch. Environ. Health* **15,** 455–461.

Levi, L. (1974). Stress, distress, and psychosocial stimuli. *In* "Occupational stress" (A. A. McLean, ed.), pp. 31–46. C. C. Thomas, Springfield.

Levy, L. and Herzog, A. N. (1974). Effects of population density and crowding on health and social adaptation in the Netherlands. *J. Health Soc. Behav.* **15,** 228–240.

Lieberman, M. A. (1982). The effects of social supports on responses to stress. *In* "Handbook of Stress" (L. Goldberger and S. Breznitz, eds), pp. 765–783. Free Press, New York.

Lin, N., Simeone, R. S., Ensel, W. M. and Kuo, W. (1979). Social support, stressful life events, and illness: A model and an empirical test. *J. Health Soc. Behav.* **20,** 108–119.

Lindvall, T. and Radord, E. P., eds (1973). Measurement of annoyance due to exposure to environmental factors. *Envir. Res.* **6,** 1–36.

Locke, E. A. (1976). The nature and causes of job satisfaction. *In* "Handbook of Industrial and Organizational Psychology" (M. D. Dunnette, ed.), pp. 1297–1349. Rand McNally, Chicago.

Lundberg, U. (1976). Urban commuting: Crowdedness and catecholamine excretion. *J. Hum. Stress* **2,** 26–32.

McCord, C. P. (1948). Life and death by the minute. *Industr. Med.* **17,** 377–382.

McGrath, J. E. (1970). A conceptual formualation for research on stress. *In* "Social and Psychological Factors in Stress" (J. E. McGrath, ed.), pp. 10–21. Holt, Rhinehart and Winston, New York.

McGrath, J. E. (1976). Stress and behavior in organizations. *In* "Handbook of Industrial and Organizational Psychology" (M. D. Dunnette, ed.), pp. 1351–1395. Rand McNally, Chicago.

McLean, A. A. (1979). "Work Stress." Addison-Wesley, Reading, Mass.

McLean, A. A. (1981). "How to Reduce Occupational Stress." Addison-Wesley, Lexington, Mass.

McQueen, D. V. and Siegrist, J. (1982). Social factors in the etiology of chronic disease: An overview. *Soc. Sci. Med.* **16,** 353–367.

Manton, K. G. and Myers, G. C. (1977). The structure of urban mortality. A methodological study of Hannover, Germany, Part II. *Int. J. Epidemiol.* **6,** 213–223.

Margolis, B. L. (1973). Stress is a work hazard, too. *Industr. Med. Surg.* **42,** 20–23.

Marmot, M. G., Rose, G., Shipley, M. and Hamilton, P. J. J. (1978). Employment grade and coronary heart disease in British civil servants. *J. Epid. Comm. Health* **32,** 244–249.

Medalie, J. H. and Goldbourt, U. (1976). Angina pectoris among 10 000 men. II. Psychosocial and other risk factors as evidenced by a multivariate analysis of a five year incidence study. *Am. J. Med.* **60,** 910–921.

Melick, M. E. (1978). Life change and illness: Illness behavior of males in the recovery period of a natural disaster. *J. Health Soc. Behav.* **19,** 335–342.

Minkler, M. (1981). Research on the health effects of retirement: An uncertain legacy. *J. Health Soc. Behav.* **22,** 117–130.

Mitchell, R. (1971). Some social implications of high density. *Am. Sociol. Rev.* **36,** 18–29.

Moos, R. H., ed. (1977). "Coping with Physical Illness." Plenum Press, New York.

Moos, R. H. (1979). Social-ecological perspectives on health. *In* "Health Psychology—A Handbook" (G. C. Stone, F. Cohen and N. E. Adler, eds), pp. 523–547. Jossey-Bass, San Francisco.

Morris, J. N., Heady, J. A. and Barley, R. G. (1952). Coronary heart disease in medical practitioners. *Br. J. Med.* **1,** 503–520.

Mossey, J. M. and Shapiro, E. (1982). Self-rated health: a predictor of mortality among the elderly. *Am. J. Pub. Health* **72,** 800–808.

Mott, P. E., Mann, F. C., McLaughlin, Q. and Warwick, D. P. (1965). "Shift Work: The Social, Psychological, and Physical Consequences." The University of Michigan Press, Ann Arbor.

Paffenbarger, R. S., Jr., Wolf, P. A., Notkin, J. and Thorne, M. C. (1966). Chronic disease in former college students. I. Early precursors of fatal coronary heart disease. *Am. J. Epidemiol.* **83,** 314–328.

Pearlin, L. I, and Schooler, C. (1978). The structure of coping. *J. Health Soc. Behav.* **19,** 2–21.

Pell, S. and D'Alonzo, C. A. (1963). Acute myocardial infarction in a large industrial population. *J. Am. Med. Ass.* **185,** 831–838.

Pflanz, M. (1971). Epidemiological and sociocultural factors in the etiology of duodenal ulcer. *In* "Advances in Psychosomatic Medicine, Vol. 6: Duodenal Ulcer" (H. Weiner, ed.), pp. 121–151. Karger, Basel.

Pinter, E. J., Tolis, G., Guyda, H. and Katsarkas, A. (1979). Hormonal and free fatty acid changes during strenuous flight in novices and trained personnel. *Psychoneuroendocrinology* **4,** 79–82.

Porritt, D. (1979). Social support in crisis: quantity or quality? *Soc. Sci. Med.* **13,** 218–222.

Power, J. G. P. (1970). Health aspects of vertical living in Hong Kong. *Comm. Health* **1,** 316–320.

Quinlan, C. B. and Barrow, J. G. (1966). Prevalence of coronary heart disease in Trappist and Benedictine monks. *Circulation* **33–34** (Suppl. III), 193.

Rentos, G. P. and Shepard, R. D., eds (1976). "Shift Work and Health, A Symposium." DHEW (NIOSH) Publication No. 76–203, Washington, D.C.

Reynolds, R. C. (1974). Community and occupational influences in stress at Cape

Kennedy: relationships to heart disease. *In* "Stress and the Heart" (R. S. Eliot, ed.), pp. 33–49. Futura Publishing, Mt. Kisco, N.Y.

Rissler, A. (1977). Stress reactions at work and after work during a period of quantitative overload. *Ergonomics* **20**, 13–16.

Roman, J. A. (1963). Cardiorespiratory functioning in flight. *Aerospace Med.* **34**, 322–337.

Rose, R. M. (1980). Endocrine responses to stressful psychological events. *Psychiat. Clin. N. Am.* **3** (2), 251–276.

Rose, R. M., Hurst, M. W., Kreger, B. E., Jenkins, C. D., Herd, J. A. and Kavanagh, M. J. (1978a). Predictors of hypertension in air traffic controllers: a prospective study. *Psychosom. Med.* **40**, 86.

Rose, R. M., Jenkins, C. D. and Hurst, M. W. (1978). "Air Traffic Controller Health Change Study." A Report to the FAA, Contract No. DOT-FA 73WA-3211, Boston, University School of Medicine.

Rowland, K. F. (1977). Environmental events prediciting death for the elderly. *Psychol. Bull.* **84**, 349–372.

Rubin, R. T. (1974). Biochemical and endocrine response to severe psychological stress. *In* "Life Stress and Illness" (E. K. E. Gunderson and R. H. Rahe, eds), pp. 227–241. C. C. Thomas, Springfield.

Russek, H. I. (1962). Emotional stress and coronary heart disease in American physicians, dentists and lawyers. *Am. J. Med. Sci.* **243**, 716–725.

Russek, H. I. (1965). Stress, tobacco, and coronary disease in North American professional groups. *J. Am. Med. Ass.* **192**, 189–194.

Sales, S. M. and House, J. S. (1971). Job dissatisfaction as a possible risk factor in coronary heart disease. *J. Chron. Dis.* **23**, 861–873.

Schorr, A. L. (1963). "Slums and Social Insecurity." Social Security Administration Research Report No. 1, Washington, D.C.

Shaffer, J. W., Duszynski, K. R. and Thomas, C. B. (1982). Family attitudes in youth as a possible precursor of cancer among physicians: A search for explanatory mechanisms. *J. Behav. Med.* **5**, 143–163.

Singer, R. and Rutenfranz, J. (1971). Attitudes of air traffic controllers at Frankfurt airport towards work and the working environment. *Ergonomics* **14**, 633–639.

Smith, H. P. R. (1967). Heart rate of pilots flying aircraft on scheduled airline routes. *Aerospace Med.* **38**, 1117–1119.

Smith, M. J., Colligan, M. J. and Hurrell, J. J., Jr. (1978). Three incidents of industrial mass psychogenic illness. *J. Occup. Med.* **20**, 399–400.

Smith, R. C. (1973). Comparison of job attitudes of personnel in three air traffic control specialities. *Aerospace Med.* **44**, 919–927.

Spivey, G. H. and Raddford, E. P. (1979). Inner-city housing and respiratory disease in children: a pilot study. *Arch. Envir. Health* **34**, 23–30.

Stevenson, A., Martin, E. and O'Neill, J. (1967). "High Living: A Study of Family Life in Flats." Melbourne University Press, London.

Stokols, D. and Novaco, R. W. (1981). Transportation and well-being: An ecological perspective. *In* "Human Behaviour and Environment, Vol. 5; Transportation Environments" (I. Altman, J. Wohlwill and P. Everett, eds), pp. 82–130. Plenum Press, New York.

Susser, M. (1967). Causes of peptic ulcer: a selective epidemiologic review. *J. Chron. Dis.* **20**, 435–456.

Susser, M. (1981). Widowhood: a situational life stress or a stressful life event? *Am. J. Pub. Health* **71**, 793–795.

Tarnapolsky, A., Watkins, G. and Hand, D. J. (1980). Aircraft noise and mental health: I. Prevalence of individual symptoms. *Psychol. Med.* **10**, 683–698.

Tasto, D. and Colligan, M. (1978). "Health Consequences of Shift Work." DHEW (NIOSH) Publication No. 78–154, Washington, D.C.

Theorell, T. and Floderus-Myrhed, B. (1977). 'Workload' and risk of myocardial infarction—A prospective psychosocial analysis. *Int. J. Epidemiol.* **6**, 17–21.

Thiis-Evensen, E. (1958). Shift work and health. *Industr. Med. Surg.* **27**, 493–497.

Thomas, C. B. and Greenstreet, R. L. (1973). Psychological characteristics in youth as predictors of five disease states: suicide, mental illness, hypertension, coronary heart disease, and tumor. *Johns Hopikins Med. J.* **132**, 16–43.

Thomas, C. B., Duszynski, K. R. and Shaffer, J. W. (1979). Family atttitudes reported in youth as potential predictors of cancer. *Psychosom. Med.* **41**, 287–302.

Timio, M. and Gentili, S. (1976). Adrenosympathetic overactivity under conditions of work stress. *Br. J. Prev. Soc. Med.* **30**, 262–265.

Tobin, S. S. and Lieberman, M. A. (1976). "Last Home for the Aged." Jossey-Bass, San Francisco.

Torsvall, L. and Akerstedt, T. (1980). A diurnal type scale: Construction, consistency and validation in shift work. *Scand. J. Work, Envir. Health* **6**, 283–290.

Turner, B. F., Tobin, S. S. and Lieberman, M. A. (1972). Personality traits as predictors of institutional adaptation among the aged. *J. Gerontol.* **27**, 61–68.

Ward, S. K. (1975). Methodological considerations in the study of population density and social pathology. *Hum. Ecol.* **3**, 275–286.

Wardwell, W. I., Hyman, M. and Bahnson, C. B. (1968). Socio-environmental antecedents to coronary heart disease in 87 white males. *Soc. Sci. Med.* **2**, 165–183.

Watkins, G., Tarnapolsky, A. and Jenkins, L. M. (1981). Aircraft noise and mental health: II. Use of medicines and health care services. *Psychol. Med.* **11**, 155–168.

Weiner, H. (1977). "Psychobiology and Human Disease." Elsevier, New York.

Whittemore, A. S. (1981). Air pollution and respiratory disease. *Ann. Rev. Pub. Health* **2**, 397–429.

Wilner, D. M., Walkley, R. P., Pinkerton, T. C. and Tayback, M. (1962). "The Housing Environment and Family Life." Johns Hopkins Press.

Wingard, D. L., Berkman, L. F. and Brand, R. J. (1982). A multivariate analysis of health-related practices. A nine-year mortality follow-up of the Alameda County Study. *Am. J. Epidemiol.* **116**, 765–775.

Winget, C. M., Hughes, L. and LaDou, J. (1978). Physiological effects of rotational work shifting: A review. *J. Occup. Med.* **20**, 204–210. Winnbust, J. A. M., Marcelissen, F. H. G. and Kleber, R. J. (1982). Effects of social support in the stressor-strain relationship: A Dutch sample. *Soc. Sci. Med.* **16**, 475–482.

Wolf, S., Almy, T. P., Bachrach, W. H., Spiro, H. M., Sturdevant, R. A. L. and Weiner, H. (1979). The role of stress in peptic ulcer disease. *J. Hum. Stress* **5**, 27–37.

Zimbardo, P. G. (1982). Shyness and the stresses of the human connection. *In* "Handbook of Stress" (L. Goldberger and S. Breznitz, eds), pp. 466–481. Free Press, New York.

Zorn, E. W., Harrington, J. M. and Goethe, H. (1977). Ischemic heart disease and work stress in West German sea pilots. *J. Occup. Med.* **19**, 762–765.

3
Psychophysiological Processes in Disease
ANDREW STEPTOE

The evidence linking cultural and psychosocial experiences with ill-health has been outlined in Chapters 1 and 2. It would appear that, despite certain conceptual and empirical reservations, the association has ample support. In this chapter, the mechanisms that translate adverse life experience into pathological dysfunctions will be explored. In keeping with the orientation of this volume, the emphasis is on non-psychiatric disorders. Unfortunately, most of the research on psychophysiological processes has been focused on the traditional "psychosomatic" diseases, such as bronchial asthma, migraine and essential hypertension. The fact that these disorders loom large in the ensuing discussion does not imply that psychophysiological mechanisms are relevant only to these problems; rather, it reflects current and past research biases. Later in the chapter, the general arguments concerning psychophysiological processes will be illustrated still more specifically by examination of ischaemic heart disease (IHD) and essential hypertension.

There are at least three basic processes through which adverse psycho-social experiences may lead to ill-health: influences on subjective symptomatology, behaviours with adverse health consequences, and psycho-physiological mechanisms. The first two will be described only briefly, but they must be considered in the interpretation of any research into psychoso-cial factors in disease aetiology.

1. Influences on Subjective Symptomatology and Complaint Behaviour
Individuals differ in their perception and acknowledgement of symptoms, and in their decisions about how to manage these symptoms and when to consult medical services. These are components of illness behaviour (Mechanic, 1968). It is possible that in response to adverse life experience, people may complain of more illness and seek medical attention for

HEALTH CARE AND HUMAN BEHAVIOUR
ISBN 0–12–666460–9

conditions that might otherwise have been ignored or treated with non-medical remedies. The problems that this process introduces into the investigation of life events have been discussed by Craig and Brown (Chapter 1). Such patterns are often considered methodological embarrassments by researchers, since they imply that life events or chronic harassments do not affect the disease process *per se*. However, they deserve consideration in their own right, for there are numerous instances of social or psychological factors affecting the subjective symptomatology of organic conditions. For example, House *et al.* (1979) investigated the concordance between subjective and objective health data in a sample of male industrial workers. Subjective symptoms of itchy skin and rash, and complaints of persistent cough and sputum were associated with reported job pressures, such as excessive work load and rôle conflict, but neither dermatological nor pulmonary condition was correlated with these parameters of psychosocial distress. It appears that adverse life experiences magnified (or may even have caused) the respondents' subjective symptomatology above the level warranted by their objective condition. Enduring individual differences may also be relevant to this pattern. Barsky and Klerman (1983) have argued that some people have an "amplifying somatic style", monitoring their bodily sensations carefully, scrutinizing trivial or transitory symptoms, and interpreting these in terms of physical disease; such tendencies may be increased by adverse life experiences.

This association between psychosocial experience and subjective symptomatology may have two consequences. Firstly, it can lead to more vigorous treatment than might otherwise have been provided. Although systematic physiological or biochemical tests are available for many organic disorders, treatment is often determined by the physician's perception of the patient's distress and discomfort. This is well recognized in the management of chronic pain, where treatment decisions are sometimes made almost entirely on the basis of pain behaviour (Fordyce, 1976). But the influence of subjective symptomatology is evident in conditions such as bronchial asthma as well. Kinsman *et al.* (1973, 1977) have developed an asthma symptom checklist, and have identified a number of symptom clusters that are experienced by asthmatic patients during episodes of wheezing. The symptom checklist was administered to a large cohort of hospitalized asthmatics, 72% of whom were discharged on maintenance doses of corticosteroids. Patients reporting high panic/fear symptoms were more frequently prescribed steriods than others, irrespective of objective pulmonary function measures. The association was mediated by the "sensitivity" of physicians as rated by their seniors. Sensitive physicians were swayed by patients' panic/fear behaviour, to the extent that correlations between prescription and pulmonary function were not significant.

Low sensitivity physicians on the other hand prescribed according to function tests, and did not provide more intensive treatment in the face of overt fear and distress.

The pattern of subjective symptomatology may even lead to drastic treatments such as surgery. This is one interpretation of Creed's (1981) data relating life events to appendectomy. The study (see Chapter 1) showed that the pattern of severely threatening events was different in patients with and without acutely inflamed appendices. The rate of severe life events was only elevated among patients who were subsequently discovered, on histological examination, to have normal or minimally inflamed appendices. It is possible that the experience of severe life events promoted a pattern of abdominal pain to which physicians responded with appendectomy. These patients also reported persisting abdominal pain over the post-operative year more frequently than those in the acute inflammation group. Severe life events evidently had little impact on the appendix itself.

Spurious associations between life experience and ill-health may therefore arise if treatment parameters are used as outcome variables in research. Similar problems arise in the study of psychological interventions and outcome of surgery as noted by Mathews and Ridgeway (Chapter 8). A second consequence of the association between subjective symptomatology and psychosocial factors is that it may result in the detection and diagnosis of genuine clinical conditions that would otherwise escape medical attention. This is well documented in the case of essential hypertension. Essential hypertension has no consistent symptoms, and many cases goes undiagnosed in the community. Stamler et al. (1976) found through a screening project that 78% of people aged 40 or less with elevated blood pressure (BP) had not had the problem detected previously. However, people who consult their physicians with non-specific symptoms frequently have their BP recorded; hence, "new" cases of hypertension will be identified through medical attention seeking. This can lead to the observation of spurious connections between high BP and psychological characteristics. This factor may account for some of the inconsistencies in psychological studies of essential hypertensives (see Steptoe et al., 1982; Steptoe, 1983a). It is important to recognize that such patterns may also confound the study of other medical disorders.

2. Alterations in Habitual Behaviours that carry Health Risks

Actions such as cigarette smoking, alcohol consumption, recreational exercise, dietary habits and the maintenance of personal hygiene have complex psychosocial determinants. They in turn affect the risk of contracting infections, developing ischaemic heart disease, malignancies and other diseases. If their frequency is modified by adverse life experience, they may mediate between psychosocial pressures and clinical disorder.

Systematic demonstrations of the impact of life events and other experiences on risk behaviours are surprisingly sparse. Clinical observation and popular opinion suggest that excessive alcohol intake is associated with periods of distress, yet few studies have been performed (Peyser, 1982). Lindenthal et al. (1982) have recently shown that life events increase levels of cigarette smoking, but only among people who are also psychiatrically impaired. Bereavement in young adults is associated with reported changes in appetite, cigarette smoking and alcohol intake (Parkes and Brown, 1972). As Kasl has noted (Chapter 2), the relationship between the "stressfulness" of medical specialities and IHD observed by Russek (1965) may be mediated by cigarette smoking.

It is worth emphasizing that the presence of behavioural mediators does not negate the link between psychological factors and illness. Cigarette smoking, exercise and eating are voluntary activities, not pathological dysfunctions, and must be treated as such. In terms of management, behavioural approaches are often very profitable. On the other hand, such mechanisms should always be taken into account, since they may render the search for more immediate psychophysiological mediators redundant.

3. Effects on Psychophysiological Processes

These processes describe the effects of stimulation from the brain on the autonomic nervous system, endocrine and immunological functions. They are relevant to disease in two ways. Firstly, sustained alterations of psychophysiological function may lead to pathological disturbances in the long-term; the research on essential hypertension and IHD described below is founded on this notion. Secondly, psychophysiological mechanisms may trigger or precipitate clinical events in people with pre-existing chronic disease. Their role here is acute rather than chronic. Lown et al. (1980) suggest this process may be relevant to sudden cardiac death and serious problems of ventricular electrical instability in the heart.

Such mechanisms are of central interest to researchers in psychosomatics and behavioural medicine. In part this is because psychophysiological investigations are conceptually interesting, as they bridge the gap between psychosocial factors and pathophysiology (Henry and Stephens, 1977). This chapter is principally concerned with psychological effects on autonomic nervous function, since Anisman and Sklar (Chapter 4) summarize the evidence on neuroendocrine and immunological parameters. The discussion will concentrate on the rôle of these processes in long-term aetiology, rather than in the acute precipitation of clinical events. But before considering this literature, some caveats about the experimental strategy are perhaps appropriate.

Many of the disorders thought to be related to psychosocial factors take several years to develop. In contrast, psychophysiological experiments in humans are commonly acute, and seldom concern reactions of a clinically significant size and duration. Attempts are made to understand pathological disorders by cross-sectional comparisons, as in the study of cardiovascular responses in essential hypertensives and normotensives. However, this design is inherently unsatisfactory, since cause and effect relationships are obscured. The absence of longitudinal data has hindered critical analysis of theoretical formulations in psychophysiology. It is presumed that patterns of reactivity displayed in acute settings parallel autonomic and neuroendocrine disturbances outside the laboratory, but this assumption may not rest on strong foundations (Steptoe, 1981). In animals too, there are marked variations in response pattern with chronicity of stressors, as Anisman and Sklar demonstrate in Chapter 4. Kasl (Chapter 2) has pointed out similar problems in relation to epidemiological studies of chronicity, emphasizing the ability of humans to cope and adapt. The advent of sophisticated ambulatory monitoring techniques may soon provide clarification of this issue. Yet, until more data are available from physiological and biochemical monitoring in long-term experiments or natural settings, detailed analyses based on acute psychophysiological studies must remain tentative.

PSYCHOPHYSIOLOGICAL MODELS OF DISEASE

Theoretical formulations of psychophysiological processes in disease need to satisfy two main requirements. Firstly, they must demonstrate how the physiological reactions associated with psychosocial stimulation lead to pathological end points. Secondly, they must account for individual differences in response: why only some people succumb to organic disease following abrasive life stress, and why the type of disease varies from person to person.

Simple stress hypotheses are unsatisfactory on two counts. Firstly, as Kasl has noted (Chapter 2), the notion of stress is theoretically vague and has serious methodological limitations. Secondly, it does not account adequately for variations in response (Steptoe, 1980). Individual differences are accommodated within the psychodynamic formulations elaborated by Dunbar (1943), Alexander (1950) and others, but these theories are scientifically unsound. Lachman (1972) has argued that learning theory offers a useful basis for the understanding of psychophysiological disorders. Emotional responses have autonomic and neuroendocrine concomitants, and salient environmental cues may acquire the status of discriminative stimuli through a process of conditioning. The appearance of these stimuli will repeatedly provoke physiological reactions that may in turn lead to pathological dysfunction. Within the learning framework, Levey and Martin (1981) have examined the role of classical conditioning, emphasizing Corson's (1971) observations on individual differences in visceral conditioned responses among dogs. They conclude that classical conditioning is unlikely to account for the development of organic disorders, although it may be relevant to the precipitation of serious episodes in a chronic complaint.

Unfortunately, demonstrations of the conditioning of sustained physiological disturbances are rare (e.g., Harris and Brady, 1977). It is also difficult for learning theory to account for the specificity of symptoms or the nature of the acquired disorder. Most theorists agree that psychological formulations are inadequate in isolation, and that interactional models are needed in order to allow for individual variations in biological predisposition and vulnerability. These are generally termed stress–diathesis models, in which psychosocial pressures combine with biological susceptibilities to produce organic reactions that may act as precursors of disease.

The scheme outlined in Fig. 1 is derived from Kagan and Levy (1974), and is typical of the stress–diathesis formulation. It is argued that psychosocial stimulation may or may not elicit emotional or physiological responses (stress mechanisms), depending on the perceptions and behaviour patterns of the individual (the psychobiological programme). The latter are determined by constitutional factors, including inherited characteristics, and by earlier environmental influences. For example, Ader (1976) has shown that experiences such as early handling or separation in animals alter sensory capacities, and may ultimately modify susceptibility to gastrointestinal

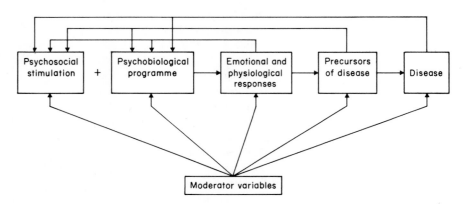

Fig. 1 Stress–diathesis model (after Kagan and Levi, 1974) for psychosocially mediated disease.

disorder and certain malignancies. The coping resources of the individual are also relevant at this stage (Holroyd and Lazarus, 1982). After the mobilization of emotional and physiological responses, the biological element of the diathesis (organ weakness or vulnerability) determines whether acute reactions are transformed into more serious and sustained dysfunctions. In some people, disease-specific reaction patterns may develop, and these will in turn lead to disease itself. In more robust individuals, reactions will dissipate with no ill-effects. The model is conceived as a cybernetic system with continuous feedback. The moderator variables include factors that promote disease, such as physical environmental hazards (noise, malnutrition, etc.), and those that protect or buffer the victim against the whole process (social supports etc).

Individual variations in disease susceptibility may be accounted for at a number of different stages in this type of model. The first possibility is that the nature of the psychosocial stimulation is responsible; exposure to particular forms of challenge may lead to specific disease endpoints. Until recently, this hypothesis has received little support. It has generally been presumed that psychosocial stimuli act in an essentially non-specific fashion. Adverse life experience lowers the threshold for ill health non-directively. However, current investigations of life events indicate that they do not act indiscriminately in the promotion of psychiatric disorder. Particular types of experience (e.g., loss of parent) predispose to particular outcomes (depression; Brown et al., 1977). Events that promote a sense of threat or danger may in contrast be associated with anxiety (Finlay-Jones and Brown, 1981). Similar arguments have been presented in the case of psychophysiological disorders. Henry (1976, 1982) has suggested that reactions mediated by the pituitary-adrenocortical system are linked with behavioural loss of control, withdrawal, subordination and depression. Catecholamines and sympathetic nervous system reactions on the other hand are mobilized when the individual retains control under challenge, responding actively in the face of adversity. Extensive evidence from studies of animals and humans supports this distinction (Steptoe, 1983b). Since different disease end-points may be promoted by these different pathways, the nature of the psychosocial stimulation may indeed influence pathology in a broad sense. For example, heightened steroid release from the adrenal cortex may be associated with the proliferation of infections and malignancy, either through direct anti-inflammatory processes or through alterations in immunological function (see Chapter 4). High blood pressure, and ventricular fibrillation leading to sudden cardiac death, may on the other hand be linked with sympathetic nervous/catecholamine stimulation. However, this factor is unlikely to account for all variations in response. Moreover, these reaction patterns are not determined entirely by the form of psychosocial stimulation, as facets of the psychobiological programme (such as the tendency to respond in an individual stereotyped way) are also involved.

Another possibility is that differences in the pattern of emotional reaction are associated with varying psychophysiological mechanisms, which in turn promote specific disease states. The tendency to manifest consistent emotional reactions of a damaging nature depends on the psychological makeup of the respondent (in Fig. 1, the psychobiological programme). For instance, the potential hypertensive may respond to psychosocial stimulation by suppressing his or her hostility (Diamond, 1982). This reaction may be linked to a pattern of sympathetic nervous system activation, possibly involving stimulation of the renin–angiotensin system (Esler et al., 1977). If the reaction pattern is repeatedly evoked by the harassments of everyday life, essential hypertension may result.

This hypothesis places responsibility for differences in disease susceptibility in the psychological domain. Much of the current research on personality characteristics of patients with psychophysiological disorders is implicity related to such a sequence of events. However, it rests on two notions of dubious merit. The first is that consistent psychological characteristics can be identified in people with psychophysiological disorders, and that the profile varies between the groups suffering from different disorders. The second is that different emotions are associated with sufficiently varying patterns of psychophysiological and neuroendocrine reaction. Both assumptions require brief scrutiny. Arguments concerning the existence of specific personality profiles or psychological hallmarks pre-dating disease onset have continued for many years in psychosomatics. Weiner's (1977) exhaustive review summarizes the evidence for several disorders, and indicates that reliable, mutually exclusive patterns are rare (see also Harrison, 1975). Many characteristics may be products of chronic illness rather than predisposing features. Nevertheless, these notions continue to be tested. For example, patients with essential hypertension are said to be chronically hostile, yet overtly submissive and compliant (Diamond, 1982). Van Der Valk (1957) suggested that suppressed hostility predisposed patients to cardiovascular hyperreactivity. The data from personality tests are however highly variable, with many negative results being reported (Harrell, 1980; Sullivan et al., 1981). Essential hypertensives with high plasma renin do not differ significantly in hostility measures from those with normal renin levels, so this factor may not be relevant (Esler et al., 1977). The selection of patients and controls for personality testing has frequently introduced significant biases in hypertension research (Steptoe, 1983a).

The relationship between patterns of emotion and biological responses also has a long history. The hypothesis that distinct patterns of adrenaline and noradrenaline secretion are associated with different emotions attracted interest in the 1950s, but was based on indirect evidence from cardiovascular reactions and urinary catecholamine output. More recently, Schwartz *et al.* (1981) demonstrated different patterns of blood pressure and heart rate during happy, sad, angry or frightening imaginal scenes. However, these patterns were associated with concomitant motor activity, suggesting that the form and intensity of behavioural output elicited by the images modulated cardiovascular responses. Emotion-specific patterning of autonomic activity has also been reported by Ekman *et al.* (1983). But the magnitude of the differences is not large, so the argument that the pattern of psychophysiological activity underlying various emotions determines the pattern of specific disease vulnerabilities has yet to be substantiated.

If disease susceptibility is not determined by aspects of the psychobiological programme, then according to the stress–diathesis model it must be dependent on biological vulnerability or "organ weakness". In terms of Fig. 1, this characteristic will mediate between physiological responses and precursors of disease. People are predisposed to different disorders, depending on constitutional or acquired vulnerabilities in particular tissues or systems. This concept is all too frequently accepted without proper examination. The nature of the predisposition that leads people to develop particular disorders must be identified, for the model has limited value unless biological vulnerability can be predicted or delineated independently. It must be presumed that the state of biological vulnerability is disease-specific, yet will not promote the disease in the absence of psychosocial stimulation. If these latent vulnerability characteristics are not defined sufficiently to allow prediction of the precise conditions required for disease onset, the concepts cannot be falsified.

INDIVIDUAL DIFFERENCES AND BIOLOGICAL VULNERABILITY

A series of interrelated hypotheses have been developed to account for individual differences in psychophysiological vulnerability. "Individual–response specificity" is the tendency of an individual to respond maximally and consistently in one physiological parameter. The concept was developed by Engel (1960), who presented healthy subjects with a number of stimuli, including mental arithmetic, a proverb test and the cold pressor test. Eight physiological variables were recorded, and it was found that each subject appeared to respond maximally in a particular parameter across stimulus conditions. It has been suggested that, if these response patterns are repeatedly elicited by psychosocial stimuli, the individual may develop a disorder related to the maximally activated parameter (Gannon, 1981). Individual–response specificity may then be transformed into "symptom specificity"; for some disorders (such as essential hypertension) individual–response specificity (in blood pressure) is pathognomic (Roessler and Engel, 1977).

"Individual–response stereotypy" is a closely related concept, defined by Sternbach (1966) as a tendency to respond with a similar pattern of activation across conditions (consistent inter-response ranking within individuals). This term is often employed interchangeably with individual–response specificity. Both should be clearly distinguished from "stimulus–response specificity" (or response stereotypy), which is the hypothesis that unique autonomic response patterns are associated with different stimuli (Lacey, 1967).

Tests of individual–response specificity and stereotypy in healthy groups are surprisingly rare, considering the central place these concepts hold in psychophysiological theory (Engel, 1960; Sersen et al., 1978; Foerster et al., 1983). Gannon (1981) has detailed a number of problems in their interpretation, related to basal differences and the use of transformed response scores. The comparison of response magnitudes across physiological parameters, each of which has a particular range and sensitivity, is difficult. Foerster and Schneider (1982) and Fahrenberg et al. (1983) have concluded from multivariate studies on large groups of subjects that approximately one-third show consistent individual–response specificity across different experimental conditions. The concept cannot of course be tested properly without measurement of several autonomic response parameters; the fact, for example, that BP reactions to different tasks correlate within individuals is of little significance in the absence of data from other variables (Steptoe and Ross, 1981; Rüddel et al., 1982).

Many investigators have preferred to focus their attention on reaction patterns in disease groups. If these hypotheses are relevant to disease susceptibility, then patients with a particular disorder should share a common reaction pattern, and the parameters displaying maximal activation should be relevant pathologically to the disorder in question. It is important to distinguish predictions concerning individual–response specificity from other aspects of functional disturbance in disease groups. Many psychophysiological disorders are characterized by chronic modifications of function in the appropriate system; hence, essential hypertensives have tonically elevated blood pressure, bronchial asthmatics have raised airways resistance, temporal artery pulse amplitude is disturbed in migraine, while some patients with muscle contraction headache have high tonic electromyographic (EMG) activity (Philips, 1980). Such patterns are products of physiological dysregulation and are not psychophysiological properties; they cannot be used, therefore, to bolster psychophysiological models. They may rise for all manner of reasons that have no relation to central nervous function (such as local tissue and cellular mechanisms). Hence, the argument that some form of individual "rest specificity" (Gannon, 1981) can be identified is spurious. Furthermore, the existence of tonic differences has implications for the analysis of reactivity to psychosocial stimulation. Early studies employed "tension" scores, the highest absolute level of function attained during stimulation (Lacey et al., 1953). Such analyses are likely to confirm individual–response specificity purely as a function of baseline differences and so have little psychophysiological significance. Lability or change scores, showing the amount of displacement in activity following stimulation, are more appropriate. Here too, analysis presents problems, since changes may be assessed both in absolute or proportional (percentage or covariance-adjusted) terms.

A few tests of individual–response specificity in disease groups have yielded unequivocal results. The early studies of Malmo and Shagass (1949) did not concern people with psychophysiological disorders at all, but psychiatric patients with different patterns of somatic complaint (specifically "head complaints" and "heart complaints"). Levenson (1979) compared the responses of adult bronchial asthmatics and healthy controls to a series of disturbing films, including an industrial accident film and a sequence displaying an asthmatic child wheezing. The asthmatic group showed increases in total respiratory resistance to both stimuli, while no significant changes were apparent in non-asthmatics. By contrast, the cardiac reactivity of non-asthmatics to the accident film was more pronounced than that of asthmatic subjects.

The majority of studies of reactivity in patients with different disorders have been far less consistent. In the case of essential hypertension, blood pressure is presumed to be the relevant variable. Several investigators have failed, however, to demonstrate heightened pressor responses from hypertensives when challenged with mental arithmetic, the cold pressor, personal interviews, assertive role-playing scenes and other stimuli (Brod et al., 1959; Sullivan et al., 1981; Svensson and Theorell, 1982; Keane et al., 1982). Other experiments have shown positive results, with heightened reactivity in both systolic and diastolic BP from hypertensives compared with normotensive controls (Nestel, 1969; Schulte et al., 1981a; Jern, 1982). Steptoe et al. (1984) have argued that three factors are responsible for this mixed pattern. Firstly, the samples of hypertensive patients have not been homogenous. There is evidence that psychophysiological factors are more significant in the early than late stages of aetiology, so mild to moderate hypertensives are more likely to show appropriate disturbances (Steptoe, 1981). Secondly, patients have been selected inadequately, relying on medical referrals that may not be representative of the hypertensive population at large. Thirdly, it cannot be assumed that all psychological stimuli are equally salient. Obrist (1981) has suggested that tasks eliciting active behavioural coping will be associated with a pattern of cardiovascular reactivity mediated by the cardiac sympathetic innervation. If this pathway is involved in the initiation of the hypertensive process (see below), then it can be predicted that essential hypertensives will only display heightened reactivity when exposed to challenges requiring active behavioural coping. Responses to passive stressors will not be disturbed in essential hypertension. These predictions were confirmed in the study reported by Steptoe *et al.* (1984), some details of which are provided later in this chapter. They suggest that, in the case of essential hypertension at least, the notion of individual–response specificity requires modification. It appears that individual–response and symptom specificity are not properties of the person alone, since they cannot be identified without taking account of the eliciting conditions. Heightened BP reactivity is not a general characteristic, but emerges only with appropriate challenges. If this pattern is confirmed for other disorders, it has serious implications for any linear psychophysiological model based on stress-diathesis.

The literature on essential hypertension indicates that individual–response specificity can be documented, but only under appropriate conditions. Less satisfactory patterns have emerged for other disorders. Walker and Sandman (1977) compared patients with duodenal ulcer, rheumatoid arthritis and healthy controls in their reactions to a series of laboratory stressors. Electromyographic activity from symptomatic muscles (for arthritics) distinguished arthritic from ulcer patients and controls; the arthritis group produced higher tonic EMG levels, and also responded to the stimuli with greater increases. But results for the electrogastrogram (EGG, the symptom-specific parameter for ulcer patients) were disappointing. The ulcer group displayed tonically lower levels of EGG activity, but differences in reactivity were modest.

Negative findings have also emerged for other disease groups. Feuerstein *et al.* (1982a) failed to uncover any differences in psychophysiological reactions or recovery in children with and without recurrent abdominal pain (although in this case, the relevant autonomic parameter is uncertain). Several investigators have tested psychophysiological reactivity patterns in patients with migraine and muscle contraction headaches. In view of the pathophysiology of these conditions, it might be predicted that migraine sufferers would show disturbances in the regulation of intra- and extra-cranial blood flow during stimulation, while control of EMG in the head and neck would be impaired in muscle contraction headache. Drummond (1982) found that migraine patients responded to mental arithmetic with greater increases in temporal artery pulse amplitude than controls, although their other cardiovascular responses were indistinguishable. On the other hand, Bakal and Kaganov (1977) and Price and Tursky (1976) found that migraineurs responded with vasoconstriction to non-aversive stimuli, while Cohen *et al.* (1978) showed that migraine and non-headache controls produced similar vasomotor reactions to mental arithmetic and attentional tasks. Research on muscle contraction headache suffers from the same inconsistencies, with some studies showing reliable differences in EMG response (Vaughn *et al.*, 1977; Van Boxtell and Roosevelt, 1978). Other investigators have failed to uncover differences in the magnitude of EMG or vasomotor reactions in the two headache groups (Philips and Hunter, 1982), or between either group and headache-free controls (Martin and Mathews, 1978; Gannon *et al.*, 1981; Feuerstein *et al.*, 1982b). Individual-response specificity has not been convincingly documented for either type of headache. In the case of muscle contraction headache, research of this type has led to doubts about the aetiological role of muscle tension (Philips, 1980; see also Chapter 9 by Johnston).

Observations on patients with peptic ulcer are sparse (Stern, 1983). A number of investigators have examined the secretion of gastric acid in relation to emotional states in patients with gastric fistulae (Wolf, 1965; Engel *et al.*, 1956). Although associations are observed their significance is unclear, and the absence of control subjects makes it impossible to determine whether the patterns of secretion are unique to ulcer patients (Weiner, 1977). Many investigators assume that other parameters of physiological activity are more relevant than gastric acid output (Hölzl and Whitehead, 1983).

An extension of the individual–response specificity hypothesis has been put forward that might account for some of these discrepancies. It has been suggested that differences occur not in the magnitude of responses, but in recovery rate following challenge. Sternbach (1966) argued that symptoms will only emerge when individual–response stereotypy is accompanied by inadequate homeostatic restraints. These will be manifest in delays of physiological restabilization following disturbances in activity. Data on the duration of BP reactions in hypertensives are consistent with this possibility. Brod (1960) and Baumann *et al.* (1973) showed that heightened cardiovascular function was maintained for longer in hypertensives than normotensives following behavioural challenge. But a more recent test has been less successful. Anderson *et al.* (1982) compared groups of patients with essential hypertension, rheumatoid arthritis, muscle contraction headache, migraine and controls. They performed an exercise step test in session 1 and mental arithmetic in session 2, and rates of recovery in several physiological variables were monitored. No important differences in recovery were found. Patients with arthritis showed slower recovery in forehead EMG, while the diastolic BP of migraine patients did not return to basal levels within the period of experimental observation, but the significance of these findings is unclear and they may be chance effects. Unfortunately, poor matching of groups complicates the interpretation of this experiment.

The studies of individual–response specificity and symptom specificity in several different disorders are evidently highly inconsistent. The hypothesis that recovery is important has done little to retrieve the situation. Moreover, another very important factor must be borne in mind. These studies on biological vulnerability have been cross-sectional. The transformation of non-pathological individual–response specificity to symptom-specific dysfunction has not been documented. It is possible that, since physiological function is by definition disturbed in these disorders, differences in response magnitude may be secondary to organic pathology. Thus, even if patients with a particular disorder can be shown to manifest heightened reactions to psychosocial stimulation, it cannot be assumed that this pattern is of any aetiological significance.

There is strong evidence in some disorders that heightened reactivity may indeed be secondary to pathophysiological disturbance. Patients with asthma tend to show bronchial hyperreactivity, a non-specific tendency to respond with exaggerated airways narrowing to challenge from a broad range of stimuli including histamine, methacholine, sulphur dioxide, exercise and dust (Boushey et al., 1980). In the case of peptic and duodenal ulcer, increased parietal cell mass may lead to heightened gastric acid secretion irrespective of autonomic influences (Grossman, 1967; Isenberg et al., 1975). Likewise, there is evidence for disorders of haemodynamic regulation in essential hypertension, and regional vasomotor control in migraine (Folkow and Neil, 1971; Lance, 1978). This means that a psychophysiological challenge may produce a larger reaction in the appropriate parameter from disease groups, purely as a function of the peripheral morphological or systemic changes associated with the disorder.

These observations suggest that it is necessary not only to show that people with a particular disorder display abberations in reactivity when compared with controls, but that these abberations exist prior to the onset of the disorder. In the absence of such evidence, the stress–diathesis model cannot be rigorously tested.

Unfortunately, it is difficult to identify people at risk for many disorders, so the analysis of pre-morbid reactivity is logistically taxing. The significance of psychophysiological vulnerability must remain unresolved in these cases until longitudinal studies are undertaken. It is possible, however, to examine risk groups for cardiovascular disorders, and these therefore provide the best opportunity for testing psychophysiological models. Two groups in particular have been investigated: those at risk for essential hypertension on genetic or haemodynamic grounds, and people exhibiting Type A coronary-prone behaviour.

REACTIVITY PATTERNS AND TYPE A CORONARY-PRONE BEHAVIOUR

It has been suggested in previous sections that the nature of the psychosocial stimulation, its interactions with the psychobiological programme, and predispositions to physiological hyperreactivity, may all contribute to the determination of disease-specific response patterns. These arguments are elaborated in the present section by contrasting two fields of research concerned with cardiovascular reactivity.

The Type A coronary-prone behaviour pattern is now recognized as a significant coronary risk factor. The behaviour pattern, which is characterized by extreme competitiveness, striving for achievement, and a chronic sense of time urgency, has been linked prospectively and retrospectively with IHD (Brand, 1978; Zyzanski, 1978). It is associated both with new and recurrent coronary events, and acts independently of standard risk factors such as blood pressure, serum cholesterol and cigarette smoking. Preliminary evidence summarized by Langosch (Chapter 10) suggests that the modification of Type A behaviour in patients who have already suffered a myocardial infarction may reduce the risk of reinfarction. Type A is a constellation of behaviours rather than a personality trait, and may be fostered in the context of western urban materialism, where individual aspirations are channelled into occupational roles. It appears, therefore, to be a culture-bound phenomenon, and as such has less universality than standard coronary risk factors (Marmot, 1983). Investigations of children are beginning to tease out the influence of parental expectations and ambitions on subsequent coronary-prone behaviour (Matthews, 1978).

The mechanisms translating coronary-prone behaviour into coronary pathology remain obscure. The first problem is whether the behaviour pattern is linked with the development of coronary atherosclerosis (a long-term process) or clinical end-points such as infarction and angina pectoris. Zyzanski et al. (1976) showed that Type A scores were correlated with degree of stenosis, determined through coronary angiography. This has been confirmed by others (Frank et al., 1978; Blumenthal et al., 1978; Williams et al., 1980). Unfortunately, however, the data are not conclusive, since several negative angiographic studies have also been reported (Dimsdale et al., 1979; Kornitzer et al., 1982; Scherwitz et al., 1983).

The psychophysiological strategy may be valuable in delineating these mechanisms. Type A behaviour is a characteristic that precedes the onset of the disorder. If consistent patterns of psychophysiological individual-response specificity can be identified among healthy Type A people, and these duplicate the response characteristics of the diseased population, insight might be gained into pathogenesis. Studies of psychophysiological reactivity in Type A people have been carried out on four groups to date: young children, students, healthy adults and patients with IHD. The significance of the child studies is uncertain, since the relevance of the behaviours examined in children for later IHD is not known (Lawler et al., 1981; Lundberg, 1983). The studies of students may suffer from similar drawbacks.

Dembroski and his associates (1977, 1978) were the first to show differences in BP and HR reactivity amongst male students classified as either Type A or Type B. Although these results have been replicated in other laboratories (Glass et al., 1980a), other reports have been negative (Scherwitz et al., 1978; Lovallo and Pishkin, 1980; Hastrup et al., 1982; Rüddel et al., 1983). Even among the positive findings there is a good deal of inconsistency. For instance, while systolic BP seems more sensitive on some occasions, Newlin and Levenson (1982) found differences in diastolic BP only. Dembroski et al., (1977), on the other hand, reported that Type Bs were more responsive than Type As in diastolic BP, and Steptoe and Ross (1981) observed a similar difference for HR. Patterns of response shown by males do not appear to replicate in female students (Manuck et al., 1978; MacDougall et al., 1981; Lane et al., 1984). Peripheral vasomotor responses are also rather variable (Lovallo and Pishkin, 1980; Van Egeren et al., 1982; Williams et al., 1982).

Two explanations have been put forward for this state of affairs. The first is that insensitive classification methods have employed. While some investigators have used the structured interview technique (as developed by Friedman and Rosenman), others prefer the student version of the Jenkins Activity Survey (JAS, Kranz et al., 1974). The relationship of this instrument to IHD has not been established, and it may indeed either be insensitive or record a different constellation of behaviours (Chesney et al., 1981). This criticism was given force by Blumenthal et al. (1983), who showed differences in systolic BP and HR reactions to a cognitive task when Type A and B students were classified on the structured interview, but not on the student JAS. Nevertheless, this cannot be the complete explanation, since some studies have failed to show differences in BP and HR reactivity even with classification by structured interview (Scherwitz et al., 1978; Williams et al., 1982; Rüddel et al., 1983).

A second possibility is that the experimental conditions have been inappropriate, placing demands on subjects that do not elicit Type A behaviours. Type A is thought to be a behaviour that emerges only when particular environmental contigencies prevail. The problem is that authorities disagree about the important features of tasks or stimuli. It is clear, for example, that making tasks very difficult or aversive is not sufficient (Hastrup *et al.*, 1982; Newlin and Levenson, 1982). Blumenthal *et al.* (1983) suggest that Type As are less sensitive to external incentives than Type Bs, but Glass *et al.* (1980b) reported that incentives had no effect on the cardiovascular responses of either group. It is to be hoped that future studies will show more consistency in identifying the salient qualities of the psychosocial environment. The Type A concept is global, and only certain components may be relevant to aetiology. In this respect, it is interesting to note the striking similarities between Type A behaviour and the description of peptic ulcer patients ("ulcer patients are always in the front line of life's activities") drawn by Davies and Wilson in 1937. However, a more important point is that the significance of the behaviour pattern in students for the development of IHD is unclear. Student life may place demands on people that evoke Type A characteristics; there are frequent deadlines to meet, the student must work on several things at once, he or she may often work in the evening or at weekends, and meals may be hurried and noisy. Unless a student progresses to a similar environment in adult life, many aspects of coronary-prone behaviour may never again be apparent. An examination of Type A characteristics in students may not, therefore, be as fruitful in the long-term as studying adults who have well-established work structures and patterns of living.

Table 1 summarizes a number of experiments that have been performed on disease-free adults. Only one study so far reported has involved women, but the male samples have come from a variety of backgrounds. For convenience, only main effects and simple interactions have been included. It can be seen that the most consistent differences are in systolic BP reactivity. Most studies have found that Type As respond with greater increases in systolic BP than Type Bs in at least some experimental conditions, particularly when the A/B classification was made by interview. The data concerning diastolic BP are generally negative while the HR results are mixed. Catecholamine responses are also variable; Friedman *et al.*, (1975) showed excessive noradrenaline but not adrenaline responses, while Glass *et al.* (1980b) and Contrada *et al.* (1982) found the reverse. The one study of women showed patterns of reactivity similar to those found in men (Lawler *et al.*, 1983).

These data indicate that, although cardiovascular and neuroendocrine hyperreactivity is associated with Type A behaviour, it is not an inevitable and stable concomitant of the behaviour pattern. Heightened reactivity is not always displayed even in the presence of demanding laboratory tasks.

Table 1 Psychophysiological reactions from Type A and Type B adults without ischaemic heart disease

Source	Population	Classification instrument	Experimental conditions	Results	Comments
Contrada et al., 1982	Policemen Age 29–53 (mean 40) $n = 87$	SI	Choice reaction time with and without control over aversive stimulation	A > B in SBP and HR No differences in DBP No consistent NAd differences A > B in Ad, except when groups have control over high intensity stimulation, when B > A	No interactions in BP or HR between A/B and behavioural control over aversive stimulation
Corse et al., 1982	Men from cardiology prevention programme Age 49.1 ± 6.9 $n = 24$	SI JAS	Concept formation, mental arithmetic, picture completion from WAIS	A > B in SBP and DBP No differences in HR No differences in BP or HR	
Dembroski et al., 1979	Non-IHD male medical patients Age 54–65 $n = 31$	SI	SI and history quiz	A > B in SBP and DBP No differences in HR	Mixed groups of ill patients
Friedman et al., 1975	Male volunteers Average age 48 $n = 30$	SI	Competitive problem-solving with distracting noise	A > B in NAd No differences in Ad	
Glass et al., 1980b	Male transport workers (i) Age 42.8 ± 6.8 $n = 22$	SI	(i) Competitive video game with and without harassment from competitor	A > B in HR A > B in SBP and Ad in harassment condition only No differences in DBP and NAd	

Study	Sample	Measure	Task	Results	Comments
	(i) Age 43.5 ± 7.4 n = 20		(ii) Video game without competition, with and without monetary incentive	A > B in SBP, DBP, HR and Ad. No differences in NAd	No incentive effects
Jennings and Choi, 1981	Male businessmen Age 48–50 n = 24	SI	Choice RT	No differences in tonic BP and HR responses	Some differences in phasic HR responses related to reaction time
Lawler et al., 1983	Unemployed females Age 25–55 (mean 40.1) n = 20	JAS	Mental arithmetic Raven's matrices	A > B in SBP and HR. No differences in DBP	Sample of younger (mean 33.5) employed professional/executive Type A women show similar reaction patterns to unemployed Type B women
Manuck et al., 1979	Male attorneys Age 34.6 ± 7.5 n = 45	JAS	Concept formation	No association between BP reactivity and JAS scores	
Rüddel et al., 1982	Male urban sample Age 36 ± 9 n = 35	SI (German version)	Mental arithmetic with distracting noise. SI.	No differences in SBP, DBP or HR	
Schmidt et al., 1982	Policemen Age 30.3 ± 2.07 n = 36	SI (German version)	SI and general knowledge quiz	A > B in SBP and HR during SI. No differences in DBP. No differences during quiz	Differences significant only on one-tailed test
Steptoe et al., 1984	Male factory workers Age 41.9 ± 6.3 n = 36	Adaptation of student JAS	Stroop test, film and non-competitive video game	B > A in DBP. No differences in HR, PTT and SBP	Some participants have essential hypertension

Abbreviations: SI = structured interview; JAS = Jenkins Activity Survey; SBP and DBP = systolic and diastolic blood pressure; HR = heart rate; Ad = plasma adrenaline; NAd = plasma noradrenaline; RT = reaction time; PTT = pulse transit time.

From studies in which different task demands were compared, it appears that harassment is important (Glass *et al.*, 1980b), while behavioural control over aversive stimulation and active behavioural coping are not (Contrada *et al.*, 1982; Steptoe *et al.*, 1984).

One problem with interpreting these results is that the relevance of the different physiological parameters is not known. We need to discover which variables are responsible for the association with IHD. Some insight may be gained by studying Type A people with manifest disease. Unfortunately, many of the participants were medicated in two of the experiments on coronary patients recently reported, so response patterns were distorted (Dembroski *et al.*, 1979; Kranz *et al.*, 1981). Corse *et al.* (1982) examined a group consisting primarily of post-infarction patients. They showed a reaction pattern similar to disease-free Type A subjects (see Table 1), with heightened modifications in systolic and diastolic BP. No biochemical measures were included, so it is not known whether pressor reactions were accompanied by catecholamine release. On the other hand, Brodner *et al.* (1983) failed to find an association between autonomic reactions and coronary-prone behaviour in a series of young (< 40 years) patients following transmural infarction.

Taking all these studies into account, BP would appear to be the parameter that is most sensitive to Type A/B differences. Yet before it can be concluded that BP reactivity is the mechanism through which Type A behaviour is translated into cardiac pathology, a parallel literature must be considered.

ESSENTIAL HYPERTENSION AND AUTONOMIC REACTIVITY

A number of cardiovascular reactivity studies have been performed in the search for factors pre-dating the onset of essential hypertension. The work in this area rests on firmer foundations than the coronary-prone behaviour studies, since the physiological parameters relevant to aetiology are better established.

Essential hypertension is a multifactorial disorder, and various mechanisms differ in their importance according to the severity and duration of the condition. In severe hypertension of long standing, elevated BP is maintained by increased systemic peripheral resistance. Renal and vascular processes help sustain altered function (Folkow and Neil, 1971). Under these circumstances, high BP may be maintained irrespective of any influences from the central nervous system. On the other hand, in many cases of early mild hypertension, elevated BP results from increased cardiac output, and a disturbance of the factors balancing cardiac output with total peripheral resistance (Julius and Esler, 1975). Disturbed autonomic nervous regulation may be responsible, involving either overactivity of sympathetic (particularly β-adrenergic) pathways, reduced vagal activity or a combination of the two. The central nervous neurochemical changes related to essential hypertension are detailed in Chapter 4.

A number of investigators have proposed that psychophysiological processes are responsible for the autonomic disturbance. It has already been noted that patients with mild or moderate hypertension display heightened BP reactions when confronted with tasks demanding active coping behaviour. This is consistent with an autonomic aetiology, but does not provide a direct demonstration, since aberrant haemodynamic regulation may be a consequence rather than a cause. Studies have, therefore, been carried out on groups at high risk for developing the disorder. Two markers of risk have been employed: family history and marginal or transient BP elevations in the patient's own records.

The involvement of genetic factors in the essential hypertension has been well documented (Pickering, 1968). Table 2 summarizes studies of autonomic reactiviy in children or young adults with (PH+) or without (PH−) a parental history of essential hypertension. In reviewing these investigations, a number of points should be borne in mind. The first is the problem of baseline levels. If two groups differ in resting levels of BP or HR, then it is possible that differences in reactivity arise purely as a result of tonic differences. Some of the studies shown in Table 2 reported differences in cardiovascular function that were present throughout baseline and stimulation periods, with no differences in reactivity *per se*. Secondly, parental histories have not always been collected with great rigour. Investigators have relied on reports from students about their parents (Jorgenson and Houston, 1981) or reports from parents without documentation from physicians (Hastrup *et al.*, 1982). Thus, misclassifications are likely, since much hypertension is undetected in the community.

Nevertheless, the experiments summarized in Table 2 show a consistent pattern. With few exceptions, experiments using demanding behavioural or cognitive tasks have produced greater cardiovascular reactions from PH+ people. On the other hand, no differences have been recorded in studies using mildly challenging tasks or passive stressors such as the cold pressor (Remington *et al.*, 1960; Ohlsson and Henningsen, 1982).

The cardiovascular parameters sensitive to parental history differ somewhat between studies. Systolic and diastolic BP and HR have successfully distinguished groups in some experiments but not all. There is at present insufficient research on which to base fine distinctions in the cardiovascular correlates of different demanding tasks. However, it appears that cardiac sympathetic pathways may be especially sensitive to alert reaction time

TABLE 2 Cardiovascular reactions to behavioural tasks and parental history of essential hypertension

	Population	Experimental conditions	Results	Comments
Falkner et al., 1979	M and F children Age 14.3 ± 0.3 $n = 58$	Mental arithmetic under harassment	PH+ > PH− in DBP and HR No difference in SBP	Subgroups of PH+ show increased SBP responses (labile group excluded)
Hastrup et al., 1982	M students Age 18–27 (median 19) $n = 103$	Shock avoidance RT	PH+ > PH− in SBP and HR No difference in DBP	Baseline (relaxation day) difference in SBP and HR
Holroyd and Gorkin, 1983	M student Age 18–22 (mean 19.3) $n = 35$	Assertive role play	PH+ > PH− in SBP and DBP No difference in HR	Baseline difference in HR
Jorgensen and Houston 1981	M and F students Age not given $n = 58$	Stroop test, mental arithmetic and digit span	PH+ > PH− in DBP and HR PH+ > PH− in SBP in women only	Interaction between PH and Type A/B classification
Lane et al., 1984	F students Age not given $n = 29$	Mental arithmetic	No differences in BP, HR or forearm blood flow	
Lawler and Allen, 1981	M and F children Age 11–13 $n = 39$	Anagrams and RT with incentive	No differences in BP or HR	Baseline difference in SBP Marginal PH+ > PH− in DBP

Study	Subjects	Stress test	Results	Comments
Light et al., 1983	M students Age 18–22 n = 24	Competitive tasks in pairs	No differences in BP or HR Risk subjects with high HR reactions show reductions in urine flow and sodium excretion	Risk group includes some borderline hypertensives as well as PH+
Manuck et al., 1981	M students Age 17–21 n = 69	Concept formation task	PH+ >PH− in SBP No differences in DBP or HR	
Manuck and Proietti, 1982	M students Age 18.8 n = 36	Concept formation and mental arithmetic	PH+ >PH− in SBP No differences in DBP or HR	Baseline differences in HR
Ohlsson and Henningsen, 1982	M adults Age 34 ± 10.8 n = 41	Choice RT and cold pressor	No difference in BP, cardiac index or peripheral resistance	Probands with two generations of hypertension
Remington et al., 1960	M and F children Age 12.7 n = 50	Cold pressor	No differences in BP or HR	Baseline differences in SBP
Schulte et al., 1981b	M adults Age 34.4 ± 8.4 n = 46	Mental arithmetic with distracting noise	PH+ >PH− in SBP and DBP No differences in HR	

Physical stress tests were included in some of these investigations, but the results are not summarized here.

Abbreviations: PH+/PH− = Parental history positive and negative; SBP and DBP = Systolic and diastolic blood pressure; HR = Heart rate; RT = reaction time.

performance under conditions of uncertainty about response outcome, while more general cardiovascular activation occurs with other tasks. It is interesting that HR differences emerge in many studies, since elevated HR reactivity may not be characteristic of essential hypertensives (Steptoe *et al.*, (1984); possibly heightened HR reactivity constitutes a very early stage of the process, developing before BP reactivity is disturbed. Recently, Light *et al.* (1983) have tested the possibility that behavioural challenge may induce sodium retention in people at genetic risk. Urine flow and sodium excretion were recorded during control periods and after subjects performed competitive tasks for one hour. PH+ subjects who displayed high HR reactions showed significant reductions in sodium excretion (mean 27%) and fluid output (mean 35%), with no change in the other groups. Within the PH+ group, sodium retention correlated reliably with HR reactions ($r = -.64$). Renal mechanisms are, therefore, also implicated in the psychophysiological process.

Some limitations of parental history studies should be borne in mind. Although PH+ subjects are at higher risk, their chances of developing essential hypertension are still not great (Julius and Schork, 1978). The PH+ groups may, therefore, contain a proportion of people who will remain normotensive in later years. Secondly, the groups may be distinguished on organic factors that could be responsible for reactivity differences. For example, Parfrey *et al.* (1981) have demonstrated differences in BP responses to dietary sodium and potassium among PH+ and PH− normotensive students, and differences in resistance vessel smooth muscle behaviour may also be present. In addition, it is possible that autonomic processes may be more important in those without genetic predispositions, operating in men and women who have no hereditary leanings to essential hypertension.

Irrespective of parental history, perhaps the most significant marker of future hypertension is initial BP level. People with slightly elevated BP in childhood and early adult life are more likely to develop hypertension than others (Paffenbarger *et al.*, 1968; Rabkin *et al.*, 1982). Epidemiological studies suggest that psychosocial factors may contribute to the gradient of BP increase with age (Marmot and Khaw, 1982). Some psychophysiological experiments have therefore been performed, comparing groups at different levels in the "normotensive" population distribution (Falkner *et al.*, 1979; Price *et al.*, 1979). For example, Light and Obrist (1980) divided a group of male student volunteers into those who displayed at least one casual systolic BP (from physicians' records or self-monitoring) over 135 mm, and others. The two groups differed significantly in systolic and diastolic BP during subsequent relaxation, and tasks involving both active and passive coping.

Unfortunately, such studies do not unequivocally demonstrate antecedent heightened reactivity, since the disease process may have already commenced in these people, even though they do not fall within the conventional (arbitrary) criteria for essential hypertension. However, a closely related marker of risk is the presence of occasional high BP readings in records of people who do not differ from controls in average BP. This situational or transient hypertension may indeed show the psychophysiological elements of aetiology in action, since the periodic high readings may occur only under behaviourally demanding conditions.

Steptoe and his colleagues (1984) included a group with this characteristic in a recent study, comparing them both with normotensives and mild hypertensives. The transient hypertension group showed high BP on screening, but this subsequently fell to normotensive levels on re-examination. Three groups of 12 men were compared during performance of two tasks involving active behavioural coping (the Stroop colour/word interference test and a video game) and one passive stressor (a distressing film, previously employed in a study of essential hypertensives by Melville and Raftery, 1981). Figure 2 illustrates some of the BP results. Compared with normotensives, mild hypertensives showed significantly greater systolic and diastolic BP reactions to the two tasks demanding active behavioural coping. In contrast, BP reactions to the passive conditions were indistinguishable, although both groups responded with small increases. Reactions to passive stressors appear not to be associated with clinical status, and may be of little aetiological significance (Voudoukis, 1978).

The behaviour of the transient hypertensives shared some features with the mild hypertension group. Their diastolic BP reactions during active coping were significantly greater than those of normotensives; indeed in percentage terms they are closer to mild hypertensives (13.6% and 14.1%). But when systolic BP reactions were assessed as changes from the stress session baseline, a different pattern emerged. The modifications during active coping were no greater than those of normotensives. The explanation for this finding may lie in baseline fluctuations. It is evident from Fig. 2 that the transient hypertensives respond substantially to the stress session itself. This situational reactivity confirms that in the presence of appropriate psychosocial stimuli, disturbed cardiovascular regulation is manifest in this risk group.

Another important aspect of psychophysiological risk may be the pattern of HR change. The transient hypertensives showed significantly greater increases during active coping (18.0 b.p.m.) than normotensives (11.4 b.p.m.), and their reactions were also greater than those of mild hypertensives (10.6 b.p.m.). Cardiac hyperreactivity was, therefore, characteristic of the risk group alone, rather than confirmed hypertensives. This

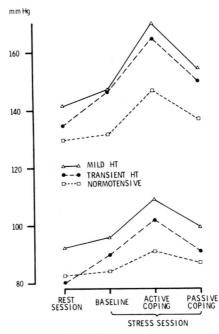

Fig. 2 Mean systolic and diastolic blood pressure in three groups of male factory workers. Rest session BPs represent the average of four readings taken at the end of a 20 minute rest session in which no tasks were performed. The baseline of the stress session is averaged from BP readings taken before, after and between three experimental stress conditions. (HT, hypertension.)

possibility has been put forward previously by Light and Obrist (1980), and has implications for the early identification and management of essential hypertensives. It may be possible to introduce prophylactic measures at a very early stage of the disease process.

There are many similarities between the strands of research relating cardiovascular reactivity to essential hypertension and coronary-prone behaviour. It is all the more surprising, therefore, that the two appear to be unrelated. Cross-sectional epidemiological studies indicate that Type A people are no more likely to have essential hypertension than Type Bs (Shekelle *et al.*, 1976; Brand, 1978). The two are independent risks for IHD. Unless some hitherto undisclosed interaction is discovered, it seems that similar psychophysiological processes are implicated in two quite different end-points: the development of essential hypertension and the appearance of IHD in people displaying Type A behaviour. This paradox will only be resolved by more detailed research, but at least three factors may be involved.

The first is that the conditions and contingencies eliciting heightened cardiovascular reactivity may be different in the two cases. Future pathology may depend on the nature of the environmental challenges to which the individual is chronically exposed. The postulated hypertensive aetiology is linked with active coping, and one aspect of this is behavioural control over sources of environmental stress. As has already been noted, however, control does not seem relevant to the cardiovascular responses of Type A men (Contrada *et al.*, 1982). Differences in sensitivity to environmental challenges may, therefore, be relevant to disease end-points.

The second possibility is that, although psychophysiological reactivity is relevant to both conditions, the physiological parameters mediating the association are different. Although BP is sensitive in both cases, it may be the accompanying neuroendocrine changes that are responsible for the pathology associated with Type A behaviour (Williams *et al.*, 1982). Alternatively, the mechanisms underlying BP change may be different, with selective involvement of cardiac and peripheral vasomotor processes in the two cases.

Lastly, it must always be borne in mind that these cardiovascular problems are multifactorial disorders. Parallel non-behavioural mechanisms may account for the differential susceptibility of people to essential hypertension and IHD. Perhaps active coping behaviour and its autonomic concomitants only increase the risk of essential hypertension in those with biological vulnerabilities (such as genetic risk or vasomotor lability). Type A individuals are no more likely to possess these characteristics than Type Bs, and so do not develop essential hypertension at a higher rate. This hypothesis reaffirms the notions of stress-diathesis (Fig. 1), albeit in an elaborated form.

CONCLUSIONS

This discussion of cardiovascular disorders has been presented in order to highlight the relevance of psychophysiological theory to disease. Some general conclusions are therefore in order. It is unlikely that many of the results outlined here can be attributed to the first process (subjective symptomatology) linking psychosocial stimuli to ill health, described at the beginning of the chapter. However, it is difficult to rule out mediation by behaviour changes (process 2), and these may contribute to many associations between adverse life experience and disease. Psychophysiological processes may have primary or secondary roles. In several disorders, such as bronchial asthma, pathophysiological dysfunctions are present. These may be stimulated both by physical challenges (exercise, air-borne substances) and psychosocial factors. Under these circumstances, psychophysiological mechanisms are of secondary importance, being relevant only in so far as the patient is confronted by appropriate psychological challenges, relative to the frequency of provocation by other stimuli.

The stress–diathesis model provides a useful starting point for disorders in which psychophysiological processes play a more prominent role. However, recent investigations emphasize that the model is interactive to such an extent that the significant facets of each component cannot be identified without reference to others. The hypothesis that psychosocial stimuli have non-specific effects cannot be maintained, for the patterns of physiological response generated by engaging in different forms of coping behaviour may have selective effects on different pathologies. Inasmuch as coping behaviours depend not only on external stimulation but the person's tendency to respond psychologically in a certain fashion, stimulus–response specificity fails to account for psychophysiological regularities. Conversely, individual–response specificity in relation to disease is not a general characteristic of the person, but may only be demonstrated under appropriate environmental challenge. This complexity has a positive aspect, since it implies that the negative results concerning individual–response specificity for many disease groups may have emerged from the presentation of inappropriate stimuli.

Several areas are in urgent need of development. The damaging aspects of behavioural coping have been emphasized in this chapter, but coping has important positive benefits that may be relevant to physiological reactivity patterns. Psychophysiological components of disease aetiology can only convincingly be demonstrated in prospective designs. The use of risk groups goes some way to clarifying cause and effect relationships, but again these must be followed longitudinally to see if predictions are fulfilled. Research in real life settings is also essential in order to establish the validity of laboratory paradigms.

Psychophysiological theories hold out exciting prospects for the future; none more so perhaps than the possibility or predicting risk of disease and markers of vulnerability. It may become possible to identify future sufferers from essential hypertension and other disorders before any clinical signs of disturbance. Allied to this is the opportunity of developing behavioural techniques for intervention and prevention. These might be based on a greater awareness of psychophysiological mechanisms than hitherto, enabling precise tailoring of treatments to conditions. Attempts have already been made for example to devise behavioural techniques for managing excessive cardiovascular reactivity (Steptoe, 1982; see Chapter 9). Behavioural procedures may come to play an important role in the early management of functional disorders, before disturbances have progressed so far that pharmacological or other medical treatments are required.

REFERENCES

Ader, R. (1976). Psychosomatic research in animals. *In* "Modern Trends in Psychosomatic Medicine, Vol. 3" (O. W. Hill, ed.), pp. 21–41. Butterworth, London.

Alexander, F. (1950). "Psychosomatic Medicine." Naughton, New York.

Anderson, C.D., Stoyva, J. M. and Vaughn, L. J. (1982). A test of delayed recovery following stressful stimulation in four psychosomatic conditions. *J. Psychosom. Res.* **26**, 571–580.

Bakal, D. A. and Kaganov, J. A. (1977). Muscle contraction and migraine headache: a psychophysiological comparison. *Headache* **17**, 208–215.

Barsky, A. J. and Klerman, G. L. (1983). Overview: hypochondriasis, bodily complaints and somatic styles. *Am. J. Psychiat.* **140**, 273–283.

Baumann, R., Ziprian, H., Godicke, W., Hartrodt, W., Naumann, E. and Lauter, J. (1973). The influence of acute psychic stress situations on biochemical and vegetative parameters of essential hypertensives at the early stages of the disease. *Psychother. Psychosom.* **22**, 131–140.

Blumenthal, J. A., Williams, R. B., Kong, Y., Schanberg, S. M. and Thompson, L. W. (1978). Type A behavior pattern and coronary atherosclerosis. *Circulation* **58**, 634–639.

Blumenthal, J. A., Lane, J. D., Williams, R. B., McKee, D. C., Haney, T. and White, A. (1983). Effects of task incentive on cardiovascular response in Type A and Type B individuals. *Psychophysiology* **20**, 63–70.

Boushey, H. A., Holtzmann, M. J., Sheller, J. R. and Nadel, J. A. (1980). Bronchial hyperreactivity. *Am. Rev. Resp. Dis.* **121**, 289–413.

Brand, R. J. (1978). Coronary-prone behavior as an independent risk factor for coronary heart disease. *In* "Coronary-prone Behavior" (T. M. Dembroski, S. M. Weiss, J. L. Shields, S. G. Haynes and M. Feinleib, eds), pp. 11–24. Springer-Verlag, New York.

Brod, J. (1960). Essential hypertension. Haemodynamic observations with a bearing on its pathogenesis. *Lancet* **ii**, 773–778.

Brod, J., Fencl., V., Hejl., Z. and Jirka, J. (1959). Circulatory changes underlying blood pressure elevation during acute emotional stress in normotensive and hypertensive subjects. *Clin. Sci.* **18**, 269–279.

Brodner, G., Langosch, W. and Brocherding, H. (1983). Psychophysiological reactivity and Type A behaviour pattern in young myocardial infarction patients. Paper presented to the VIIth World Congress of the International College of Psychosomatic Medicine, Hamburg.

Brown, G. W., Harris, T. and Copeland, J. R. (1977). Depression and loss. *Br. J. Psychiat.* **130**, 1–18.

Chesney, M. A., Black, G. W., Chadwick, J. H. and Rosenman, R. H. (1981). Psychological correlates of the Type A behavior pattern. *J. Behav. Med.* **4**, 217–229.

Cohen, M. J., Rickles, W. H. and MacArthur, D. L. (1978). Evidence for physiological response stereotypy in migraine headache. *Psychosom. Med.* **40**, 344–354.

Contrada, R. J., Glass, D. C., Krakoff, L. R., Krantz, D. S., Kehoe, K., Isecke, W., Collins, C. and Elting, E. (1982). Effects of control over aversive stimulation and Type A behavior on cardiovascular and plasma catecholamine responses. *Psychophysiology* **19**, 408–419.

Corse, C. D., Manuck, S. B., Cantwell, J. D., Giordani, B. and Matthews, K. A. (1982). Coronary-prone behavior pattern and cardiovascular response in persons with and without coronary heart-disease. *Psychosom. Med.* **44**, 449–459.

Corson, S. A. and Corson, E. O-L. (1971). Psychosocial influences on renal function—implications for human pathophysiology. *In* "Society, Stress and Disease" (L. Levi, ed.), Vol. 1, pp. 338–351. Oxford University Press, London.

Creed, F. (1981). Life events and appendicectomy. *Lancet* **i**, 1381–1385.

Davies, D. T. and Wilson, A. T. M. (1937). Observations on the life-history of chronic peptic ulcer. *Lancet* **ii**, 1353–1360.

Dembroski, T. M., MacDougall, J. M. and Shields, J. L. (1977). Physiologic reactions to social challenge in persons evidencing the Type A coronary-prone behavior pattern. *J. Hum. Stress* **3**(3), 2–10.

Dembroski, T. M., MacDougall, J. M., Shields, J. L., Petitto, J. and Lushene, R. (1978). Components of the coronary-prone behavior pattern and cardiovascular responses to psychomotor performance challenge. *J. Behav. Med.* **1**, 159–176.

Dembroski, T. M., MacDougall, J. M. and Lushene, R. (1979). Interpersonal interaction and cardiovascular response in Type A subjects and coronary patients. *J. Hum. Stress* **5**(4), 28–36.

Diamond, E. L. (1982). The rôle of anger and hostility in essential hypertension and coronary heart disease. *Psychol. Bull.* **92**, 410–433.

Dimsdale, J. E., Hackett, T. P., Catanzano, D. M. and White, P. J. (1979). The relationship between diverse measures of Type A personality and coronary angiographic findings. *J. Psychosom. Res.* **23**, 289–294.

Drummond, P. D. (1982). Extracranial and cardiovascular reactivity in migrainous subjects. *J. Psychosom. Res.* **26**, 317–332.

Dunbar, H. F. (1943). "Psychosomatic Diagnosis." Hoeber, New York.

Ekman, P., Levenson, R. W. and Friesen, W. (1983). Autonomic nervous system activity distinguishes among emotions. *Science* **221**, 1208–1210.

Engel, B. T. (1960). Stimulus–response and individual–response specificity. *Arch. Gen. Psychiat.* **2**, 305–313.

Engel, G. L., Reichsman, F. and Segal, H. L. (1956). Study of an infant with a gastric fistula, 1. Behavior and the rate of total hydrochloric acid secretion. *Psychosom. Med.* **18**, 374–398.

Esler, M. D., Julius, S., Zweifler, A., Randall, O., Harburg, E., Gardiner, H. and De Quattro, V. (1977). Mild high-renin essential hypertension: a neurogenic human hypertension? *New Engl. J. Med.* **296**, 405–411.

Fahrenberg, J., Walschburger, P., Foerster, F., Myrtek, M. and Müller, W. (1983). An evaluation of trait state and reaction aspects of activation processes. *Psychophysiology* **20**, 188–195.

Falkner, B., Onesti, G., Angelakos, E. T., Fernanadez, M. and Langman, C. (1979). Cardiovascular response to mental stress in normal adolescents with hypertensive parents. *Hypertension* **1**, 23–30.

Feuerstein, M., Barr, R. G., Francouer, T. E., Houle, M. and Rafman, S. (1982a). Potential bio-behavioral mechanisms of recurrent abdominal pain in children. *Pain* **13**, 287–298.

Feuerstein, M., Bush, C. and Corbisiero, R. (1982b). Stress and chronic headache: a psychophysiological analysis of mechanisms. *J. Psychosom. Res.* **26**, 167–182.

Finlay-Jones, R. and Brown, G. W. (1981). Types of stressful life event and the onset of anxiety and depressive disorders. *Psychol. Med.* **11**, 803–815.

Foerster, F. and Schneider, H. J. (1982). Individualspezifische, stimulusspezifische, ünd motivationsspezifische Reaktionsmuster im zweimal wiederholten Aktivierungsexperiment. *Z. Exp. Ang. Psychol.* **29**, 598–612.

Foerster, F., Schneider, H. J. and Walschburger, P. (1983). "Psychophysiologische Reaktionsmuster." Minerva, Munich.

Folkow, B. and Neil, E. (1971). "Circulation." Oxford University Press, London.

Fordyce, W. (1976). "Behavioral Methods for Chronic Pain and Illness." Mosby, St Louis.

Frank, K. A., Heller, S. S., Kornfeld, D. S., Sporn, A. A. and Weiss, M. B. (1978). Type A behavior pattern and coronary angiographic findings. *J. Am. Med. Ass.* **240**, 761–763.

Friedman, M., Byers, S., Diamant, J. and Rosenman, R. H. (1975). Plasma catecholamine response of coronary-prone subjects (Type A) to a specific challenge. *Metabolism* **24**, 205–210.

Gannon, L. (1981). The psychophysiology of psychosomatic disorders. In "Psychosomatic Disorders" (S. N. Haynes and L. Gannon, eds), pp. 1–31. Praeger, New York.

Gannon, L., Haynes, S. N., Safranek, R. and Hamilton, J. (1981). A psychophysiological investigation of muscle-contraction and migraine headache. *J. Psychosom. Res.* **25**, 271–280.

Glass, D. C., Krakoff, L. R., Finkleman, J., Snow, B., Contrada, R., Kehoe, K., Mannucci, E. G., Iseke, W., Collins, C., Hilton, W. F. and Elting, E. (1980a). Effect of task overload on cardiovascular and plasma catecholamine responses in Type A and B individuals. *Basic Appl. Soc. Psychol.* **1**, 119–218.

Glass, D. C., Krakoff, L. R., Contrada, R., Hilton, W. F., Kehoe, K., Mannucci, E. G., Collins, C., Snow, B., And Elting, E. (1980b). Effect of harassment and competition upon cardiovascular plasma catecholamine responses in Type A and Type B individuals. *Psychophysiology* **17**, 453–463.

Grossmann, M. I. (1967). Neural and hormonal stimulation of acid secretion. In "Handbook of Physiology, Section 6, Alimentary Canal, Vol. II" (edited by American Physiological Society). Williams and Wilkins, Baltimore.

Harrell, J. P. (1980). Psychological factors and hypertension: a status report. *Psychol. Bull.* **87**, 482–501.

Harris, A. H. and Brady, J. V. (1977). Long-term studies of cardiovascular control in primates. In "Biofeedback: Theory and Research" (G. E. Schwartz and J. Beatty, eds), pp. 243–264. Academic Press, London, Orlando and New York.

Harrison, R. H. (1975). Psychological testing in headache: a review. *Headache* **15**, 177–185.

Hastrup, J. L., Light, K. C. and Obrist, P. A. (1982). Parental hypertension and cardiovascular response to stress in healthy young adults. *Psychophysiology* **19**, 615–622.

Henry, J. P. (1976). Mechanisms of psychosomatic disease in animals. *Adv. Vet. Sci. Comp. Med.* **20**, 115–145.

Henry, J. P. (1982). The relation of social to biological processes in disease. *Soc. Sci. Med.* **16**, 369–380.

Henry, J. P. and Stephens, P. M. (1977). "Stress, Health and the Social Environment." Springer-Verlag, New York.

Holroyd, K. A. and Lazarus, R. S. (1982). Stress, coping and somatic adaptation. In "Handbook of Stress" (L. Goldberger and S. Breznitz, eds), pp. 21–35. The Free Press, New York.

Holroyd, K. A. and Gorkin, L. (1983). Young adults at risk for hypertension: effects of family history and anger management in determining responses to interpersonal conflict. *J. Psychosom. Res.* **27**, 131–138.

Hölzl, R. and Whitehead, W. E. (1983). "Psychophysiology of the Gastrointestinal Tract." Plenum Press, New York.

House, J. S., McMichael, A. J., Wells, J. A., Kaplan, B. H. and Landerman, L. R. (1979). Occupational stress and health among factory workers. *J. Health. Soc. Behav.* **20**, 139–160.

Isenberg, J. I., Grossman, M. I., Maxwell V. and Walsh, J. H. (1975). Increased sensitivity to stimulation of acid secretion by pentagastrin in duodenal ulcer. *J. Clin. Invest.* **55**, 330–337.

Jennings, J. R. and Choi, S. (1981). Type A components and psychophysiological responses to an attention-demanding performance task. *Psychosom. Med.* **43**, 475–487.

Jern, S. (1982). Psychological and haemodynamic facors in borderline hypertension. *Acta. Med. Scand.* **662**, (suppl.).

Jorgensen, R. S. and Houston, B. K. (1981). Family history of hypertension, gender, and cardiovascular reactivity and stereotypy during stress. *J. Behav. Med.* **4**, 175–189.

Julius, S. and Esler, M. D. (1975). Autonomic nervous cardiovascular regulation in borderline hypertension. *Am. J. Cardiol.* **36**, 685–696.

Julius, S. and Schork, M. A. (1978). Predictors of hypertension. *Ann. N.Y. Acad. Sci.* **304**, 38–52.

Kagan, A. R. and Levi, L. (1974). Health and environment—psychosocial stimuli: a review. *Soc. Sci. Med.* **8**, 225–241.

Keane, T. M., Martin, J. E., Berler, E. S., Wooten, L. S., Fleece, L. and Williams, J. G. (1982). Are hypertensives less assertive? A controlled evaluation. *J. Consult. Clin. Psychol.* **50**, 499–508.

Kinsman, R. A., Luparello, T., O'Banion, K. and Spector, S. (1973). Multidimensional analysis of the subjective symptomatology of asthma. *Psychosom. Med* **35**, 250–257.

Kinsman, R., Dahlen, N., Spector, S. and Staudenmayer, H. (1977). Observations on subjective symptomatology, coping behavior and medical decisions in asthma. *Psychosom. Med.* **39**, 102–119.

Kornitzer, M., Magotteau, V., Degre, C., Kittel, F., Struyvn, J. and Van Thiel, E. (1982). Angiographic findings and the Type A pattern assessed by means of the Bortner Scale. *J. Behav. Med.* **5**, 313–320.

Krantz, D. S., Glass, D. C. and Snyder, M. L. (1974). Helplessness, stress level, and the coronary-prone behavior pattern. *J. Abnorm. Psychol.* **10**, 284–300.

Krantz, D. S., Schaefer, M. A., Davia, J. E., Dembroski, T. M., MacDougall, J. M. and Schaffer, R. T. (1981). Extent of coronary atherosclerosis, Type A behavior and cardiovascular response to social interaction. *Psychophysiology* **18**, 654–664.

Lacey, J. I. (1967). Somatic response patterning and stress: some reformulations of activation theory. *In* "Psychological Stress—issues in research" (M. H. Appley and R. Trumball, eds), pp. 14–44. Appleton-Century-Crofts, New York.

Lacey, J. I., Bateman, D. E. and Van Lehn, R. (1953). Autonomic response specificity: an experimental study. *Psychosom. Med.* **15**, 8–21.

Lachman, S. J. (1972). "Psychosomatic Disorders: a Behavioristic Interpretation." Wiley, New York.

Lance, J. W. (1978). "Mechanism and Management of Headache." Butterworths, London.

Lane, J. D., White, A. D. and Williams, R. B. (1984). Cardiovascular effects of mental arithmetic in Type A and Type B females. *Psychophysiology* **21**, 39–46.

Lawler, K. A. and Allen, M. T. (1981). Risk factors for hypertension in children: their relationship to psychophysiological responses. *J. Psychosom. Res.* **25**, 199–204.

Lawler, K. A., Allen, M. T., Critcher, E. C. and Standard, B. A. (1981). The relationship of physiological responses to the coronary prone behavior pattern in children. *J. Behav. Med.* **4**, 203–216.

Lawler, K. A., Rix, S. E. A. and Allen, M. T. (1983). Type A behavior and psychophysiological responses in adult women. *Psychophysiology* **20**, 343–350.

Levenson, R. W. (1979). Effects of thematically relevant and general stressors on specificity of response in asthmatic and non-asthmatic subjects. *Psychosom. Med.* **41**, 28–39.

Levey, A. B. and Martin, I. (1981). The relevance of classical conditioning to psychosomatic disorder. *In* "Foundations of Psychosomatics" (M. Christie and P. Mellett, eds), pp. 259–282. Wiley, Chichester.

Light, K. C. and Obrist, P. A. (1980). Cardiovascular reactivity to behavioral stress in young males with and without marginally elevated casual systolic pressure. *Hypertension* **2**, 802–808.

Light, K. C., Koepke, J. P., Obrist, P. A. and Willis, P. W. (1983). Psychological stress induces sodium and fluid retention in men at high risk for hypertension. *Science* **220**, 429–431.

Lindenthal, J. J., Myers, J. K. and Pepper, M. P. (1982). Smoking, psychological status and stress. *Soc. Sci. Med.* **6**, 583–591.

Lovallo, W. R. and Pishkin, V. (1980). A psychophysiological comparison of Type A and B men exposed to failure and uncontrollable noise. *Psychophysiology* **17**, 29–36.

Lown, B., De Silva, R. A., Reich, P. and Murawski, V. J. (1980). Psychophysiologic factors in sudden cardiac death. *Am. J. Psychiatry* **137**, 1325–1335.

Lundberg, U. (1983). Notes on Type A behaviour and cardiovascular responses to challenge in 3–6-year-old children. *J. Psychosom. Res.* **27**, 39–42.

MacDougall, M., Dembroski, T. M. and Krantz, D. S. (1981). Effects of types of challenge on pressor and heart rate responses in Type A and B women. *Psychophysiology* **18**, 1–9.

Malmo, R. B. and Shagass, C. (1949). Physiologic study of symptom mechanisms in psychiatric patients under stress. *Psychosom. Med.* **11**, 25–29.

Manuck, S. B., Craft, S. and Gold, K. J. (1978). Coronary-prone behavior and cardiovascular response. *Psychophysiology* **15**, 403–411.

Manuck, S. B., Giordani, B., McQuaid, K. J. and Garrity, S. J. (1981). Behaviorally-induced cardiovascular reactivity amongst the sons of reported hypertensive and normotensive parents. *J. Psychosom. Res.* **25**, 261–269.

Manuck, S. B. and Proietti, J. M. (1982). Parental hypertension and cardiovascular response to cognitive and isometric challenge. *Psychophysiology* **19**, 481–490.

Marmot, M. G. (1983). Stress, social and cultural variations in heart disease. *J. Psychosom. Res.* **27**, 377–384.

Marmot, M. G. and Khaw, K-T. (1982). Implications for population studies of the age trend in blood pressure. *Contr. Nephrol.* **30**, 101–107.

Martin, P. R. and Mathews, A. M. (1978). Tension headaches: psychophysiological investigations and treatment. *J. Psychosom. Res.* **22**, 389–399.

Matthews, K. A. (1978). Assessment and developmental antecedents of the coronary-prone behavior pattern in children. In "Coronary-prone Behavior" (T. M. Dembroski, S. M. Weiss, J. L. Shields, S. G. Haynes and M. Feinleib, eds), pp. 207–215. Springer-Verlag, New York.

Mechanic, D. (1968). "Medical Sociology: a selective view." The Free Press, New York.

Melville, D. I. and Raftery, E. B. (1981). Blood pressure changes during acute mental stress in hypertensive subjects using the Oxford Intra-Arterial system. *J. Psychosom. Res.* **25**, 487–498.

Nestel, P. J. (1969). Blood pressure and catecholamine excretion after mental stress in labile hypertension. *Lancet* **i**, 692–694.

Newlin, D. B. and Levenson, R. W. (1982). Cardiovascular responses of individuals with Type A behavior pattern and parental coronary heart disease. *J. Psychosom. Res.* **26**, 393–402.

Obrist, P. A. (1981). "Cardiovascular Psychophysiology." Plenum Press, New York.

Ohlsson, O. and Henningsen, N. C. (1982). Blood pressure, cardiac output and systemic vascular resistance during stress, muscle work, cold pressor test and psychological stress. *Acta Med. Scand.* **212**, 329–336.

Paffenbarger, R. D., Thorne, M. C. and Wing, A. L. (1968). Chronic disease in former college students, VIII: Characteristics in youth predisposing to hypertension in later years. *Am. J. Epidemiol.* **88**, 25–32.

Parfrey, P. S., Condon, K., Wright, P., Vandenberg, M. J., Holly, J. M. P., Goodwin, F. J., Evans, S. J. W. and Ledingham, J. M. (1981) Blood pressure and hormonal changes following alteration in dietary sodium and potassium in young men with and without a familial predisposition to hypertension. *Lancet* **i**, 113–117.

Parkes, C. M. and Brown, R. J. (1972). Health after bereavement: a controlled study of young Boston widows and widowers. *Psychosom. Med.* **34**, 449–461.

Peyser, H. (1982). Stress and alcohol. In "Handbook of Stress" (L. Goldberger and S. Breznitz, eds), pp. 285–298. The Free Press, New York.

Philips, C. (1980). Recent developments in tension headache research: implications for understanding and management of the disorder. In "Contributions to Medical Psychology" (S. Rachman, ed.), Vol. 2., pp. 113–130. Pergamon Press, Oxford.

Philips, H. C. and Hunter, M. S. (1982). A psychophysiological investigation of tension headache. *Headache* **22**, 173–179.

Pickering, G. W. (1968). "High Blood Pressure" 2nd ed. Churchill, London.

Price, K. P. and Tursky, B. (1976). Vascular reactivity of migraineurs and non-migraineurs: a comparison of responses to self-control procedures. *Headache* **16**, 210–217.

Price, K. P., Lott, G., Fixler, D. E. and Browne, R. H. (1979). Cardiovascular responses to stress in adolescents with elevated blood pressures. *Psychosom. Med.* **41**, 74.

Rabkin, S. W., Mathewson, F. A. L. and Tate, R. B. (1982). Relationship of blood pressure in 20–39-year-old men to subsequent blood pressure and incidence of hypertension over a 30-year observation period. *Circulation* **65**, 291–296.

Remington, R. D., Lambarth, B., Moser, M. and Hoobler, S. W. (1960). Circulatory reactions of normotensive and hypertensive subjects and the children of normal and hypertensive patients. *Am. Heart J.* **59**, 58–70.

Roessler, R. and Engel, B. T. (1977). The current status of the concepts of physiological response specificity and activation. In "Psychosomatic Medicine: current trends and clinical applications" (Z. J. Lipowski, D. R. Lipsitt and P. C. Whybrow, eds), pp. 50–57. Oxford University Press, New York.

Rüddel, H., Langewitz, W., Neus, H., Schiebener A., Schmieder, R. and Schulte, W. (1982). Cardiovascular reactivity during mental stress testing, the Type A interview, and exercise testing in healthy male subjects. *Activ. Nerv. Sup. (Praha)* **3**(suppl.), 268–273.

Rüddel, H., Gogolin, E., Friedrich, G., Neus, H. and Schulte, W. (1983). Coronary-prone behavior and blood pressure reactivity in laboratory and life stress. In "Biobehavioral Bases of Coronary Heart Disease" (T. M. Dembroski, T. H. Schmidt and G. Blümchen, eds), pp. 185–196. Karger, Basel.

Russek, H. I. (1965). Stress, tobacco and coronary disease in North American professional groups. *J. Am. Med. Ass.* **192**, 189–194.

Scherwitz, L., Berton, K. and Leventhal, H. (1978). Type A behavior, self-involvement and cardiovascular response. *Psychosom. Med.* **40**, 593–609.

Scherwitz, L., McKelvain, R., Laman, C., Patterson, J., Dutton, L., Yusim, S., Lester, J., Kraft, I., Rochelle, D. and Leachman, R. (1983). Type A behavior, self-involvement and coronary atherosclerosis. *Psychosom. Med.* **45**, 47–57.

Schmidt, T. H., Undeutsch, K., Dembroski, T. M., Langosch, W., Neus, H. and Rüddel, H. (1982). Coronary-prone behaviour and cardiovascular reactions during the German version of the Type A interview and during a quiz. *Activ. Nerv. Sup. (Praha)* **3**(suppl.), 241–251.

Schulte, W., Neus, H. and Von Eiff, A. W. (1981a). Blutdruckreaktivität unter emotionalen Stress bei unkomplizierten Formen des Hochdrucks. *Klin. Wochenschr.* **59**, 1243–1249.

Schulte, W., Neus, H. and Rüddel, H. (1981b). Zum blutdruckverhalten unter emotionalen Stress bei Normotonikern mit familiärer Hypertonieanamnese. *Med. Welt* **32**, 1135–1137.

Schwartz, G. E., Weinberger, D. A. and Singer, J. A. (1981). Cardiovascular differentiation of happiness, sadness, anger and fear following imagery and exercise. *Psychosom. Med.* **43**, 343–364.

Sersen, E. A., Clausen, J. and Lidsky, A. (1978). Autonomic specificity and stereotypy revisited. *Psychophysiology* **15**, 60–67.

Shekelle, R. B., Schoenberger, J. A. and Stamler, J. (1976). Correlates of the JAS Type A behaviour pattern score. *J. Chron. Dis.* **29**, 381–394.

Stamler, J., Stamler, B., Riedlinger, W., Algera, G. and Roberts, T. (1976). Hypertension screening of 1 million Americans. *J. Am. Med. Ass.* **235**, 2299–2306.

Steptoe, A. (1980). Stress and medical disorders. In "Contributions to Medical Psychology" (S. Rachman, ed.), Vol. 2, pp. 55–77. Pergamon Press, Oxford.

Steptoe, A. (1981). "Psychological Factors in Cardiovascular Disorders." Academic Press, London, Orlando and New York.

Steptoe, A. (1982). Control of cardiovascular reactivity and the treatment of hypertension. In "Behavioral Treatment of Disease (R. S. Surwit, R. B. Williams, A. Steptoe, R. Biersner, eds), pp. 159–172. Plenum Press, New York.

Steptoe, A. (1983a). Communication to the Editor. *J. Psychosom. Res.* **27**, 85–86.

Steptoe, A. (1983b). Stress, helplessness and control: the implications of laboratory studies. *J. Psychosom. Res.* **27,** 361–368.

Steptoe, A. and Ross, A. (1981). Psychophysiological reactivity and the prediction of cardiovascular disorders. *J. Psychosom. Res.* **25,** 23–32.

Steptoe, A., Melville, D. and Ross, A. (1982). Essential hypertension and psychological functioning: a study of factory workers. *Br. J. Clin. Psychol.* **21,** 303–311.

Steptoe, A., Melville, D. and Ross, A. (1984). Behavioural response demands, cardiovascular reactivity and essential hypertension. *Psychosom. Med.* **45,**

Stern, R. M. (1983). Responsiveness of the stomach to environmental events. In "Psychophysiology of the Gastrointestinal Tract" (R. Hölzl and W. E. Whitehead, eds), pp. 181–207. Plenum Press, New York.

Sternbach, R. A. (1966). "Principles of Psychophysiology." Academic Press, Orlando, New York and London.

Sullivan, P., Schoentgen, S., De Quattro, V., Procci, W., Levine, D., Van der Meulen, J. and Bonheimer, J. (1981). Anxiety, anger and neurogenic tone at rest and in stress in patients with primary hypertension. *Hypertension* **3,** II-119–II-123.

Svensson, J. C. and Theorell, T. (1982). Cardiovascular effects of anxiety induced by interviewing young hypertensive male subjects. *J. Psychosom. Res.* **26,** 359–370.

Van Boxtel, A. and Roozeveld van der Ven, J. (1978). Differential EMG activity in subjects with muscle contraction headaches related to mental effort. *Headache* **17,** 233–237.

Van der Valk, J. M. (1957). Blood pressure changes under emotional influences in patients with hypertension and control subjects. *J. Psychosom. Res.* **2,** 134–146.

Van Egeren, L. F., Sniderman, L. D. and Hoggelin, M. S. (1982). Competitive two-person interactions of Type A and Type B individuals. *J. Behav. Med.* **5,** 55–66.

Vaughn, R., Pall, M. L. and Haynes, S. N. (1977). Frontalis EMG response to stress in subjects with frequent muscle contraction headaches. *Headache* **16,** 313–317.

Voudoukis, I. J. (1978). Cold pressor test and hypertension. *Angiology* **29,** 429–439.

Walker, B. B. and Sandman, C. A. (1977). Physiological response patterns in ulcer patients: phasic and tonic components of the electrogastrogram. *Psychophysiology* **14,** 343–400.

Weiner, H. (1977). "Psychobiology and Human Disease." Elsevier North-Holland, New York.

Williams, R. B., Haney, T. L., Lee, K. L., Kong, Y., Blumenthal, J. A. and Whalen, R. E. (1980). Type A behavior, hostility and coronary atherosclerosis. *Psychosom. Med.* **42,** 539–549.

Williams, R. B., Lane, J. D., Kuhn, C. M., Melosh, W., White, A. D. and Schanberg, S. M. (1982). Type A behavior and elevated physiological and neuroendocrine responses to cognitive tasks. *Science* **218,** 483–485.

Wolf, S. (1965). "The Stomach." Oxford University Press, New York.

Zyzanski, S. J. (1978). Coronary-prone behavior and coronary heart disease: epidemiological observations. In "Coronary-prone Behavior" (T. M. Dembroski, S. M. Weiss, J. L. Shields, S. G. Haynes and M. Feinleib, eds), pp. 25–40. Springer-Verlag, New York.

Zyzanski, S. J., Jenkins, C. D., Ryan, T. J., Flessas, A. and Everist, M. (1976). Psychologic correlates of coronary angiographic findings. *Arch. Intern. Med.* **136,** 1234–1237.

4

Psychological Insults and Pathology. Contribution of Neurochemical, Hormonal and Immunological Mechanisms

HYMIE ANISMAN and LAWRENCE S. SKLAR

The prevalence of chronic disorders that cannot be attributed to exogenous or infectious disease processes has stimulated attempts to identify psychological or experiential variables that influence vulnerability to pathology (Depue et al., 1979). Indeed, greater attention is increasingly being devoted to the possibility that physical and psychological stressors may be fundamental in the provocation or exacerbation of several forms of pathology, or may increase vulnerability to illness.

It is somewhat curious that, while psychologists frequently question the contribution of psychological and physical insults to behavioural pathology (see the discussion in Anisman and Zacharko, 1982), the supposition that such factors may be fundamental in the course of immunologically related disorders is receiving progressively greater attention (see the various papers in the magnificent volume edited by Ader, 1981).

In order to assess satisfactorily the contribution of stressors to pathology, several approaches may be adopted. An attempt might be made to identify relevant substrates for the illness and to determine the conditions where stressful events influence these physiological processes. In addition, it might be desirable to determine the background conditions (including social, experiential and environmental) that lend themselves to the physiological changes induced by stressors. An alternative approach is to evaluate the consequences of stressful events on cognitive processes and to determine the conditions in which these cognitive changes are maximal. The particular method employed is governed by the predilections of the experimenter, as well as the characteristics of the pathology being examined. It is fair to say

HEALTH CARE AND HUMAN BEHAVIOUR
ISBN 0–12–666460–9

that in some instances analysis of both cognitive and physiological functioning may be fundamental for adequate determination of pathologies related to aversive life events (see Anisman and Zacharko, 1982; Chapter 1, this volume, by Craig and Brown).

Although the relationship between physical/psychological insults and illness have been evaluated in both humans and infrahumans, the present paper will be concerned primarily with research concerning infrahuman subjects.

Methodological considerations inherent in human experiments have frequently limited the conclusions that can be derived from this research (Rabkin and Streuning, 1976). Nevertheless, these shortcomings should not lead one to reject the supposition that stressful events are related to pathology, but only that caution should be exercised in evaluating the literature pointing to such a relationship. Indeed, research involving infrahuman subjects has largely supported the contention that stressful events may increase vulnerability to some forms of pathology. However, some inconsistent results have been reported in this respect, and often the source for these contradictions cannot be readily deduced. In the sections that follow, we will describe some of the physiological changes precipitated by stressors, as well as the limiting conditions in order that these changes occur. These physiological changes will then be related to pathology, with particular emphasis devoted to neoplastic disease.

STRESS-INDUCED NEUROCHEMICAL CHANGE

Considerable evidence is available suggesting that the central nervous system may modulate or initiate immune responses (see Spector and Korneva, 1981; Hall & Goldstein, 1981; Stein et al., 1981). Likewise, it appears that interrelationships exist between neurochemical and hormonal activity (Ganong, 1980; Terry and Martin, 1978), as well as hormonal and immunological responses (Maclean and Reichlin, 1981). Accordingly, in assessing the effects of stressors on some pathologies, it is appropriate to consider the interactive effects of these processes.

Variations in the lability of central nervous system neurotransmitters have been assessed following exposure to a number of different stressors, including footshock, restraint (immobilization), cold exposure, forced exercise, swim, rotation, etc. To a large extent, these stressors have yielded qualitatively similar effects on neurochemical activity, differing as a function of stress severity. In the case of cold exposure, some differences have been noted from other stressors, but these are minimized if animals are shaved prior to stress application or if cold is applied following water immersion.

Upon exposure to aversive stimulation the synthesis and utilization of noradrenaline (NA) is increased in several brain regions, including locus coeruleus, hippocamus, cortex and hypothalamus (Thierry, 1973; Thierry, et al., 1968, 1971; see reviews in Anisman, 1978; Stone, 1975). These effects have been witnessed in several different species. Soon after stress inception an actual rise of NA concentrations may occur, thereby assuring adequate supplies of the amine, at least in the short run (Welch and Welch, 1970). If the stressor is sufficiently severe and protracted the utilization of brain NA may exceed the rate of synthesis, and NA reductions of approximately 20–30% may occur (Thierry, 1973; Weiss et al., 1975; Anisman, 1978). On the basis of disappearance rates of ^{3}H-NA exogenously administered or synthetized from ^{3}H-tyrosine or ^{3}H-DOPA, it was suggested that moderate stress results in NA release from the functional storage pools, whereas severe stress calls upon release from the functional and main storage pools (Thierry, 1973; Thierry et al., 1971).

Although reductions of NA have been reported from several brain regions it appears that the reductions are more readily seen in some brain regions than others. For instance, Nakagawa et al. (1981) found that NA reductions in hypothalamus can be induced more readily than in hippocampus. In fact, we have found that stress severity that does not provoke reductions of hippocampal NA may elicit a 20% reduction in hypothalamic NA concentrations (Anisman, Beauchamp, Irwin and Zacharko, unpublished report). It should be emphasized that within the hypothalamus the NA reductions actually occur in only a limited number of nuclei, namely the lateral ventromedial nucleus, supraoptic nucleus (Kvetnansky et al., 1976) and the arcuate nucleus (Kobayashi et al., 1976). However, given the relationship between the hypothalamus and hormonal secretion from the pituitary and the fact that only some hypothalamic nuclei appear to influence immune functioning, it is important to specify the restricted hypothalamic nuclei in which NA is depleted after exposure to a stressor.

One apparently essential feature in determining whether or not the NE depletion will occur concerns the organism's ability to deal with the stress through behavioural means (Anisman et al., 1980; Weiss et al., 1970, 1981). In our own experiments, mice were exposed to 60 shocks of 150 μA applied at 60 s intervals. Mice could escape the shock by jumping over a low hurdle separating the two compartments of the shuttle box. Among these mice, no reduction of NA levels are observed (see Fig. 1), although we have observed an increase of NA turnover. A second group received yoked inescapable shock. That is, shock onset occurred for these animals at the same time as it did for the escape animals; however, shock offset was independent of the responses made by the yoked animal. When the animal in the escape group made the appropriate response the shock terminated for this animal and its

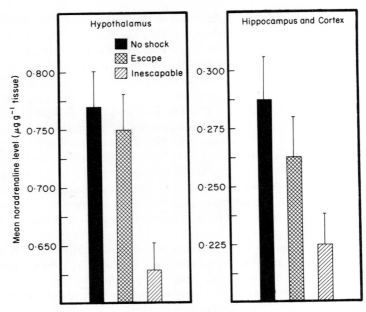

Fig. 1 Mean (± SEM) concentrations of noradrenaline in hypothalamus and in hippocampus among mice exposed to 60 escapable shocks, 60 inescapable shocks applied in a yoked paradigm or no shock (from Anisman *et al.*, 1980, with permission).

yoked partner. As seen in Fig. 1, among mice that received the inescapable shock, a substantial reduction of NA was observed in the hypothalamus and the hippocampus and cortex. Since mice in both groups received an equivalent amount and severity of stress, the shock *per se* was not responsible for the NA lability. Rather, it appears that the psychological dimension of "coping" with the stressor was responsible for the NA alterations. Along the same lines, Stolk *et al.* (1974) found that the NA alterations that are provoked by inescapable shock were modified if rats were shocked in pairs and permitted to fight. In fact, the extent of the amine alterations were inversely proportional to the number of fighting bouts in which rats had engaged. Inasmuch as a similar manipulation was found to limit stress-induced gastric ulceration (Weiss *et al.*, 1976), it is not unreasonable to suspect that fighting acted as a coping mechanism much in the same way as escaping from shock did.

It has been our contention that the response to aversive stimuli reflects adaptive changes in order to meet environmental demands. When faced with an aversive stimulus, the organism attempts to deal with the stressor through behavioural means (in humans this would include social support systems, cognitive strategies, and so forth). Concurrently, several physiological changes occur, including neurochemical, hormonal and immunological, which may diminish some of the adverse consequences of the insult. That is, they may blunt the physical or psychological impact of the aversive stimulation, enhance the organism's ablility to take evasive actions, or even protect the organism from health threats. Initially the heightened NA levels assure a transient supply of the amine, while the increased synthesis and utilization may be essential for coping attempts.

When behavioural control over the aversive stimuli is possible, the burden of coping is shared between behavioural and physiological mechanisms. However, when behavioural methods of dealing with stress are not available, then the burden is, by default, placed more fully on endogenous processes. Under such conditions, physiological systems may become excessively taxed, ultimately leading to coping failure. We previously suggested (Anisman, 1982; Anisman and Zacharko, 1982; Sklar and Anisman, 1981a) that failure of adaptive systems (in this instance, NA synthesis keeping pace with utilization) may be one factor that increases vulnerability to illness.

The adaptability of neurochemical systems following the application of aversive stimuli does not end with depletion of the neurotransmitter. Several investigators reported that if the stressor is applied for a sufficiently long duration, or is repeated on successive days, the NA depletion that ordinarily occurs after a single stress will be absent (Kvetnansky et al., 1976; Weiss et al., 1975). Figure 2, for example, shows the effects of acute and chronic stress on NA levels in several brain regions (Bowers et al., 1982). Whereas reductions of brain NA are seen in hypothalamus following a single session of shock (60 shocks, $150 \mu A$, 6 s on each day), the depletion is absent among mice that received 15 stress sessions previously. Indeed, in several brain regions in which acute stress did not produce NA reductions (although increase turnover was evident) the chronic regimen provoked an increase of amine levels, which actually exceeded levels seen in non-shocked mice. In contrast to brain NA, adaptation was not seen with respect to the corticosterone changes induced by the footshock. The increased serum corticosterone seen after a single shock session was fully evident following 15 stress sessions.

The increased levels of NA following chronic stress appears to result from the increased activity of synthetic enzymes, tyrosine-hydroxylase and dopamine-β-hydroxylase (Kvetnansky et al., 1976; Weiss et al., 1975). Moreover, it was indicated that chronic exposure to shock led to a decrease in the rate of NA re-uptake (Weiss et al., 1975). Although the levels of NA after chronic stress approach that of naive animals, one should not be misled

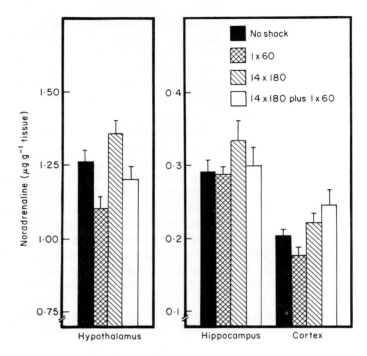

Fig. 2 Mean (± SEM) concentrations of noradrenaline in several brain regions among mice that received either no shock, a single session of 60 shocks and decapitated immediately thereafter (group 1 × 60), 14 sessions of 180 shocks and decapitated 24 h after the last shock session (group 14 × 180), or 14 sessions of 180 shocks followed by a single session of 60 shocks immediately prior to decapitation (group 14 × 180 plus 1 × 60) (from Bowers *et al.*, 1982, with permission).

in believing that this, in fact, implies functional equivalence. Although levels of NA are comparable in the two conditions, the rate of synthesis and utilization among chronically stressed mice is appreciably greater than that of naive (non-stressed) animals. Indeed, it has been argued that the increased amine activity may be fundamental to the provocation of some forms of psychological pathology (e.g. Stone, 1979a). However, it appears that the increased NA turnover is followed by still other adaptive changes. Specifically, it seems that following chronic exposure to a stressor, the sensitivity of β-NA receptors may be reduced, presumably as an adaptive response to the heightened NA activity that follows repeated aversive stimulation (Stone, 1979a,b; U'Prichard and Kvetnansky, 1981). It is conceivable that malfunction in any one of the many adaptive changes in neurochemical lability could potentially contribute to one form of pathology or another.

The consequences of psychological and physical insults are not limited to alterations of noradrenaline. Owing to the low concentrations of adrenaline in the brain, determination of the effects of stress awaited the development of sensitive assay techniques. The recent development of such methods has, in fact, revealed that stressors influence the rate of adrenaline synthesis and utilization in brain. Immobilization for 150 min was found to increase the activity of the synthetic enzyme, phenylethanolamine–N–methyltransferase (PNMT), in the locus coeruleus, nucleus tractus solitarus and the A2 region (medial portion of the nucleus tractus solitarus). After several stress sessions applied on consecutive days, the PNMT activity approached control values, although the increase of PNMT activity was still evident in the A2 region (Saavedra, 1980; Saavedra and Torda, 1980). Concentrations of adrenaline have also been found to vary as a function of stress severity. Following 20 min of immobilization stress, a reduction of adrenaline was found in the anterior hypothalamus and the nucleus commisuralis, while increased concentrations were evident in the median eminence. Following 240 min of immobilization, reductions of adrenaline were seen in the anterior hypothalamus and in the periventricular and ventromedial nucleus, as well as in the nucleus tractus solitarus, nucleus commisuralis and the A1 and A2 regions (Saavedra, 1980; Saavedra et al., 1979). In view of the finding that the anterior hypothalamus lesions may result in hypertension, owing to catecholamine release from the adrenal, Saavedra (1980) raised the possibility that the effects of stress on hypothalamic noradrenaline and adrenaline may be related to hypertension. As will be seen later, the possibility also exists that these catecholamine changes may be important in the regulation of immune responsitivity.

The effects of stress on dopamine (DA) neurones are less extensive than on NA neurones. Typically, stress will not influence DA levels when assays are performed on relatively large tissue samples, such as the whole hypothalamus. Likewise, reductions of DA are not observed in DA rich areas such as the substantia nigra. However, alterations in the activity of this amine can be detected in relatively discrete brain regions (see review by Anisman et al., 1982). Reductions of DA have been reported in the arcuate nucleus of the hypothalamus after exposure to acute stress (Kobayashi et al., 1976; Kvetnansky et al., 1976). Given that the arcuate nucleus may play a fundamental role in hormone secretion from the pituitary, the effects of stress on this brain region may prove to be particularly important in the analysis of stress related pathology, particularly those pathologies involving hormonal changes (see later discussion). In other brain regions, such as the nucleus accumbens and the frontal mesocortex, several experiments have reported that stressors will increase the turnover of DA (Fekete et al., 1981; Tissari et al., 1979; Blanc et al., 1980; Thierry et al., 1976; Fadda et al., 1978).

Moreover, reductions of DA levels have been observed in the mesocortex (Hervé et al., 1979; Blanc et al., 1980). It has been reported (Fadda et al., 1978) that stress decreased DA levels in substantia nigra, but without an increase in the concentrations of the DA metabolite (DOPAC).

The contribution of stress controllability to the DA changes has not been examined extensively. It seems that researchers interested in determining the contribution of stress controllability have evaluated the DA alterations in fairly large tissue samples or in regions where DA concentrations are typically not altered, whereas investigators that evaluated the DA altera-tions in discrete brain regions have not considered the role of coping factors. Recently, Cherek et al. (1980) reported that in the frontal mesolimbic cortex, uncontrollable stress increased DA receptor binding relative to rats that had received controllable shock.

Exposure to aversive stimulation has reliably been shown to influence the activity of serotonin (5-HT) neurones, although it seems that the stress severity necessary to induce these changes may be greater than that required to provoke NA alterations (see Thierry, 1973). Increased synthesis and utilization of 5-HT were repeatedly shown to follow a variety of stressors (Anisman, 1982). Evaluation of whole hypothalamus, as well as several individual nuclei within this structure, indicated that 150 min of immobi-lization stress resulted in increased concentrations of 5-HT (Culman et al., 1980). Soon after exposure to more protracted stress (300 min of immobi-lization), reductions of the amine were evident in several brain regions, including cingulate cortex, median eminence, suprachiasmatic nucleus, amygdala and dorsal raphe nucleus (Palkovits et al., 1976). Within 30–90 min of stress termination, levels of 5-HT approach control values (Palkovits et al., 1976; Telgedy and Vermes, 1976). Among animals that received repeated exposure to the stressor, an increase of tryptophan hydroxylase activity was seen in the dorsal raphé nucleus, possibly in response to the amine depletion engendered by the stressor (Palkovits et al., 1976).

The data concerning the contribution of coping factors to 5-HT changes induced by stress are somewhat enigmatic. Weiss et al. (1981) reported that in the locus coeruleus, uncontrollable shock reduced 5-HT concentrations relative to that seen among non-shocked animals. In the brainstem (exclud-ing the locus coeruleus) uncontrollable shock was without effect, but controllable shock resulted in an increase in this amine. When the accumula-tion of the 5-HT metabolite, 5-hydroxyindoleacetic acid, was examined, Sherman and Petty (1980) reported that uncontrollable shock reduced the accumulation of the metabolite in hippocampus, septum and entorhinal cortex, relative to that of rats that received controllable shock or no shock, suggesting decreased utilization of serotonin. Differences in regions ex-amined between studies, as well as differences in the stress procedures employed, do not permit conclusions to be drawn concerning the differential outcomes observed. Weiss *et al.* (1981) have suggested, however, that the increased levels of 5-HT seen in brainstem of rats exposed to controllable shock may reflect amine changes in response to performing the coping response, whereas reductions of NA that occur in the inescapable group reflect the stressfulness of the procedures.

Turning briefly to the effects of variations of acetylcholine (ACh) induced by stressors, it seems that several different physical insults will increase levels of this transmitter. It has been reported that the increase of ACh is not evident until about 40 min after stress exposure, and was preceded by a reduction in levels of the transmitter (Zajaczkowska, 1975). As in the case of other transmitters, it also appears that the effectiveness of stress in modifying ACh activity varies with brain region and severity (duration) of stress application. For example, it was found that 20–25 min after cold exposure for 1 h, turnover of ACh is reduced in the frontal cortex. Following cold exposure for either 4 or 24 h, the decreased turnover was absent. In hypothalamus the reduced ACh turnover was evident after either 1 or 24 h of stress (Costa *et al.*, 1980). Limited data are available concerning the contribution of stress controllability to the ACh changes, but data from independent experiments conducted by Karczmar *et al.* (1973) suggested that the increase of ACh levels may be produced more readily among rats exposed to uncontrollable stress. Moreover, Cherek *et al.* (1980) found that uncontrollable stress was more effective in increasing muscarinic ACh receptor binding.

THE CONTRIBUTION OF ORGANISMIC AND ENVIRONMENTAL VARIABLES TO NEUROCHEMICAL CHANGES

Vulnerability to stress-induced neurochemical changes may be affected by several organismic and environmental factors. For example, it has been reported that the NA depletion induced by stress is less readily achieved among young mature rats (3 months) than among older animals (8 months). Moreover, recovery of amine levels was achieved more readily in the younger rats (Ritter and Pelzer, 1978). It also was suggested that in response to stressors, young rats rely principally on newly synthesized amines, whereas the older animals are more reliant on amines previously synthesized (Ritter and Pelzer, 1980).

As in the case of age, it has been observed that social housing conditions will influence the response to aversive stimulation. Several investigators (Modigh, 1976; Thoa *et al.*, 1977; Welch and Welch, 1970) reported that turnover of brain NA was reduced among animals housed individually relative to group-housed animals. Furthermore, it seems that reductions of NA levels can be attained more readily among individually-housed mice than in group-housed animals (Anisman and Sklar, 1981). Likewise, Blanc et al. (1980) reported that DA activity in mesofrontal cortex was reduced among mice housed individually than in group-housed mice.

Considerable evidence is also available indicating pronounced strain differences in basal levels of several transmitters, as well as neurochemical changes in response to a stressor. For instance, Wimer et al. (1974) found that stress reduced 5-HT concentrations in one strain of mouse but had little effect in a second strain, whereas NA was reduced in the second strain but not the first. Hervé et al. (1979) likewise reported that DA activity in mesocortical neurones following footshock varied considerably between strains of mice. Similarly, it has been shown that strains of rats differ in 5-HT levels and turnover following stress and these neurochemical changes may be related to the behavioural output of these animals (Ray and Barrett, 1975). Finally, Sudakov et al. (1980) reported differences in catecholamine concentration in August and Wistar rats after exposure to immobilization stress. Interestingly, within each stock of rat the catecholamine response to immobilization was related to cardiovascular responsivity and might be related to hypertension.

Thus the response to aversive stimulation will vary behaviourally and neurochemically across strains, and as such it might be expected that the pathological consequences of a stressor might likewise vary in a corresponding manner.

It should be clear from the data described thus far that stressors profoundly influence neurochemical lability. It is inappropriate, however, to consider the putative effects of aversive stimulation in a narrow context. Not only will behavioural coping influence the course of neurochemical change, but the chronicity of the stressor has profound effects as well. Moreover, vulnerability to neurochemical change is subject to age, strain and social factors. Clearly, the effects of a stressor in one subject may have somewhat different effects in a second subject. Indeed, it appears that subjects may differ appreciably with respect to the particular neurochemical most influenced by a given stressor. In attempting to extrapolate from infrahumans to humans, it will be recognized that a given stressor may be perceived or interpreted differently across individuals. Moreover, other things being equal, it might be expected that a given stressor may engender diverse neurochemical consequences across individuals. Accordingly, if one accepts that stressors may increase vulnerability to pathology owing to neurochemical change, it must likewise be assumed that a particular stressor may also have quantitatively different consequences, that might actually result in interindividual differences in the pathological state that ensues.

TIME COURSE AND SENSITIZATION

Exposure to traumatic stressors may have long-term neurochemical repercussions, in that vulnerability to later stress-provoked neurochemical
changes may be increased. Typically, the reductions of NA that occur after
stress exposure are fairly transient, persisting for a matter of only a few
hours. As seen in Fig. 3, exposure to 60 and 180 shocks (60 s duration,
150 μA) reduced NA by approximately equivalent amounts. In both
instances, concentrations of the amine approach control values with 3 h of
stress termination, but the recovery rate was somewhat slower with the
more severe stressor. Using more extensive stressors, others have found the
NA reductions to be somewhat more persistent. Weiss et al. (1981) found
that hypothalamic NA concentrations were reduced as long as 48 h after
stress exposure, while reductions in the locus coeruleus persisted for 72 h. It
should also be noted at this juncture that amine levels vary as a function of
time of day, and we have also observed that the NA reductions provoked
by a stressor are more pronounced between 08:00 and 13:00 than between
15:00 and 18:00 h (Irwin et al., 1982).

Despite the transience of the NA reductions provoked by a stressor, it
seems that a traumatic experience may result in the conditioning or
sensitization of systems governing neurochemical lability. For example,
Anisman and Sklar (1979) found that although the NA depletion was absent
24 h after exposure to 60 footshocks (see Fig. 4), re-exposure to 10 shocks, a
treatment that typically has either no effect or produces a small rise of NA
levels, effectively reinstated the amine depletion. Similarly, Cassens et al.
(1980) reported that presentation of a cue that had previously been explicitly
paired with shock increased the accumulation of MHPG, a metabolite of
NA. Evidently, re-exposure to a stressor or even cues associated with the
stressor will effectively increase the release of brain NA.

The conditioning or sensitization of neurotransmitters does not appear to
be limited to NA. Indeed, two recent reports support the supposition that
cues associated with stress will increase turnover of DA in some brain
regions (Burns et al., 1981; Herman et al., 1981). Moreover, it has been
shown that a cue explicitly paired with shock will increase ACh levels
(Hingtgen, 1976), while the stimulus complex associated with aversive
stimulation may increase endorphin activity (Chance et al., 1978).

Taken together, it appears that exposure to a stressor will have an
immediate effect on catecholamine activity, and dysfunction of adaptive
changes may contribute to pathology. In addition, it seems that application
of a traumatic stressor may increase vulnerability to later amine alterations,
and as such may also represent an important dimension in determining
vulnerability to pathology. Unfortunately, the available data concerning the

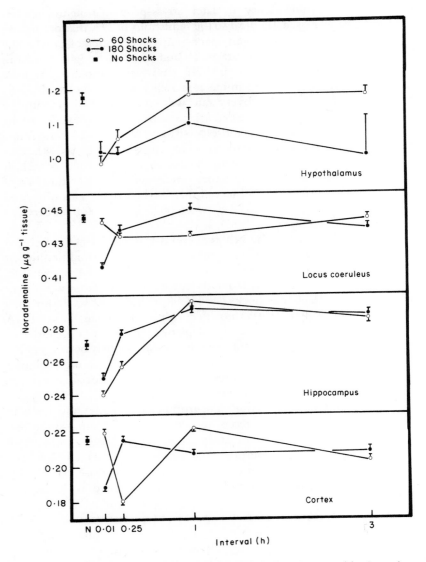

Fig. 3 Mean (± SEM) concentrations of noradrenaline in several brain regions at various intervals after exposure to 60 or 180 shocks. N denotes levels in non-shocked control animals.

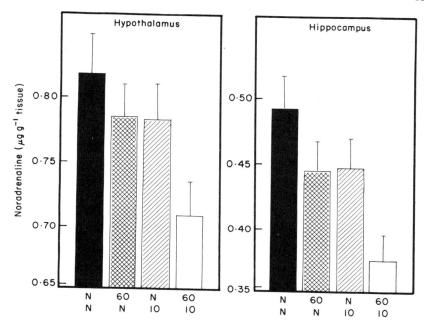

Fig. 4 Mean (± SEM) concentrations of noradrenaline in hypothalamus and in hippocampus as a function of the stress treatment mice received on two consecutive days. Mice received either no shock on each of the two days (group N/N), 60 shocks on the first day and no shock on the second day (group 60/N), no shock treatment on the first day and 10 shocks on the second day (group N/10), or 60 shocks on the first day followed by 10 shocks on the second day (group 60/10).

sensitization to stress are relatively sparse, and among other things, the time course for the sensitization effect is not known. Nevertheless, it is possible that in humans exposure to trauma will have considerable ramifications in terms of the response to later aversive experiences. In the case of affective illnesses, there is reason to suspect that early life stress increases vulnerability to illness in adulthood (Lloyd, 1980), particularly among individuals that again encounter stressful events in adulthood (Brown, 1979). It is certainly conceivable that similar processes are pertinent in the analysis of other forms of pathology.

STRESS-INDUCED NEUROENDOCRINE CHANGE

There is a great deal of evidence indicating that the secretion of pituitary hormones may be determined by variations in hypothalamic amine activity (see reviews in Guillemin, 1978; Ganong, 1980; Terry and Martin, 1978; Van Loon, 1976). It is not surprising, therefore, that stress will alter hormonal release and influence serum steroid concentrations (Yuwiler, 1976). Several forms of stress were shown to increase secretion of adreno-corticotrophic hormone (ACTH) and to increase the concentration of plasma corticosterone (e.g. Bassett and Cairncross, 1975; Coover et al., 1973; Keim and Sigg, 1976; Rossier et al., 1977). Similarly, stressors have been shown to increase release of thyrotropin and thyroid hormone (Martin and Reichlin, 1970; Taché et al., 1978), as well as prolactin (McCann et al., 1978) and β-endorphin (Rossier et al., 1977). Finally, it is well established that physical insults will increase the synthesis and release of peripheral adrenaline and noradrenaline (Kvetnansky and Mikulaj, 1970; Kvetnansky, 1980; Kopin et al., 1980; McCarty et al., 1978).

As in the case of the neurochemical consequences of stressors, hormonal changes vary as a function of stress chronicity. The increases of corticoster-oids, ACTH and β-endorphin ordinarily provoked by acute stress were diminished among animals that received repeated stress exposure (Feldman and Brown, 1976; Keim and Sigg, 1976; Kvetnansky, 1980; Mikulaj et al., 1976; Taché et al., 1978). Similar effects have been seen in the case of secretion of growth hormone and thyrotropic hormone (Martin, 1974). To some extent, it seems that coping factors also contribute to the extent of hormonal change. Although controllable and uncontrollable shock were both found to increase serum corticosterone, the extent of the increase was greater following uncontrollable shock (Weiss, 1971).

STRESS-INDUCED IMMUNOLOGICAL CHANGE

It has become increasingly more apparent that alterations of central nervous system functioning will come to influence immunological activity. For example, it has been reported that lesions of the anterior hypothalamus will inhibit both B- and T-lymphocyte activity (Stein et al., 1976, 1981). It was reported (Macris et al., 1970) that anterior hypothalamic lesions were associated with reduced antibody titres to the hapten, picrylchloride, whereas lesions to other portions of the hypothalamus were without effect. Similarly, depression of ovalbumin production was observed in rats after anterior hypothalamic lesions (Tyrey and Nalvandov, 1972). As in the case of humoural immunity, there is evidence that cell-mediated immunity is modifiable by hypothalamic manipulations (see Solomon and Amkraut, 1981; Spector and Korneva, 1981; Stein et al., 1981). For instance, it has been shown that anterior hypothalamic lesions will depress lymphocyte stimulation by phytohaemaglutinin (Keller *et al.*, 1980), as well as modifying delayed hypersensitivity to an antigen (see Stein *et al.*, 1981).

Substantial evidence is available indicating that hormonal variations will profoundly influence immunological functioning (see MacLean and Reichlin, 1981; Besedovsky and Sorkin, 1981; Rogers *et al.*, 1979). It is known, for instance, that corticosteroids will result in immunosuppression (Balow and Rosenthal, 1973; Riley, 1981), and several hormones have been shown to influence intracellular nucleotides (cAMP and cGMP), which have been reported to affect antibody formation, cellular immunity and phagocytosis (see discussion in Besedovsky and Sorkin, 1981). Moreover, receptors for corticosteroids, growth hormone, oestradiol, testosterone and β-endorphin have been found to be present in lymphoid cells (Cake and Litwak, 1975; Werb *et al.*, 1978; Arrenbrecht, 1974; Gillette and Gillette, 1979; Abraham and Bug, 1976; Hazum *et al.*, 1979). Finally, in their review of the literature, Besedovsky and Sorkin (1981), as well as Hall and Goldstein (1981), indicated in some detail that peripheral neurochemical modification will modify immune responsivity.

Inasmuch as hormonal changes influence immune responsivity, and hormonal secretion is itself regulated by central neurotransmitters, it is not surprising that neurochemical manipulations will influence immunological activity. It has been reported that treatments that result in 5-HT stimulation depressed the immune response (Bliznakov, 1980; Idova and Devoino, 1972), whereas reductions of 5-HT enhanced antibody production (Eremina and Devoino, 1973; Segall and Timiras, 1976). Depletion of catecholamines has been found provoke immunosuppression (Dukor *et al.*, 1966), whereas DA receptor stimulation produced augmented immune functioning (Cotzias and Tang, 1977; Tang *et al.*, 1974).

Just as manipulation of central neurotransmitter functioning may affect immunological activity, it appears that altering immune activity will affect central nervous system functioning. It has been reported that the presence of an antigen was associated with a substantial increase in the activity of neurones in the ventromedial hypothalamus (Besedovsky *et al.*, 1977; see also Besedosky and Sorkin, 1981). Likewise, reduction of hypothalamic NA was found to be associated with the latent phase of antibody production (Vekshina and Magaeva, 1974). These data are consistent with the proposition that hypothalmic functioning is integrally related with immunological activity. Of course, this relationship cannot be taken as a causal one simply on the basis of the aforementioned data.

Several sources of evidence have indicated that stressful events may influence immunological functioning, and might thus lead to provocation or exacerbation of pathological states. Several papers have summarized this literature recently, and consequently only a very abbreviated review will be presented here (Monjan, 1981; Palmblad, 1981; Sklar and Anisman, 1981; Solomon and Amkraut, 1979; Riley et al., 1979, 1981). Exposure to physical or psychological insults have been shown to increase the response to virus challenge such as herpes simplex (Rasmussen et al., 1957), poliomyelitis (Teodoro and Schwartzman, 1956; Johnsson and Rasmussen, 1965), vesicular stomatitis (Jensen and Rasmussen, 1963), trincella spirals (Davis and Read, 1958), rabies (Soave, 1964) and coxsackie B-2 (Friedman et al., 1965; Johnsson et al., 1963). Consistent with the proposition that stressors may decrease immunoreactivity, it was reported that aversive physical stimulation in the form of avoidance training increased resistance to passive anaphylaxis, an acute hypersensitivity reaction (Rasmussen et al., 1959; Treadwell et al., 1959; Jensen and Rasmussen, 1963). Overcrowding reduced the antibody response to salmonella flagellin (Solomon, 1969) and reduced granuloma formation to subcutaneously implanted cotton pellets (Christian and Williamson, 1958). Trauma in the form of burns depressed graft-versus-host response, enhanced tumour growth (Munster et al., 1972, 1977) and increased susceptibility to mortality following pseudomonas infection (McEuen et al., 1976). Likewise, stress associated with surgery was found to reduce intravasculaphagocytosis (Saba and DiLuzio, 1969). Recently, Toge et al. (1981) also reported that surgical stress not only resulted in depression of the proliferative response to phytohaemagglutinin, but also provoked depression of natural killer cell activity. Indeed, such an effect was evident as long as 7 days following laparothoracotomy.

As might be expected, exposure to uncontrollable shock, as well as stressors related to housing conditions or shipment of animals, was found to reduce blood lymphocyte levels (Nieburgs et al., 1979), decrease immune reactivity of peritoneal and spleen B-cells (Gisler et al., 1971) and suppress antibody and T-cell functioning (Folch and Waksman, 1974; Lundy et al., 1979). More recently, Keller et al. (1981) reported that a series of graded stressors provoked a progressive increase in the suppression of lymphocyte function as indicated by the number of circulating lymphocytes and phytohaemagglutinin stimulation of lymphocytes.

The alterations of immune functioning engendered by stressors appear to be dependent on the chronicity of the stress regimen employed. The studies mentioned in the preceding paragraphs uniformly indicate that stress acutely applied will provoke immunosuppression. However, when administered chronically, some of these stressors have been shown to either leave immune functioning relatively unimpaired or may even lead to immunofacilitation (see Monjan, 1981). For instance, Amkraut and Solomon (1972) found that footshock applied for 3 days prior to injection of Moloney murine sarcoma virus provoked immunofacilitation, whereas stress application after virus inoculation provoked immunosuppression. Moreover,

Solomon and Amkraut (1979) reported that interferon production was enhanced if subjects were stressed prior to virus inoculation. In a similar fashion, Monjan and Collector (1977) reported that within the first 2 weeks of repeated stress application (noise for 3 h day^{-1}) immunological functioning was depressed; however, by 3 weeks enhancement of immune functioning was evident.

The background conditions on which a stressor is applied appears to be an important determinant of the extent of immunological change. Monjan (1981) reported that retro-orbital bleeding had profound effects on lymphocytes in culture (Splenic removal occurred within 3 min of bleeding). A more pronounced and longer lasting effect was evident among mice that had undergone up to 8 days of sound stress. Beyond 8 days, however, the lymphocyte activity was decreased. In a similar fashion, Riley and his associates (Riley et al., 1981; Riley and Spackman, 1977) found that corticosterone levels and incidence of mammary tumours were dependent on housing conditions, and the effects of a stressor on tumour growth may be altered by the conditions under which mice had been housed. Likewise, Sklar and Anisman (1980) found that inescapable shock may differentially influence the size of tumours among mice housed individually and in small groups. It seems, in fact, that even the stress of transporting animals from the breeders may affect lymphocyte activity, and may alter the immune response to experimental stressors (Nieburgs et al., 1979).

A particularly interesting aspect of immune system functioning was noted in a series of studies conducted by Ader and his associates (see Ader and Cohen 1975, 1981; Wayner et al., 1978). These investigators demonstrated that, if animals were permitted to consume a saccharine solution followed by administration of the immunosuppressant, cyclophosphamide, re-exposure to the saccharine solution resulted in diminished antibody response to sheep red blood cells. In effect, pairing a stimulus with an immunosuppressive treatment provoked a (conditioned) depression of the immune response. Moreover, it does not appear to be the case that the conditioning effects were secondary to alterations of plasma steroids (see Ader and Cohen, 1981). In accordance with the results reported by Ader and Cohen, it was reported (Bovbjerg et al., 1980) that a cellular immune response was conditionable. It was found that multiple (3) doses of cyclophosphamide was effective in suppressing a graft-vs-host response. As might have been expected, a suppressant effect almost as great was observed when the conditioned stimulus (saccharine) was substituted for the cyclophosphamide injection on the three days after cellular graft.

As in studies involving infrahuman subjects, it appears that aversive events may influence immune functioning in humans (see Palmblad, 1981). Depressed lymphocyte functioning was found to be associated with bereavement (Bartrop *et al.*, 1977; Pees, 1977). Likewise, Locke *et al.* (1978) found that natural killer cell activity varied as a function of the interaction between life changes and self-reported psychiatric symptoms. Further, Nieburgs *et al.* (1979) reported a change in the percentage of small and large lymphocytes among patients awaiting bronchoscopy, possibly reflecting the emotional stress in anticipation of this procedure. Finally, in a series of experiments, Palmblad and associates (1976, 1979a, 1979b) found that stress of sleep deprivation initially reduced lymphocyte and granulocyte function, and was followed by an increase of interferon production. Taken together, these data suggest that stressors will induce reduction of lymphocyte activity in humans, although increased immune functioning may be expected soon after the stress. Whether the varied immunological changes are secondary to neurotransmitter and hormonal alterations remains to be fully determined.

STRESS AND CANCER

A number of reports involving human and infrahuman subjects, have evaluated the relationship between stressful events and the occurrence of neoplastic disease. While suggestive of such a relationship, the human studies can be considered as only highly provisional and are subject to alternative interpretations (see critique in Fox, 1978). Nonetheless, there appears to be reason to believe that stressful events and the individual's ability to cope with the stress effectively may be fundamental to the incidence or course of the disease (Sklar and Anisman 1981a and Chapter 11 by Grossarth-Maticek and colleagues).

Studies involving infrahuman subjects indicated that physical and psychological insults may influence tumour development; however, results between laboratories have not been uniformly consistent. Among other things, researchers have assessed different tumour systems, stressors that differ qualitatively and quantitatively and in time of application, and have used either acute or chronic regimens. As a result, it is often difficult to determine the source for between-laboratory differences that have been reported (see Sklar and Anisman, 1981a; Riley, 1979). However, it seems that some of variables that contribute to the effects of stress on tumour development can be identified. For example, stress controllability and chronicity, as well as the organism's social history appear to be critical factors in governing the nature of the tumour changes that occur.

In studies involving carcinogen-induced tumours, a considerable period of time may elapse between neoplastic cell transformation and detection of the tumour. As a result, it is difficult to identify the time period that might be most sensitive to the potential influence of a stressor. Accordingly, it is not surprising that researchers have tended to employ procedures in which animals are repeatedly exposed to a stressor. Experiments which employed repeated application of restraint, footshock, electroconvulsive shock and sound stress indicated reduced incidence of mammary tumours induced by 7,12,dimethylbenz(a)anthracene (DMBA) (Newberry et al., 1976; Pradham and Ray, 1974; Ray and Pradham, 1974). Although comparisons have not been conducted of the effects of single vs. multiple stress sessions, Nieburgs et al. (1979) reported that stress applied over 90 days (5 min stress at 96 h intervals) increased the number of tumours, whereas 150 days of the stress regimen reduced both the size and number of tumours.

The timing of stress application, like the chronicity, appears to be an essential variable in determining tumour development, just as it was fundamental in determining immunological change. Newberry (1978) found stress to inhibit tumour development when applied after DMBA administration, but had little effect if applied prior to or during carcinogen treatment. Similar effects were found concerning the effects of cold exposure on radiation-induced tumours (Baker and Jahn, 1976). It appears that a critical period exists, during which chronic application of stress will inhibit tumour incidence. Indeed, it was suggested that stress application reduced cell proliferation rates but did not influence the initial neoplastic change (Newberry, 1978; Newberry and Sengbusch, 1979).

It is not clear what mechanisms are operative in determining the tumour inhibition. On the one hand, reductions of food intake during repeated stress may be fundamental to the tumour changes, while on the other hand, increases in the rate of neurotransmitter turnover in either the central or peripheral nervous system directly or indirectly may be responsible for the inhibition. Likewise, it is possible that chronicity or timing of the stressor affected a critical developmental phase of the tumour (e.g. angiogenesis), thus altering the course of development.

In contrast to carconigen-induced tumours, the effects of both acute and chronic stress were evaluated on the development of viral-induced and transplanted tumours. Such studies revealed that acute stress may increase the development of tumours, as well as increase the incidence of tumours in mice that received a Take-Dose$_{50}$, i.e., where 50% of subjects develop a tumour (Amkraut and Solomon 1972; Jamasbi and Netesheim 1977; Peters 1975; Peters and Kelly 1977; Sklar and Anisman 1979, 1980). It was suggested (Riley et al., 1981) that acute stress will only enhance tumours that are ordinarily under partial or total control of the T- and B-immune systems. That is, stress is thought to release the tumour from the inhibiting influence of the immune system owing to the immunosuppression induced by stress provoked corticosterone release. Indeed, it was demonstrated that rotational stress enhanced the growth of a lymphosarcoma in a C3H substrain of mice where the tumour and host were non-histocompatible, but had little effect where they were histocompatible. Moreover, within a single strain of mice, exposure to LDH virus accelerated the development of a non-pigmented melanoma (see Riley et al., 1981). While these results are consistent with the interpretation offered by Riley, it should be considered that factors other than histocompatibility may be responsible for the observed outcome. For instance, different strains may have responded differently to the stressor in terms of emotionality, as well as neurochemically. Furthermore, the rate of development of the pigmented and non-pigmented tumours differed even in the absence of stress, and the effects of the stressor may have been obscured in the more rapidly developing line.

There is, in fact, some evidence suggesting that the effects of stress on tumour growth might not be related either to corticoid changes or variations in the immune response. Several of the previously mentioned studies showing stress-provoked tumour enhancement involved transplantation of non-immunogenic cells synegeic with the host animals (transplants between genetically identical organisms), suggesting that alterations of the T- and B-lymphocyte immune systems were not responsible for the stress effects. Furthermore, irradiation stress was found to enhance TD_{50} provided that the treatments were applied within 24 h of one another, despite the fact that the immunosuppressive effects of irradiation persisted for as long as 2 weeks. Furthermore, the stress-provoked enhancement of TD_{50} was not influenced by immunologic reconstitution of syngeneic spleen cells (Jamasbi and Nettesheim, 1977). It was also shown (Peters and Kelly, 1977) that the effect of surgical stress on tumour growth was not affected by adrenalectomy, although ACTH or dexamethasone treatment did influence tumour development.

In addition to modifying the development of transplanted cells, it should be added as well that stressors have been shown to influence tumour metastasis. Not only will stressors increase the TD_{50}, but they will increase the incidence of liver and pulmonary tumours following intravenous injections of malignant cells (Fisher and Fisher, 1959; Saba and Antikatzides, 1976; Van Der Brenk et al., 1976). The incidence of tumours was increased by irradiation stress, even after injection of a single lymphosarcoma cell (Maruyama and Johnson, 1969). Moreover, using spontaneously metastasizing tumour, Lundy et al. (1979) found that surgical stress increased the frequency of metastases.

Consistent with human experiments, there is reason to believe that psychological variables may influence tumour development. For instance, Kavetsky et al. (1966) found that the application of chronic signalled shock increased rather than inhibited spontaneous tumours in C3H/A mice and

DMBA tumours in rats. A similar, although not statistically significant effect, was also observed by Newberry *et al.* (1972). Inasmuch as stress predictability is a cogent variable in determining the aversiveness of the stimulus, it is not surprising that such a variable would influence tumour growth.

A series of experiments conducted in our laboratory revealed that the animals' ability to cope behaviourally with a stressor may appreciably influence tumour development. When animals were exposed to 60 escapable shocks 24 h after transplantation of P815 cells, no enhancement of tumour size was evident relative to non-shocked mice. As seen in Fig. 5, an identical amount of inescapable shock applied in a yoked paradigm resulted in an enhancement of tumour size (see Sklar and Anisman, 1979; Sklar *et al.*, 1981). It seems that the shock *per se* was not responsible for the tumour enhancement, but rather not having control over shock was associated with the tumour change. It will be recalled that the noradrenaline depletion was also seen exclusively after uncontrollable stress. Of course, this does not necessarily imply a causal relationship; however, this possibility needs to be considered.

As observed in the case of carcinogen-induced tumours, chronic exposure to a stressor will have an inhibitory effect on the development of trans-planted and virus-induced tumours. As seen in Fig. 5, the tumour enhance-ment seen after a single session of uncontrollable shock is absent after 5 or 10 sessions. Sklar *et al.* (1981), in fact, found that the enhanced tumour development ordinarily evident after a single session of inescapable shock was absent after repeated exposure, regardless of whether the chronic stressor was applied prior to or after cell transplantation. Other investiga-tors likewise reported chronic stress to produce inhibition of several different types of neoplasia, including L1210 leukaemia, Ehrlich carcinoma, 256-Walker carcinosarcoma and 4-M carcinoma (Gershben *et al.*, 1974; Pradham and Ray, 1974).

Social stressors, like psychological stressors, will influence tumour growth. Chronic isolation (Andervont, 1944; DeChambre and Gosse, 1973) and social disruption (Henry *et al.*, 1975) were found to increase the incidence of spontaneously occurring tumours. In immature animals, handling and intermittent separation inhibited (Ader and Friedman, 1965; LaBarba and White, 1971) or exacerbated (Ader and Friedman, 1965; Levine and Cohen, 1959) tumour growth. It is likely that in the case of the latter studies the developmental period during which the stress was applied was critical in determining the nature of the change which occurred. It might also be noted that social factors may influence the effects of other stressors on tumour growth, and vice versa. For instance, although both isolation and shock stress enhance growth of a P815 mastocytoma, the combination

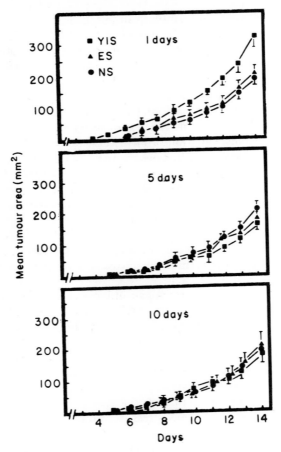

Fig. 5 Mean (± SEM) tumour size among mice that received no shock (NS), 60 escapable shocks per day (ES) or yoked inescapable shock (YIS). Independent groups of mice received either a single stress session 24 h after tumour cell transplantation, 5 such sessions, or 10 sessions on successive days commencing 24 h after cell transplantation (from Sklar *et al.*, 1981, with permission).

of treatments results in tumour inhibition (Sklar and Anisman, 1980). It will be recalled that the combination of stress treatments will also eliminate the immunosuppressant effects of either treatment alone.

Aggressive behaviour, it seems, will also modify the course of tumour growth. Both DeChambre and Gosse (1973) and Sklar and Anisman (1980) found that changes in social condition will enhance tumour growth. Sklar and Anisman (1980), however, found that when mice were transferred from individual to group housing conditions, the tumour enhancement was not evident among mice that engaged in fighting. Similarly, Amkraut and Solomon (1972) found increased resistance to Moloney-murine sarcoma virus among animals that engaged in fighting. As discussed earlier, fighting might possibly act as a coping response to stresses associated with the environmental conditions.

CONCLUSIONS

Exposure to aversive stimuli will profoundly influence central and peripheral neurochemical activity, hormonal secretion and immunological functioning. Factors such as stress controllability and chronicity, as well as social conditions, largely determine the nature and extent of the neurochemical changes. Similarly, it seems that stressful events will influence the development of several forms of tumours. Moreover, some of the same variables that modify central neurochemical activity also influence the variations in tumour development. Indeed, it does seem that manipulations of central nervous system neurotransmitters, particularly in hypothalamus, will affect immunological functioning. Thus, it has been our contention (Sklar and Anisman, 1981b) that the effects of physical and psychological insults on neoplasia may be directly or indirectly influenced by the effects of the insults on central neurotransmitters.

In accordance with the aforementioned hypothesis, it has been demonstrated that catecholamine stimulants will inhibit development of transplanted and carcinogen-induced tumours (Driscoll et al., 1978; Quadri et al., 1973a; Wick 1977, 1978a,b, 1979), whereas catecholamine antagonists will have an opposite effect (Lacassagne and Duplan, 1959; Lapin, 1978; Quadri et al., 1973b; Sklar and Anisman, 1981b; Welsch and Meites, 1970). Of course, mechanisms other than neurochemical–immunological interactions might be responsible for the observed effects. Wick (1979), for example, argued that the effects of the catecholamine stimulant, L-DOPA, on tumour development was due to inhibition of enzymes associated with DNA synthesis. Furthermore, in considering the nature of the immunological consequences of stressors, it is not necessarily the case that T- and B-lymphocytes govern the course of tumour development. Given that macrophages and natural killer cells may be fundamental to the host defence against neoplasia (see review in Herberman and Ortaldo, 1981), effects of aversive events on these mechanisms (Pavlidis and Chirigos, 1980; Toge et al., 1981) might be responsible for the alterations in tumour growth that occur after stress exposure. Finally, it is certainly possible that metabolic changes induced by stressors affect the course of neoplasia.

Clearly, considerable research will be necessary to identify the conditions and mechanisms associated with stress related pathology. It seems fairly certain that a more comprehensive understanding of the processes that increase vulnerability to illness as well as its prognosis requires that greater attention be devoted to the role of psychological factors on neurochemical and immunological processes.

ACKNOWLEDGEMENTS

Supported by Grants A9845 and MT6486 from the Natural Sciences and Engineering Research Council and the Medical Research Council of Canada. We are indebted to R. Zacharko, Angela Corradini, Wayne Bowers, Jill Irwin, Venera Bruto and Christine Beauchamp for their assistance and comments.

REFERENCES

Abraham, A. D. and Bug, G. (1976). H-testosterone distribution and binding in rat thymus cells *in vivo*. *Mol. Cell. Biochem.* **13**, 157–163.

Ader, R. (1981). "Psychoneuroimmunology." Academic Press, Orlando, New York and London.

Ader, R. and Cohen, N. (1975). Behaviorally conditioned immunosuppression. *Psychosom. Med.* **37**, 333–340.

Ader, R. and Cohen, N. (1981). Conditioned immunopharmacologic response. *In* "Psychoneuroimmunology" (R. Ader, ed.), pp. 281–319. Academic Press, Orlando, New York and London.

Ader, R. and Friedman, S. B. (1965). Differential early experiences and susceptibility to transplanted tumor in the rat. *J. Comp. Physiol. Psychol.* **59**, 361–364.

Amkraut, A. and Solomon, G. F. (1972). Stress and murine sarcoma virus (maloney) induced tumors. *Cancer Res.* **32**, 1428–1433.

Andervont, E. B. (1944). Influence of environment on mammary cancer in mice. *J. Nat. Cancer Inst.* **4**, 579–591.

Anisman, H. (1978). Neurochemical changes elicited by stress. *In* "Psychopharmacology of aversively motivated behavior" (H. Anisman and G. Bignami, eds), pp. 119–172. Plenum Press, New York.

Anisman, H. (1983). Vulnerability to depression. *In* "Neurobiology of Mood Disorders" (R. M. Post and J. C. Ballenger, eds), pp. 1063–1112. Williams and Wilkins, Baltimore.

Anisman, H. and Sklar, L. S. (1979). Catecholamine depletion in mice upon re-exposure to stress: Mediation of the escape deficits produced by inescapable shock. *J. Comp. Physiol. Psychol.* **93**, 610–625.

Anisman, H. and Sklar, L. S. (1981). Social housing conditions influence escape deficits produced by uncontrollable stress: Assessment of the contribution of norepinephrine. *Behav. Neur. Biol.* **32**, 406–427.

Anisman, H. and Zacharko, R. M. (1982). Depression: The predisposing influence of stress. *Behav. Brain Sci.* **5**, 89–137.

Anisman, H., Pizzino, A. and Sklar, L. S. (1980). Coping with stress, norepinephrine depletion and escape performance. *Brain Res.* **191**, 583–588.

Arrenbrecht, S. (1974). Specific binding of growth hormone to thymocytes. *Nature,* **252**, 255–257.

Baker, D. G. and Jahn, A. (1976). The influence of a chronic environment stress on radiation carcinogenesis. *Rad. Res.* **68**, 449–458.

Balow, J. E. and Rosenthal, A. S. (1973). Glucocorticoid suppression of macrophage migration inhibiting factor. *J. Exp. Med.* **137**, 1031–1041.

Bartrop, R. W., Lazarus, L., Luckhurst, E., Kiloh, L. G. and Penny, R. (1977). Depressed lymphocyte function after bereavement. *Lancet* **i**, 834–836.

Bassett, J. R. and Cairncross, K. D. (1975). Time course for plasma 11-hydrocorticosteroid elevations in rats during stress. *Pharm. Biochem. Behav.* **3**, 139–142.

Besedovsky, H. O. and Sorkin, E. (1981). Immunologic-neuroendocrine circuits: Physiological approaches. *In* "Psychoneuroimmunology" (R. Ader, ed.), pp. 281–319. Academic Press, Orlando, New York and London.

Besedovsky, H. O., Sorkin, E., Felix, D. and Haas, H. (1977). Hypothalamic changes during the immune response. *Eur. J. Immunol.* **7**, 325–328.

Blanc, G., Hervé, D., Simon, H., Lisporawski, A., Glowinski, J. and Tassin, J. P. (1980). Response to stress of mesocortico-frontal dopaminergic neurones in rats after long-term isolation. *Nature* **284**, 265–267.

Bliznakov, E. G. (1980). Serotonin and its precursors as modulators of the immunological responsiveness in mice. *J. Med.* **11**, 81–105.

Bovbjerg, E. H., Cohen, N. and Ader, R. (1980). Conditioned suppression of a cellular immune response. *Psychosom. Med.* **42**, 73.

Bowers, W. J., Beauchamp, D., Irwin, P. J., Zacharko, R. M. and Anisman, H. (1982). Behavioral and neurochemical consequences of acute and chronic stress. Paper presented at the meeting of the Canadian Psychological Association, Montreal.

Brown, G. W. (1979). The social etiology of depression—London studies. *In* "The Psychobiology of Depressive Disorders" (R. A. Depue, ed.), pp. 263–289. Academic Press, Orlando. New York and London.

Burns, P. K., Sands, M. P., Cherek, D. R., Smith, J. E. and Lane, J. D. (1981). Monoamine changes following conditioned emotional response. *Soc. Neurosci. Abstr.* **7**, 155.

Cake, M. H. and Litwack, G. (1975). The glucocorticoid receptors. *In* "Biochemical Actions of Hormones" (G. Litwack, ed.), Vol. 3, pp. 317–390. Academic Press, Orlando, New York and London.

Cassens, G., Roffman, M., Kuruc A., Orsulak, P. J. and Schildkraut, J. J. (1980). Alterations in brain norepinephrine metabolism induced by environmental stimuli previously paired with inescapable shock. *Science* **209**, 1138–1140.

Chance, W. T., White, A. C., Krynock, G. M. and Rosecrans, J. A. (1978). Conditional fear-induced antinociception and decreased binding of [³H]N-Leu-enkephalin to rat brain. *Brain Res.* **141**, 371–374.

Cherek, D. R., Lane, J. D., Freeman, M. E. and Smith, J. E. (1980). Receptor changes following shock avoidance. *Soc. Neurosci. Abstr.* **6**, 543.

Christian, J. J. and Williamson, H. O. (1958). Effect of crowding on experimental granuloma formation in mice. *Proc. Soc. Exp. Biol. Med.* **99**, 385–387.

Coover, G. D., Ursin, H. and Levine, S. (1973). Plasma corticosterone levels during active avoidance learning in rats. *J. Comp. Physiol. Psychol.* **82**, 170–174.

Costa, E., Tagliomonte, A., Brunello, N. and Cheney D. L. (1980). Effect of stress on the metabolism of acetylcholine in the cholinergic pathways of extrapyramidal and limbic systems. *In* "Catecholamines and Stress: Recent Advances" (E. Usdin, R. Kvetnansky and I. J. Kopin, eds), pp. 59–68. Elsevier, New York.

Cotzias, G. C. and Tang, L. (1977). An adenylate cyclase of brain reflects propensity for breast cancer in mice. *Science* **197**, 1094–1096.

Culman, J., Kvetnansky, R., Kiss, A., Mezey, E. and Murgas, K. (1980). Interacting serotonin and catecholamines in individual brain nuclei in adrenocortical activity regulation during stress. *In* "Catecholamines and stress: Recent advances" (E. Usdin, R. Kvetnansky and I. J. Kopin, eds), pp. 69–74. Elsevier, New York.

Davis, D. E. and Read, C. P. (1958). Effect of behavior on development of resistance in trichionosis. *Proc. Soc. Exp. Biol. Med.* **99**, 269–272.

DeChambre, R. P. and Gosse, C. (1973). Individual versus group caging of mice with grafted tumors. *Cancer Res.* **33**, 140–144.

Depue, R. A., Monroe, S. M. and Shackman, S. L. (1979). The psychobiology of human disease: Implications for conceptualizing the depressive disorders. *In* "The Psychobiology of the Depressive Disorders" (R. A. Depue, ed.), pp. 3–20. Academic Press, Orlando, New York and London.

Driscoll, J. S., Melnick, N. R., Quinn, F. R., Davignon, J. P., Ing, R., Abbott, B. J., Congleton, G. and Dudeck, L. (1978). Psychotropic drugs as potential antitumor agents: A selective screening study. *Cancer Treat. Rep.* **62**, 45–73.

Dukor, P., Salvin, S. B., Dietrich, F. M., Glezer, J., Hess, R. and Loustalot, P. (1966). Effect of reserpine on immune reactions and tumor growth. *Eur. J. Cancer* **2**, 253–261.

Eremina, O. F. and Devoino, L. V. (1973). Production of humoral antibodies in rabbits with destruction of the nucleus of the midbrain raphe. *Bull. Exp. Biol. Med.* **75**, 149–151.

Fadda, F., Argiolas, A., Melis, M. R., Tissari, A. H., Onali, P. L. and Gessa, G. L. (1978). Stress-induced increase in 3,4-dihydroxyphenylacetic acid (DOPAC) levels in the cerebral cortex and in nucleus accumbens: Reversal by diazepam. *Life Sci.* **23**, 2219–2224.

Fekete, M. I. K., Szentendrei, T., Kanyicska, B. and Palkovits, M. (1981). Effects of anxiolytic drugs on the catecholamine and DOPAC (3,4-dihydroxyphenylacetic acid) levels in brain cortical areas and on corticosterone and prolactin secretion in rats subjected to stress. *Psychoneuroendocrinology* **6**, 113–120.

Feldman, J. and Brown, G. M. (1976). Endocrine responses to electric shock and avoidance conditioning in the rhesus monkey: Cortisol and growth hormone. *Psychoneuroendocrinology* **1**, 231–242.

Fisher, B. and Fisher, E. R. (1959). Experimental studies of factors influencing hepatic metastases: II. Effect of partial hepatectomy. *Cancer* **12**, 929–932.

Folch, H. and Waksman, B. H. (1974). The splenic suppressor cell: I. Activity of thymus-dependent adherent cells. Changes with age and stress. *J. Immunol.* **113**, 127–137.

Fox, B. H. (1978). Premorbid psychological factors as related to cancer incidence. *J. Behav. Med.* **1**, 45–133.

Friedman, S. B., Ader, R. and Glasgow, L. A. (1965). Effects of psychological stress in adult mice inoculated with Coxsackie B virus. *Psychosom. Med.* **27**, 361–368.

Ganong, W. F. (1980). Participation of brain monoamines in the regulation of neuroendocrine activity under stress. *In* "Catecholamines and Stress: Recent

Advances" (E. Usdin, R. Kvetnansky and I. J. Kopin, eds), pp. 115–124. Elsevier, New York.

Gershben, L. L., Benuck, I. and Shurrager, P. S. (1974). Influence of stress on lesion growth and on survival of animals bearing parenteral and intracerebral leukemia L1210 and Walker tumors. *Oncology* **30**, 429–435.

Gillette, S. & Gillette, R. W. (1979). Changes in thymic estrogen receptor expression following orchidectomy. *Cell. Immunol.* **42**, 194–196.

Gisler, R. H., Bussard, A. E., Mazie, J. C. and Hess, R. (1971). Hormonal regulation of the immune response: I. Induction of an immune response *in vitro* with lymphoid cells from mice exposed to acute systemic stress. *Cell. Immunol.* **2**, 634–645.

Guillemin, R. (1978). Peptides in the brain: The new endocrinology of the neuron. *Science* **202**, 390–402.

Hall, N. R. and Goldstein, A. L. (1981). Neurotransmitters and the immune system. *In* "Psychoneuroimmunology" (R. Ader, ed.), pp. 521–543. Academic Press, Orlando, New York and London.

Hazum, E., Chang, K. J. and Cuatrecases, P. (1979). Specific non-opiate receptors for β-endorphin. *Science* **205**, 1033–1035.

Henry, J. P., Stephens, P. M. and Watson, F. M. C. (1975). Force breeding, social disorder and mammary tumor formation in CBA/USC mouse colonies: A pilot study. *Psychosom. Med.* **37**, 277–283.

Herberman, R. B. and Ortaldo, J. R. (1981). Natural killer cells: Their role in defenses against disease. *Science* **214**, 24–30.

Herman, J. P., Guillonneau, D., Dantzer, R., Mormède, P., Simon, H. and LeMoal, M. (1981). Differential activation of limbic and cortical dopaminergic systems to stress and anticipation of stress. *Soc. Neurosci. Abstr.* **7**, 155.

Hervé, D., Tassin, P., Barthelemy, C., Blanc, G., Lavielle, S. and Glowinski, J. (1979). Differences in the reactivity of the mesocortical dopaminergic neurones to stress in the Balb/c and C57 BL/6 mice. *Life Sci.* **25**, 1659–1664.

Hingtgen, J. N., Smith, J. E., Shea, P. A., Aprison, M. H. and Gaff, T. M. (1976). Chronic changes during conditioned suppression in rats. *Science* **193**, 332–334.

Idova, G. V. and Devoino, L. V. (1972). Dynamics of formation of VM- and V6-antibodies in mice after administration of serotonin and its precursor 5-hydroxytryptophan. *Bull. Exp. Biol. Med.* (Engl. trans.) **73**, 294–296.

Irwin, J., Beauchamp, C., Bowers, W., Zacharko, R. M. and Anisman, H. (1982). Cross-stressor effects of uncontrollable shock: Escape performance and norepinephrine concentration. Paper presented at the Meeting of the Canadian Psychological Association, Montreal.

Jamasbi, R. J. and Nettesheim, P. (1977). Non-immunological enhancement of tumor transplantability in x-irradiated host animals. *Br. J. Cancer* **36** 723–729.

Jensen, M. M. and Rasmussen, A. F., Jr. (1963). Stress and susceptibility to viral infection. I. Response of adrenals, liver, thymus, spleen and peripheral leukocyte counts to sound stress. *J. Immunol.* **90**, 17–20.

Johnsson, T. and Rasmussen, A. F., Jr. (1965). Emotional stress and susceptibility to poliomyelitis virus infection in mice. *Arch. Gesmate Virusforsch* **18**, 393–396.

Johnsson, T., Lavender, J. F., Hultin, E. and Rasmussen, A. F. (1963). The influence of avoidance-learning stress on resistance to Coxsackie B virus in mice. *J. Immunol.* **91**, 569–575.

Karczmar, A. G., Scudder, C. L. and Richardson, D. L. (1973). Interdisciplinary approach to the study of behavior in related mice types. *In* "Chemical Approaches to Brain Function" (S. Ehrenpreis and I. J. Kopin, eds). Academic Press, Orlando, New York and London.

Kavetsky, R. E., Turkevich, N. M. and Balitsky, K. P. (1966). On the psychophysiological mechanism of the organism's resistance to tumor growth. *Ann. N.Y. Acad. Sci.* **125**, 933–945.

Keim, K. L. and Sigg, E. B. (1976). Physiological and biochemical concomitants of restraint stress in rats. *Pharmacol. Biochem. Behav.* **4**, 289–297.

Keller, S. E., Weiss, J. M., Schleifer, S. J., Miller, N. E. and Stein, M. (1980). Suppression of immunity by stress: Effect of a graded series of stressors on lymphocyte stimulation in the rat. *Science* **213**, 1397–1400.

Kobayashi, R. M., Palkovits, M., Kizer, J. S., Jacobowitz, D. M. and Kopin, I. J. (1976). Selective alterations of catecholamines and tyrosine hydroxylase activity in the hypothalamus following acute and chronic stress. *In* "Catecholamines and Stress" (E. Usdin, R. Kvetnansky and I. J. Kopin, eds), pp. 29–38. Pergamon Press, Oxford.

Kopin, I. J., McCarty, R., Torda, R. and Yamaguchi, I. (1980). Catecholamines in plasma and responses to stress. *In* "Catecholamines and Stress: Recent Advances" (E. Usdin, R. Kvetnansky and I. J. Kopin, eds), pp. 197–204. Elsevier, New York.

Kvetnansky, R. (1980). Recent progress in catecholamine under stress. *In* "Catecholamines and Stress: Recent Advances" (E. Usdin, R. Kvetnansky and I. J. Kopin, eds), pp. 7–20. Elsevier, New York.

Kvetnansky, R. and Mikulaj, L. (1970). Adrenal and urinary catecholamines in rats during adaptation to repeated immobilization stress. *Endocrinology* **87**, 738–743.

Kvetnansky, R., Mitro, A., Palkovits, M., Brownstein, M., Torda, T., Vigas, M. and Mikulaj, L. (1976). Catecholamines in individual hypothalamic nuclei in stressed rats. *In* "Catecholamines and Stress" (E. Usdin, R. Kvetnansky and I. J. Kopin, eds), pp. 39–50. Elsevier, New York.

LaBarba, R. C. and White, J. L. (1971). Maternal deprivation and the response to Ehrlich carcinoma in BALB/c mice. *Psychosom. Med.* **33**, 458–460.

Lacassagne, A. and Duplan, J. F. (1959). Le mécanisme de la cancérisation de la mammelle chex les souris, considéré d'après les résultats d'expériences au moyen de la réserpine. *C. R. Hebd. Séanc. Acad. Sci., Paris* **249**, 810–812.

Lapin, V. (1978). Effects of reserpine on the incidence of 9,10-dimethyl-1,2-benzanthracene-induced tumors in pinealectomised and thymectomised rats. *Oncology* **35**, 132–135.

Levine, S. and Cohen, C. (1959). Differential survival to leukemia as a function of infantile stimulation in DBA/2 mice. *Proc. Soc. Exp. Biol. Med.* **102**, 53–54 (summary).

Lloyd, C. (1980). Life events and depressive disorder reviewed. II. Events as precipitatory factors. *Arch. Gen. Psychiat.* **37**, 541–548.

Locke, S. E., Hurst, M. W., Williams, R. M. and Heisel, I. S. (1978). The influence of psychosocial factors on human cell-mediated immune function. Presented at the meeting of the American Psychosomatic Society, Washington, D.C.

Lundy, J., Lovett, E. J., Wolinsky, S. M. and Conran, P. (1979). Immune impairment and metastatic tumor growth. *Cancer* **43**, 945–951.

McCann, S. M., Krulich, L., Ojeda, S. R. and Vijayan, E. (1978). Control of prolactin release by putative synaptic transmitters. *In* "Progress in Prolactin Physiology and Pathology" (C. Robyn and M. Harter, eds). Elsevier, Amsterdam.

McCarty, R., Chiueh, C. C. and Kopin, I. L. (1978). Behavioral and cardiovascular responses of spontaneously hypertensive and normotensive rats to inescapable footshock. *Behav. Biol.* **22**, 405–410.

McEuen, D. D., Blair, P., Delbene, V. E. and Eurenius, K. (1976). Correlation between pseudomonas burn wound infection and granulocyte antibacterial activity. *Infect. Immunol.* **13**, 1360–1362.

MacLean, D. and Reichlin, S. (1981). Neuroendocrinology and the immune process. *In* "Psychoneuroimmunology" (R. Ader, ed), pp. 475–520. Academic Press, Orlando, New York and London.

Macris, N. T., Schiavi, R. C., Camerino, M. S. and Stein, M. (1970). Effect of hypothalamic lesions on immune processes in the guinea pig. *Am. J. Physiol.* **229**, 1205–1209.

Martin, J. B. (1974). Regulation of pituitary-thyroid axis. *In* "Endocrine Physiology" (S. M. McCann, ed.), pp. 67–107. Butterworth, London.

Martin, J. B. and Reichlin, S. (1973). Neural regulation of the pituitary-thyroid axis. *In* "Proceedings of the Sixth Midwest Conference on Thyroid" (A. D. Kenny and R. R. Anderson, eds). University of Columbia Press, New York.

Maruyama, Y. and Johnson, E. A. (1969). Quantitative study of isologous tumor cell inactivation and effective cell fraction for the LSA mouse lymphoma. *Cancer* **23**, 309–312.

Mikulaj, L., Kvetnansky, R., Murgas, K., Parsikova, J. and Vencel, P. (1976). Catecholamines and corticosteroids in acute and repeated stress. *In* "Catecholamines and Stress" (E. Usdin, R. Kvetnansky and I. J. Kopin, eds), pp. 445–455. Pergamon Press, Oxford.

Modigh, K. (1976). Influence of social stress on brain catecholamine mechanisms. *In* "Catecholamines and Stress" (E. Usdin, R. Kvetnansky and I. J. Kopin, eds), pp. 17–28. Pergamon Press, Oxford.

Monjan, A. A. (1981). Stress and immunologic competence: Studies in animals. *In* "Psychoneuroimmunology" (R. Ader, ed.), pp. 185–228. Academic Press, Orlando, New York and London.

Monjan, A. A. and Collector, M. I. (1977). Stress-induced modulation of the immune response. *Science* **196**, 307–308.

Munster, A. M., Eurenius, K., Mortenson, R. F. and Mason, A. D., Jr. (1972) Ability of splenic lymphocytes from injured rats to induce a graft-versus-host reaction. *Transplantation* **14**, 106–108.

Munster, A. M., Gale, G. R. and Hunt, H. H. (1977). Accelerated tumor growth following experimental burns. *J. Trauma* **17**, 373–375.

Nakagawa, R., Tanaka, M., Kohno, Y., Noda, Y. and Nagasaki, N. (1981). Regional responses of rat brain noradrenergic neurones to acute intense stress. *Pharmacol. Biochem. Behav.* **14**, 729–732.

Newberry, B. H. (1978). Restraint-induced inhibition of 7,12-dimethylbenz(a)anthracene-induced mammary tumors: Relation to stages of tumor development. *J. Nat. Cancer Inst.* **61**, 725–729.

Newberry, B. H., Frankie, G., Beatty, P. A., Maloney, B. D. and Gilchrist, J. C. (1972). Shock stress and DMBA-induced mammary tumors, *Psychosom. Med.* **34**, 295–303.

Newberry, B. H., Gildow, J., Wogan, J. and Reese, R. L. (1976). Inhibition of Huggins tumors by forced restraint, *Psychosom. Med.* **38**, 155–162.

Newberry, B. H. and Sengbush, L. (1979). Inhibitory effects of stress on experimental mammary tumors, *Cancer Detect. Preven.* **2**, 255–233.

Nieburgs, H. E., Weiss, J., Navarrete, M., Strax, P., Teirstein, A., Grillione and Sidlecki, B. (1979). The role of stress in human and experimental oncogenesis, *Cancer Detect. Preven.* **2**, 307–336.

Palkovits, M., Brownstein, M., Kizer, J. S., Saavedra, J. M. and Kopin, I. J. (1976). Effect of stress on sertonin and tryptophan hydroxylase activity of brain nuclei. *In* "Catecholamines and Stress" (E. Usdin, R. Kvetnansky and I. J. Kopin, eds), pp. 51–60. Pergamon Press, Oxford.

Palmblad, J. (1981). Stress and immunologic competence: Studies in man. *In* "Psychoneuroimmunology" (R. Ader, ed.), pp. 281–319. Academic Press, Orlando, New York and London.

Palmblad, J., Cantell, K., Strander, J., Tröberg, J., Karlsson, C.-G., Levi, L., Granström, M and Unger, P. (1976). Stressor exposure and immunological response in man: Interferon-producing capacity and phagocytosis. *J. Psychosom. Res.* **20**, 193–199.

Palmblad, J., Karlsson, C. G., Levi, L. and Lidberg (1979a). The erythrocyte sedimentation rate and stress. *Acta Med. Scand.* **205**, 517–520.

Palmblad, J., Petrini, B., Wasserman, J. and Akerstedt, T. (1979b). Lymphocyte and granulocyte reactions during sleep deprivation. *Psychosom. Med.* **41**, 273–278.

Pavlidis, N. and Chirigos, M. (1980). Stress-induced impairment of macrophage tumoricidal function. *Psychosom. Med.* **42**, 47–54.

Pees, H. W. (1977). Influence of surgery and dexamethasone on cell-mediated immune responses in patients with meningiomas, *Br. J. Cancer* **35**, 537–545.

Peters, L. J. (1975). Enhancement of syngeneic murine tumor transplantation by whole body irradiation—A nonimmunological phenomenon. *Br. J. Cancer* **31**, 293–300.

Peters, L. J. and Kelly, H. (1977). The influence of stress and stress hormones on the transplantability of a nonimmunogenic syngeneic murine tumor, *Cancer* **39**, 1482–1488.

Pradhan, S. N. and Ray, P. (1974). Effects of stress on growth of transplanted and 7,12-dimethylbenz(a)anthracene-induced tumors and their modification by psychotropic drugs. *J. Nat. Cancer. Inst.* **53**, 1241–1245.

Quadri, S. K., Kledzik, G. S. and Meites, J. (1973a). Effects of L-DOPA and methyldopa on growth of mammary cancers in rats. *Proc. Soc. Exp. Biol. Med.* **142**, 759–761.

Quadri, S. K., Clark, J. L. and Meites, J. (1973b). Effects of LSD, Pargyline and Haloperidol on mammary tumor growth in rats. *Proc. Soc. Exp. Biol. Med.* **124**, 22–26.

Rabkin, J. G. and Streuning, E. L. (1976). Life events, stress and illness. *Science* **194**, 1013–1020.

Rasmussen, A. F., Marsh, J. T. and Brill, N. Q. (1957). Increased susceptibility to herpes simplex in mice subjected to avoidance-learning stress or restraint. *Proc. Soc. Exp. Biol. Med.* **96**, 183–184.

Rasmussen, A. F., Spencer E. S. and Marsh, J. T. (1959). Decrease in susceptibility of mice to passive anaphylaxis following avoidance-learning stress. *Proc. Soc. Exp. Biol. Med.* **100**, 878–879.

Ray, O. S. and Barrett, R. J. (1975). Behavioral, pharmacological and biochemical analysis of genetic differences in rats. *Behav. Biol.* **15**, 391–417.

Ray, P. and Pradhan, S. N. (1974). Growth of transplanted and induced tumors in rats under a schedule of punished behavior. *J. Nat. Cancer Inst.* **52**, 575–577.

Riley, V. (1979). Cancer and stress: Overview and critique. *Cancer Detect. Preven.* **2**, 163–195.

Riley, V. and Spackman, D. H. (1977). Cage crowding stress: Absence of effect on melanoma within protective facilities. *Proc. Am. Ass. Cancer Res.* **18,** 173.

Riley, V., Spackman, D. H., McClanahan, H. and Santisteban, G. A. (1979). The role of stress in malignancy. *Cancer Detect. Preven.* **2,** 235–255.

Riley, V., Fitzmaurice, M. A. and Spackman, D. H. (1981). Psychoneuroimmunologic factors in neoplasia: Studies in animals. *In* "Psychoneuroimmuology" (R. Ader, ed.), pp. 31–102. Academic Press, Orlando, New York and London.

Ritter, S. and Pelzer, N. L. (1978). Magnitude of stress-induced norepinephrine depletion varies with age. *Brain Res.* **152,** 170–175.

Ritter, S. and Pelzer, N. L. (1980). Age-related changes in norepinephrine neuron function during stress. *In* "Catecholamines and Stress: Recent Advances" (E. Usdin, R. Kvetnansky and I. J. Kopin, eds), pp. 107–112. Elsevier, New York.

Rogers, M. P., Dubey, D. and Reich, P. (1979). The influence of the psyche and the brain on immunity and disease susceptibility: A critical review. *Psychosom. Med.* **41,** 147–164.

Rossier, J., French, E. D., Rivier, C., Ling, N., Guillemin, R. and Bloom, F. E. (1977). Foot-shock induced stress increases beta-endorphin levels in blood but not in brain. *Nature* **270,** 618–620.

Saavedra, J. M. (1980). Brain and pineal adrenaline: Its level, synthesis and possible function in stress. *In* "Stress and Catecholamines: Recent Advances" (E. Usdin, R. Kvetnansky and I. J. Kopin, eds), pp. 37–46. Elsevier, New York.

Saavedra, J. M. and Torda, T. (1980). Increased brain stem and decreased hypothalamic adrenaline-forming enzyme after acute and repeated immobilization stress in the rat. *Neuroendocrinology* **31,** 142–146.

Saavedra, J. M., Kvetnansky, R. and Kopin, I. J. (1979). Adrenaline, noradrenaline and dopamine levels in specific brainstem areas of acutely immobilized rats. *Brain Res.* **160,** 271–280.

Saba, T. M. and Antikatzides, T. G. (1976). Decreased resistance to intravenous tumor cell challenge during reticuloendothelial depression following surgery, *Br. J. Cancer* **34,** 381–389.

Segall, P. E. and Timiras, P. S. (1976). Patho-physiologic findings after chronic tryptophan deficiency in rats: A model for delayed growth and aging. *Mech. Aging Dev.* **5,** 109–124.

Sherman, A. D. and Petty, F. (1980). Neurochemical basis of the action of anti-depressants on learned helplessness. *Behav. Neural Biol.* **30,** 119–134.

Sklar, L. S. and Anisman, H. (1979). Stress and coping factors influence tumor growth. *Science* **205,** 513–515.

Sklar, L. S. and Anisman, H. (1980). Social stress influences tumor growth. *Psychosom. Med.* **42,** 347–365.

Sklar, L. S. and Anisman, H. (1981a). Stress and cancer. *Psych. Bull.* **89,** 396–406.

Sklar, L. S. and Anisman, H. (1981b). Contributions of stress and coping to cancer development and growth. *In* "Stress and Cancer" (K. Bammer and B. H. Newberry, eds), pp. 98–136. Hogrefe, Toronto.

Sklar, L. S., Bruto, V. and Anisman, H. (1981). Adaptation to the tumor-enhancing effects of stress. *Psychosom. Med.* **43,** 331–342.

Soave, O. A. (1964). Reactivation of rabies virus in guinea pigs to the stress of crowding. *Am. J. Vet. Res.* **25,** 268–269.

Solomon, G. F. (1969). Stress and antibody response in rats. *Int. Arch. Allergy Appl. Immunol.* **35,** 97–104.

Solomon, G. F. and Amkraut, A. A. (1979). Neuroendocrine aspects of the immune response and their implications for stress effects on tumor immunity. *Cancer Detect.* **2**, 197–223.

Solomon, G. F. and Amkraut, A. A. (1981). Psychoneuroendocrinological effects on the immune response. *Ann. Rev. Microbiol.* **35**, 155–184.

Spector, N. H. and Korneva, E. A. (1981). Neurophysiology, immunophysiology and neuroimmunomodulation. *In* "Psychoneuroimmunology" (R. Ader, ed.), pp. 449–473. Academic Press, Orlando, New York and London.

Stein, M., Keller, S. and Schleifer, S. (1981). The hypothalamus and the immune response. *In* "Brain, Behavior and Bodily Disease" (H. Weiner and M. A. Hofer, eds), pp. 45–66. Raven Press, New York.

Stein, M., Schiavi, R. C. and Camerino, M. (1976). Influence of brain and behavior on the immune system. *Science* **191**, 435–440.

Stein, M., Schleifer, S. J. and Keller, S. E. (1981). Hypothalamic influences on immune responses. *In* "Psychoneuroimmunology" (R. Ader, ed.), pp. 429–447. Academic Press, Orlando, New York and London.

Stolk, J. M., Conner, R. L., Levine, S. and Barchas, J. D. (1974). Brain norepinephrine metabolism and shock-induced fighting behavior in rats: Differential effects of shock and fighting on the neurochemical response to a common footshock stimulus. *J. Pharmacol. Exp. Ther.* **190**, 193–209.

Stone, E. A. (1979a). Subsensitivity to norepinephrine as a link between adaptation to stress and antidepressant therapy: An hypothesis. *Res. Comm. Psychol. Psychiat. Behav.* **4**, 241–255.

Stone, E. A. (1979b). Reduction by stress of norepinephrine-stimulated accumulation of cyclic AMP in rat cerebral cortex. *J. Neurochem.* **32**, 1335–1337.

Stone, E. A. (1975). Stress and catecholamines. *In* "Catecholamines and Behavior" (A. J. Friedhoff, ed.), pp. 31–72. Plenum Press, New York.

Sudakov, K. V., Anokhina, I. P., Belova, T. I., Bolyakin, V. I., Ivanova, T. M., Skotzelyas, Y. G. and Yumatov, E. A. (1980). Catecholamine content in brain of rats with different resistance to emotional stress. *In* "Catecholamines and Stress: Recent Advances" (E. Usdin, R. Kvetnansky and I. J. Kopin, eds), pp. 75–78. Elsevier, New York.

Taché, Y., Ruisseau, P. D., Ducharme, J. R. and Collu, R. (1978). Pattern of adenohypophyseal hormone changes in male rats following chronic stress. *Neuroendocrinology* **26**, 208–219.

Tang, L. C., Cotzias, G. C. and Dunn, M. (1974). Changing the action of neuroactive drugs by changing brain protein synthesis. *Proc. Nat. Acad. Sci. USA* **71**, 3350–3354.

Telgedy, G. and Vermes, I. (1976). Changes induced by stress in the activity of the serotonergic system in limbic brain structures. *In* "Catecholamines and Stress" (E. Usdin, R. Kvetnansky and I. J. Kopin, eds), pp. 145–156. Pergamon Press, Oxford.

Teodoru, C. V. and Schwartzman, G. (1956). Endocrine factors in pathogenesis of experimental poliomyelitis in hamsters: Role of inoculating and environmental stress. *Proc. Soc. Exp. Biol. Med.* **91**, 181–187.

Terry, L. C. and Martin, J. B. (1978). Hypothalamic hormones: Subcellular distribution and mechanisms of release. *In* "Annual Review of Pharmacology and Toxicology" (R. George and R. Okun, eds), Vol. 18, pp. 111–123. Annual Reviews, Palo Alto, California.

Theirry, A. M. (1973). Effects of stress on the metabolism of serotonin and norepinephrine in the central nervous system of the rat. *In* "Hormones, Metabolism and Stress: Recent Progress and Perspectives" (S. Nemeth, ed.), pp. 37–53. Slovak Academy of Sciences, Bratislava, Czechoslovakia.

Thierry, A. M., Fekete, M. and Glowinski, J. (1968). Effects of stress on the metabolism of noradrenaline, dopamine and serotonin (5-HT) in the central nervous system of the rat: II. Modifications of brain serotonin metabolism. *Eur. J. Pharmacol.* **4**, 384–389.

Thierry, A. M., Blanc, G. and Glowinski, J. (1971). Effect of stress on the disposition of catecholamines localized in various intraneurotonal storage forms in the brainstem of the rat. *J. Neurochem.* **18**, 449–461.

Thierry, S. M., Tassin, J. P., Blanc, G. and Glowinski, J. (1976). Selective activation of the mesocortical DA system by stress. *Nature* **263**, 242–244.

Thoa, N. B., Tizabi, Y. and Jacobowitz, D. M. (1977). The effect of isolation on catecholamine concentration and turnover in discrete areas of the rat brain. *Brain Res.* **131**, 259–269.

Tissari, A. H., Argiolas, A., Fadda, F., Serra, G. and Gessa, G. L. (1979). Footshock stress accelerates non-stratal dopamine synthesis without activating tyrosine hydroxylase. *Arch. Pharmacol.* **308**, 155–158.

Toge, T., Hirai, T., Takiyama, W. and Hattori, T. (1981). Effects of surgical stress on natural killer cell activity, proliferative response of spleen cells, and cytostatic activity of lung macrophages in rats. *Gann* **72**, 790–794.

Treadwell, P. E., Wista, R., Rasmussen, A. F., Jr. and Marsh, J. T. (1959). The effect of acute stress on the susceptibility of mice to passive anaphylaxis. *Fed. Proc. Fed. Am. Soc. Exp. Biol.* **18**, 602.

Tyrey, L. and Nalbandov, A. V. (1972). Influence of anterior hypothalamic lesions on circulating antibody titers in the rat. *Am. J. Physiol.* **222**, 179–185.

U'Prichard, D. C. and Kvetnansky, R. (1981). Central and peripheral adrenergic receptors in acute and repeated immobilization stress. In "Catecholamines and Stress: Recent Advances" (E. Usdin, R. Kvetnansky and I. J. Kopin, eds), pp. 299–308. Elsevier, New York.

Van Den Brenk, H. A. S., Stone, M. G., Kelly, H. and Sharpington, C. (1976). Lowering of innate resistance of the lungs to the growth of blood-borne cancer cells in states of topical and systemic stress. *Br. J. Cancer* **33**, 60–78.

Van Loon, G. R. (1976). Brain dopamine beta hydroxylase activity: Response to stress, tyrosine hydroxylase inhibition, hypophysectomy and ACTH administration. In "Catecholamines and Stress" (E. Usdin, R. Kvetnansky and I. J. Kopin, eds), pp. 77–88. Pergamon Press, Oxford.

Vekshina, N. L. and Magaeva, S. V. (1974). Changes in the serotonin concentration in the limbic structures of the brain during immunization. *Bull. Exp. Biol. Med.* (English translation) **77**, 625–627.

Wayner, E. A., Flannery, G. R. and Singer, G. (1978). The effects of taste aversion conditioning on the primary antibody response to sheep red blood cells and Brucella abortus in the albino rat. *Physiol. Behav.* **21**, 995–1000.

Weiss, J. M. (1971). Effects of coping behavior with and without a feedback signal on stress pathology in rats. *J. Comp. Physiol. Psychol.* **77**, 22–30.

Weiss, J. M., Stone, E. A. and Harrell, N. (1970). Coping behavior and brain norepinephrine levels in rats. *J. Comp. Physiol. Psychol.* **72**, 153–160.

Weiss, J. M., Glazer, H. I., Pohorecky, L. A., Brick, J. and Miller, N. E. (1975). Effects of chronic exposure to stressors on avoidance-escape behavior and on brain norepinephrine. *Psychosom. Med.* **37**, 552–534.

Weiss, J. M., Pohorecky, L. A., Salman, S. and Gruenthal, M. (1976). Attenuation of gastric lesions by psychological aspects of aggression in rats. *J. Comp. Physiol. Psychol.* **90**, 252–259.

Weiss, J. M., Goodman, P. A., Losito, B. G., Corrigan, S., Charry, J. M. and Bailey, W. H. (1981). Behavioral depression produced by an uncontrollable stressor: Relationship to norepinephrine, dopamine and serotonin levels in various regions of rat brain. *Brain Res. Rev.* **3**, 167–205.

Welch, B. L. and Welch, A. S. (1970). Control of brain catecholamines and serotonin during acute stress and after d-amphetamine by natural inhibition of monoamine oxidase: An hypothesis. *In* "Amphetamines and Related Compounds" (E. Costa and S. Garattini, eds), pp. 415–445. Raven Press, New York.

Welsch, C. W. and Meites, J. (1970). Effects of reserpine on development of 7,12-dimethylbenzanthracene-induced mammary tumors in female rats. *Experientia* **26**, 1133–1134.

Werb, Z., Foley, Re. and Munck, A. (1978). Interaction of glucocorticoids with macrophages. Identification of glucocorticoid receptors in monocytes and macrophages. *J. Exp. Med.* **147**, 1684–1694.

Wick, M. M. (1977). L-dopa methyl ester as a new anti-tumor agent. *Nature* **269** 512–513.

Wick, M. M. (1978a). L-dopa methyl ester: Prolongation of survival of neuroblastoma-bearing mice after treatment. *Science* **199**, 775–776.

Wick, M. M. (1978b). Dopamine: A novel antitumor agent active against B-16 melanoma *in vivo. J. Invest. Derm.* **71**, 163–164.

Wick, M. M. (1979). Levadopa and dopamine analogs: Melanin precursors as antitumor agents in experimental human and murine leukemia. *Cancer Treat. Rep.* **63**, 991–997.

Wimer, R. E., Norman, R. and Eleftheriou, E. (1974). Serotonin levels in hippocampus: Striking variations associated with mouse strain and treatment. *Brain Res.* **63**, 397–401.

Yuwiler, A. (1976). Stress, anxiety and endocrine function. *In* "Biological Foundations of Psychiatry" (R. G. Grenell and S. Gabay, eds), pp. 889–943. Raven Press, New York.

Zajaczkowska, M. N. (1975). Acetylcholine content in the central and peripheral nervous system and its synthesis in the rat brain during stress and post-stress exhaustion. *Acta Physiologica Polska* **26**, 493–497.

Part Two

Behavioural Adjuncts to Medical Treatment

Introduction

The first section of this book has been concerned with evidence that emotional or behavioural events are linked with the onset and maintenance of physical disease states. While a number of methodological problems have been identified, we can reasonably conclude that psychological events are involved in the disease process, without the underlying mechanisms being clearly established to date. The very existence of such associations, however, indicates the possibility of reverse effects: that is, the induction of emotional or motivational states conducive to positive health or recovery from disease. Such effects may be exploited in many different ways, but we will here consider their use either as adjuncts to conventional medical treatments, or as treatment procedures in their own right. Although these two uses clearly overlap, we have chosen to employ this distinction in structuring the remaining two sections of this book.

The following section on behavioural adjuncts to medical treatment begins with a chapter by Maguire on communication skills, and the problems that can arise in social interactions between doctors and patients. No matter how effective the medical treatments available to doctors, patients cannot profit by them if they do not themselves recognize the need for medical help, and actively cooperate with treatment. As has become apparent in recent years, many patients do not obtain treatment when it would in fact benefit them, even in the presence of serious and sometimes fatal disease. The reasons for this are multiple, including not only deficiencies in the patients' own health knowledge, but also deficiencies on the doctors' part in misunderstanding or failing to use knowledge about the psychological factors involved. It is important to provide a psychological environment in which patients are free to talk about what is worrying them, since otherwise the information needed for diagnosis may not be obtained. As well as problems of obtaining information, doctors are not always skilled at providing information to patients in a reassuring way. Both these deficiencies in communication skills can have extremely serious consequences in handicapping effective health care delivery. Fortunately, however, there is also evidence that poor communication can be alleviated given appropriate training, and with growing recognition of these problems there is some hope that such training will become more widespread.

In Chapter 6, Becker and Rosenstock review the problem of compliance, or treatment adherence. As is now well known, treatments are rejected by patients on a grand scale, with between a third and two thirds failing to take medication or to follow advice correctly. Before we can make rational recommendations about the appropriate response to this finding, it is necessary to understand its origins. The health belief model is a major step in that direction. Rather than attributing non-compliance to an "uncooperative personality", the phenomenon can be understood as a rational behavioural response, resulting from an interaction between the patient's beliefs about personal vulnerability to disease, its consequences and the perceived benefits or costs of remedial action. Such a model has important theoretical and practical implications. Compliance may be improved by changing the patients own beliefs about personal vulnerability, and by increasing the benefits while decreasing the inconvenience of adherence. Indeed, as demonstrated by Haynes et al., (1976), a behavioural programme specifically tailored to the patient's existing habits, so as to minimize obstacles to taking medication, combined with the use of self-monitoring and social reinforcement, significantly improved adherence in otherwise non-compliant patients. While an educational component, such as informing patients about personal risk, is a necessary part of such programmes, it does not always seem sufficient in the absence of specific behavioural strategies.

Such interactions between educational and behavioural strategies in psychological interventions for promoting recovery are the subject of Chapter 7. Cromwell and Levenkron report on a unique study of recovery from myocardial infarction, showing that various psychological interventions and personality differences can produce significant effects on both short and long term medical outcome. Interventions such as high information and high participation with treatment had a significant impact on length of hospital stay, while personality differences had more predictive power for subsequent re-hospitalization or death. The different types of intervention appeared to interact in an informative way. Patients given extensive information only did well if it was coupled with either high participation or with high diversion/distraction. Thus, the effect of providing information appears to be crucially modulated by the methods used or resources available for processing and acting on that information. However, the mechanism whereby psychological interventions or personality variables exert their effects remains uncertain. While not ruling out possible physiological mechanisms, behavioural consequences such as sensitivity to symptoms, complaining of pain, or motivation for self-help, present themselves as likely mediating factors. Rather than diminishing the significance of the benefits achieved, however, this explanation re-emphasizes the significant part played by emotional and behavioural reactions in health or disease.

Similar considerations arise from the study of invasive or other traumatic treatment procedures. Entering hospital for surgery is a demanding and stressful experience, and it is perhaps not surprising that recovery from such invasive treatments may also be influenced by psychological factors. Mathews and Ridgeway (Chapter 8) discuss a large body of evidence showing that recovery variables, such as post-operative pain, medical complications, and return to normal activities, can be powerfully influenced by psychological interventions prior to surgery. In general, if patients are forewarned about the events and sensations that they will experience, or learn to manage their worries about surgery more effectively, their post-operative recovery is likely to be smoother. Interestingly, the consideration of mechanisms whereby such consequences can be brought about raises possibilities related to those discussed earlier. That is, while autonomic, hormonal or immunological processes may be directly influenced by psychological events, behavioural mediation may also provide an adequate and possibly more parsimonious explanation. Perhaps psychological preparation for surgery aids the patient to appraise post-surgical events and sensations in a less threatening way, and thus promote self-help behaviours that ultimately lead to a better physical recovery. A further question addressed in this chapter is how to identify patients in special need of psychological preparation, or those who might profit most by it. Consistent with the position outlined above, it does seem that individuals who characteristically use cognitive coping strategies which minimize the psychological impact of aversive information may be less in need of help than those that actively monitor their environment for threat.

All four chapters in Part II show how existing medical treatments may be either undermined, or be made optimally effective by behavioural strategies deriving from psychological research. Hence, their interest is far from being purely academic, but derives in part from the fact that general application of these results would significantly enhance the effectiveness of existing treatments. Nonetheless, all are also alike in generating important theoretical questions about the ways in which cognitive or emotional processes translate into health related behaviours and the recovery from disease. Particular symptoms or reactions to treatment may be interpreted by patients and doctors in different ways, and the manner in which this information is processed may then lead to different perceptions of the disease and behavioural intentions concerning its relief. It is crucial for clinicians to be aware of the fact that such diverse perceptions can undermine the therapeutic alliance that is essential for optimal health care.

Testing descriptive models of the manner in which patient's cognitive and emotional processes influence health related behaviour or physiological state, is an important stage in the development of more effective psychological interventions, whether aimed at modifying health beliefs, self-help behaviour, or the physical disease process itself.

REFERENCES

Haynes, R. B., Sackett, D. L., Gibson, E. S., Taylor, D. W., Hackett, B. C., Roberts, R. S. and Johnson, A. L. (1976). Improvement of medication compliance in uncontrolled hypertension. *Lancet* **i,** 1265–1268.

5

Communication Skills and Patient Care

PETER MAGUIRE

A 53-year-old woman noticed that she had a small lump in her left breast, and feared that it might be cancer, but told herself that it was probably nothing and would soon go away. Not wishing to waste her general practitioner's time she waited until it was clear that the lump was not going to disappear. She thought it it might be easier if she first mentioned that she had suffered "bad headaches" for three months following a change to a busy and stressful job, since this would be an acceptable reason for seeking help. She therefore rang the receptionist and asked for an appointment to discuss her "headaches". When she arrived the surgery was full and on entering the consulting room her doctor appeared harrassed. He clarified rapidly the nature of her headaches and their relation to tension. Before she could add anything about her lump he wrote a prescription for a tranquilliser and said he would like to see her again in a month's time. She felt flustered and left without mentioning her lump, which was later found to be cancer.

This case history illustrates one common problem of communication, resulting in a failure to identify an important problem. To be fully effective, doctors must be able to talk with patients in a way that promotes trust and the belief that they are interested in the problem. Otherwise, patients withhold information and the diagnosis and plan of treatment will then be wrongly based, as in the example above. As well as identifying problems, it is also necessary to provide an adequate explanation to patients, to reassure them, to monitor their progress and satisfaction, and to promote adherence to treatment. Failures in these other tasks are no less important. Thus, after identifying the problem, some explanation of what is wrong must be provided. This must be done in a way which enables the patient to understand the nature of his or her illness but avoids unnecessary worry. If the patient's need for information is not established and heeded, serious misunderstandings may arise which hinder recovery. For example, when

HEALTH CARE AND HUMAN BEHAVIOUR
ISBN 0–12–666460–9

faced with a postman who had had a serious attack of rheumatism and was very worried about his future, a doctor attempted to alleviate this worry by describing it as "only a moderate attack which should not occur again or affect his future". The man interpreted this as meaning he could return immediately to his normal busy life. When he did this he found it difficult to manage and caused further damage to his still inflamed joints. He also became bitter about the inappropriateness of the advice he had been given.

The explanation of what is wrong and of treatment to be given often provokes worry. It is helpful first to establish how patients feel about what they have been told and what is proposed before attempting any reassurance. If the patient's own perception and attitudes are not elicited, then any reassurance may be misplaced and ineffective. For example, a 45-year-old shopkeeper presented to his doctor with "chest pain". He said it was related to exertion and mentioned that he was worried that he would die from a heart attack because his father had done so. After a thorough examination it was explained that he had "angina" due to narrowing of the arteries in his heart, that an electrocardiograph would be carried out and he would be told the result. After the investigation the diagnosis was confirmed, but it was explained that the patient had little to worry about providing he did less in his shop and cut down his cigarette consumption. The patient left the surgery as worried as he was beforehand. His father had developed angina at the same age and was also told it was mild but had died before the age of 50 years. His shop was not doing well because of the recession and he saw no way of employing more staff to enable him to do less work.

Many illnesses and their treatments may cause substantial practical, social and psychological problems. These can hinder recovery and seriously impair the patient's and relatives' quality of life unless they are recognized and dealt with adequately. A 42-year-old woman had a colostomy performed for cancer of the large bowel. The cancer was removed completely and it was thought that she would survive for some years at least. However, she could not accept her colostomy and felt "dirty", "unclean" and "repulsive". She also noticed that her ability to enjoy sex had gone completely. She became increasingly depressed and began to feel that she had no future. She refused to go out socially, despite her husband's urging, except for follow-up visits to hospital. Discussion between her and the surgeons focused solely on the physical functioning of her colostomy and her physical health. Her emotional problems only came to light when she was admitted for psychiatric treatment following a serious attempt at suicide.

Doctors also have to ensure that they explain their plan of management so that the patient understands it, follows the advice and complies with the offered treatment. Otherwise the medical help will be rendered ineffective, as in the following example. A 27-year-old woman presented with a depressive illness. Her doctor told her she needed some tablets for her nerves and should take them regularly. She believed she had been given "tranquillisers" and declined to take them, because she had heard that people could become too dependent on them. When it was later explained that she was on "antidepressants" for her depressive illness and that there was little risk of dependence she complied fully.

It is often assumed that, despite the failures illustrated in these case histories, most doctors usually make accurate diagnosis, provide adequate explanations of what is wrong and what they plan to do, give effective reassurance, achieve a good level of compliance and monitor progress routinely. However, there is now good reason to challenged this assumption and argue that the examples of poor communication already quoted are much more common than is realized.

FAILURE TO IDENTIFY PROBLEMS

Recent studies have confirmed that a substantial proportion of the problems which patients are experiencing when they consult doctors remain undisclosed and undetected. Direct observation of 145 doctors, while they were obtaining histories from medical patients, found that they often failed to elicit some of their key physical problems (Weiner and Nathanson, 1976). Psychological and social problems appear to be missed even more often as Querido (1963) claimed. He obtained a random selection of 125 families from general practitioners' lists and then interviewed them in depth. The doctors had been accurate in their diagnoses of 95% of those suffering from serious physical illness, but had recognized only 50% of those patients who were suffering from associated social and psychological problems.

General practitioners have been found by Marks et al., (1979) to vary greatly in their ability to recognize psychiatric problems. They observed directly over 2000 consultations conducted by 55 experienced practitioners. On average, the practitioners correctly recognized half of those with problems, but the accuracy of identification by individual doctors varied from 20% to 80%. It has been suggested that psychological difficulties are especially likely to be missed when the patient presents with "somatic" symptoms, or when they occur in the setting of an established physical illness (Goldberg and Blackwell, 1970). This may explain why only half of the psychiatric disorders present in patients admitted with physical illness to two general medical wards were recognized (Maguire et al., 1974). Even when the medical patients are well known to the physicians, through being seen regularly by the same doctors in an outpatient clinic, a third of the existing psychiatric problems are missed (Brody, 1980).

A similar failure to detect such problems has been found in surgical practice. In a follow-up study of 75 women who had had a simple mastectomy followed by radiotherapy (Maguire *et al.*, 1978a) 19 (25%) were found to have developed an anxiety state and/or depressive disorder within 12 months of surgery. Only eight (42%) of these patients were recognized as having a psychological problem by the surgeons or general practitioners. A third of the women who had a satisfactory and active sex life before surgery, developed sexual problems, but none were recognized as having such difficulties during the follow-up period.

The adverse psychological sequelae of serious illness in children also commonly remain hidden. For example, in a study of 60 families who had a child under treatment for leukaemia, a quarter of the mothers developed morbid anxiety and depression. The paediatricians and practitioners were aware of this in only 17% of the mothers (Maguire *et al.*, 1979a). Such mood disturbance is even more likely to be missed if it becomes chronic (Weisman and Klerman, 1977).

This frequent failure to detect the adverse sequelae of physical illness extends to social and practical problems, and the extent to which patients have returned to their former level of functioning is often grossly over-estimated. In a study of patients who had had a colostomy for ano-rectal carcinoma, the difficulties many experienced in managing their colostomy was much greater than had been realized (Devlin *et al.*, 1971). Social isolation was also much commoner than expected. Similarly, women who have undergone mastectomy for breast cancer are often more dissatisfied with their breast prostheses and have suffered more pain and swelling than the surgeons estimate (Maguire, 1976).

The toxicity of drug treatments is also often under-estimated. In eight (40%) of 20 patients who were being treated with powerful anti-cancer drugs and developed unpleasant side effects, including vomiting and hair loss, the toxicity was not recognized by the doctors treating them (Maguire *et al.*, 1980a). Consequently, five patients dropped out of what might have been lifesaving treatment because they could not tolerate any more. Palmer *et al.* (1980) also found that clinicians under-estimated the real impact of such treatment on the patient's quality of life.

While psychological problems are less likely to be recognized when they occur in the setting of physical illness, the converse is also true. Physical illness may remain undiagnosed if the patient is already known to have a psychiatric disorder, as Maguire and Granville-Grossman (1968) found. Of 200 patients consecutively admitted to a general hospital psychiatric unit 67 (33%) were found to have a physical illness. This had been recognized by the patient's general practitioner before admission in only 33 (49%).

OTHER FAILURES OF COMMUNICATION

The task of identifying patients' perceptions and attitudes has received much less attention than the problem of hidden morbidity. However, the study by Korsch *et al.* (1968) indicated that there was much room for improvement. They used audiotape recording to monitor consultations between paediatricians working in a hospital outpatient department and mothers and their children. In 65% of mothers the doctors failed to establish what the mothers had expected from their visits, and only 24% of mothers revealed what their main concerns were about their child.

A similar study used trained observers to monitor how surgeons interacted with women suffering from breast disease (Maguire, 1976). Little attempt was made to identify the women's worries. Consequently, much of their reassurance was ineffective and the women remained very anxious. It was also noticeable that they used set strategies of reassurance which bore little relationship to the individual concerns of the women.

There has been little scrutiny of how clinicians give information to patients about their illness and treatment; most studies in the area have focused on what doctors tell patients with cancer (Sanson–Fisher and Maguire, 1980). There appears to be a considerable discrepancy between what doctors think the patients should know and the patients' desire for information. Reynolds *et al.* (1981) found that 91% of a group of cancer patients wanted to know their diagnosis, 97% wished to learn about their treatment and 88% would have liked to have been given a prognosis. In reality, their wishes were rarely recognized and met. Yet, when they were, the patients were much more satisfied with the care they were given.

Ley (1982), in a review of attempts to improve the compliance of patients given advice and medication, concluded that only an average of 50% comply. Consequently, much medical care is rendered ineffective. Brody (1980) has suggested that doctors are poor at recognizing non-compliance. He found that 79% of the under-compliance of medical outpatients went undetected by the doctors who were following them up at regular intervals.

Deficiencies in knowledge about treatment could also have serious repercussions. Muss *et al.* (1979) assessed the knowledge of patients taking anti-cancer drugs. Twenty five per cent were unable to identify a single one of the agents they were receiving. Most patients did not understand the goals of treatment, and were especially ignorant of potentially life-threatening side effects, including bleeding and infection. While communicating with patients with cancer may be especially difficult, there is little evidence that communications are much better between doctors and patients suffering from other illnesses. Instead, it is becoming increasingly clear that

medical students and doctors often lack the communication skills which are
essential for the proper fulfilment of these basic tasks.

DEFICIENCIES IN COMMUNICATION SKILLS

If medical training were effective in equipping medical students with these
key skills, those about to qualify as doctors ought to be reasonably
proficient. Direct observation using videotape recordings of 50 final year
students found that this was not the case (Maguire and Rutter 1976).
Although asked to interview patients who were willing to explain their
problems, they obtained only a third of the information that was readily
available to them.

   This failure to identify many of their patients' problems seemed linked to
serious deficiencies in their skills. Eighty per cent avoided covering more
personal issues, such as the impact of patients' illness on their personal
relationships and their attitudes to illness. A similar proportion were too
ready to accept phrases from the patient like "diarrhoea", "angina" or
"nervous breakdown" without clarifying what the patient meant. Three-
quarters of the students accepted imprecise data and failed to respond to
important verbal clues that patients gave them about their problems, even
when these were offered repeatedly. Only 8% were consistently able to
clarify exactly what the patients' symptoms had been like. Although some
students sought to excuse their poor performance on the grounds of lack of
time, it was noted that the majority wasted much time through needless
repetition of areas covered already. Over half of the students found it
difficult to keep patients to the point and only a a third asked open-ended
and brief questions. These findings were remarkably similar to those
reported by Wolf et al. (1952) nearly 25 years earlier. In a series of audiotape
recordings of fourth year students, it was found that most stuck to a rigid
list of questions that were fired rapidly at the patient in a form that invited a
"yes" or "no" answer. They often failed to notice or follow up important
leads and obtained only superficial information. Students did too much
talking and often came up with the wrong diagnosis. They allowed the
patient too much opportunity to discuss irrelevancies and appeared insensitive to patients' feelings, avoiding psychological and social aspects by
"choking off" the patient and ignoring emotional problems.

   More junior medical students have been found to display a similar pattern
of deficiencies (Pollack and Manning, 1967). They are too directive, too
easily sidetracked, and avoid psychosocial aspects. This similarity between
senior and junior medical students suggests that traditional methods of
training do little to remedy these deficiencies, and several follow-up studies

have confirmed this. Barbee and Feldman (1970) followed up 10 students for three years. Some improvement was found in the students' ability to elicit pertinent medical data, but little change in their coverage of psychosocial aspects. They were no better able to establish the patients' views of their illness or probe emotional aspects. In another small study, six students were also followed up for three years (Wright et al., 1980). Deficiencies had persisted and there was little improvement. They still failed to introduce themselves, rarely enquired about the impact of illness and were poor at clarifying the patients' key problems. Nor were they more able to elicit medical facts.

These findings have been confirmed by studies which have compared students from different years of training (Scott et al., 1975; Bishop et al., 1981). These studies have also suggested that medical students became less emphathic over time and were no better at providing reassurance. Helfer (1970) and his colleague (Helfer and Ealy, 1972) have remarked on the contrast between the innate skills and interest evident in beginning medical students and the cold, directive, machine gun like mode of questioning observed in senior medical students, who seemed much less interested in psychological and social aspects of illness. Their findings suggest that medical training may erode at least some of the students' communication skills.

Although these studies present a gloomy picture, it is heartening that when medical students are asked what aspects of relating to patients seem difficult, they are aware of their own deficiencies (McNamara, 1974). Students report feeling unable to enquire about more personal and emotional topics or to provide reassurance; and dislike asking about sexual adjustment or being asked difficult questions like "Have I got cancer?". They are uncertain about how honest they should be with patients and how to deal with silences. It might be hoped that these deficiencies would be remedied as a result of postgraduate medical training, and greater contact with patients. However, such a conclusion is not supported by the available evidence. In observing short interviews between 145 doctors in training and medical patients, Weiner and Nathanson (1976) found that they rarely allowed patients to tell their own stories. They asked too many questions and made little attempt to clarify poorly-defined complaints. They were often imprecise, wasted time and rarely answered patients' questions appropriately.

When Platt and McMath (1979) observed 300 interviews by physicians representing all levels of experience, five key defects were noted. The first concerned the "low therapeutic content". Patients were not greeted adequately or provided with explanations of what they were doing. Doctors appeared eager to close the interview and missed key leads. They were not very understanding or supportive in their comments, neglected to ask how the patient was feeling and were poor at giving reassurance. The authors concluded that doctors based their plans for treatment on a "flawed data base" because they ignored the patients' concerns, failed to check if they had any other problems or were experiencing any other stresses and found out little about their daily lives. A "failure to generate hypotheses" was noted about why particular patients or problems were found difficult to handle. Doctors also "failed to demand primary data". They accepted too easily the patient's or referring clinician's interpretation of the symptoms, instead of first clarifying for themselves exactly what the patients had experienced. Finally, Platt and McMath highlighted the doctors' "high control style". They asked too many closed and directive questions, ignored clues, tolerated silences poorly and focused too quickly on what they regarded as the main problem, so missing other important difficulties. Of particular importance was the authors' comment that "physicians at all levels who had previously been thought quite competent appeared defective in their interactions with patients."

The doctors in training assessed by Aloia and Jonas (1976) were less deficient, but still tended to ask patients little about the home and family situation, or impact of the illness. What seemed to change with experience was their ability to obtain more precise information about the medical illness and a greater knowledge of the relevant repertoires of questions they should ask.

This neglect of psychosocial aspects was also found by Duffy et al. (1980) in their study of doctors within a medical out-patient clinic. It was found that about two thirds of the doctors omitted social histories, failed to establish what the patients' understanding of their illnesses was, and did not clarify how the patients had responded emotionally.

Choice of speciality does not appear to affect the incidence of such deficiencies, for psychiatrists in training have been found to have difficulty in establishing a productive relationship, listening properly and handling emotionally loaded material (Janek et al., 1979). Similarly, surgeons appear very directive, often focus only on physical aspects, ignore important verbal and non-verbal cues, fail to clarify what the patient feels or thinks about the illness, and give reassurance too quickly and ineffectively (Maguire, 1976).

Although one might expect paediatricians to be more able to communicate, since their concern is with children, Korsch et al. (1968) found that they were also lacking in key skills. Over half of the paediatricians studied in a clinic used medical jargon. They often gave vague answers to mothers' questions and failed to heed and follow up cues. They wasted much time through not identifying and responding to the mothers' concerns and sometimes reduced the mothers to silence by giving monosyllabic replies.

While half the mothers indicated they felt guilty about their child's illness, little attempt was made to alleviate these feelings. Over one third of the mothers asked few, if any, questions.

Hospital doctors seeing new patients do not have the general practitioners' potential advantages of already knowing the patient and his or her background and being the first to hear about the problems the patient is presenting. However, the expectation that general practitioners might therefore avoid communication problems has not been confirmed by studies carried out in primary care settings.

Byrne and Long (1976) recorded over 2000 consultations carried out by general practitioners on audiotape and subjected the data to an interaction analysis. These authors concluded that the practitioners much preferred focusing on organic aspects and neglected emotional and social problems. A set sequence of questions was often followed that was little affected by what the patient needed or said. Practitioners tended to seize on the first problem mentioned and assume that it was the only one. Their behaviour suggested that they did not want to enter into any really close relationship with their patients and they often prevented or tried to stifle expressions of feeling by the patient. Few attempts were made to clarify what patients meant and they usually avoided more difficult areas. Only rarely did they check back with their patients that they had correctly identified and understood their problems. They provided little opportunity for patients to ask questions and were too inclined to attempt reassurance before they had established what their patients were concerned about.

Similar findings were reported by Verby et al., (1979), who studied 17 practitioners. Deficiencies were found in both experienced doctors and less experienced practitioners. Verby et al. (1980) also suggested that the skills of trainees in general practice worsened over time unless they were given special feedback training.

Some practitioners realize that they find certain communication tasks difficult (Bennett et al., 1978). Couples, adolescents and medically trained personnel are found hard to interview, while drug dependency, child abuse and terminal illness are seen as being especially difficult to handle. Doctors feel uncertain about how best to convey to patients that their problem is trivial or that they have a potentially fatal disease. They also admit to often finding it difficult to uncover the patients' real problems, and bring the consultation to an end.

It is clear, then, that medical students and doctors are often deficient in key communication skills and that these deficiencies remain relatively unchanged despite further experience and training. It is, therefore, worth considering why these skills are not acquired to a sufficient level by many medical students and doctors.

REASONS FOR THESE DEFICIENCIES

At the outset of their clinical training medical students are usually given a booklet on history-taking. This is commonly limited to guidance about the areas to be covered and lists of questions. The focus is on eliciting physical signs and symptoms, with little if any attention devoted to psychological and social aspects. The notes on history-taking also rarely contain any explicit advice on how to relate to patients, to begin and end interviews, the techniques that might be helpful when obtaining a history, or trying to determine a patient's perception, feelings or attitude. Nor are students usually given explicit guidance about how to give reassurance, or information about diagnosis and treatment, how to break bad news, or talk with dying patients and bereaved relatives.

One reason why this guidance is often lacking is the assumption by many medical teachers that the students will learn the relevant skills by "watching experts at work". Yet, the teachers who they are watching will rarely have received any formal training in these skills. While they may possess some of them, other skills are likely to be lacking. Clinical teachers are unlikely, therefore, to afford an optimal role model of all the essential communication skills in action. Moreover, there is a risk that students will copy undesirable rather than desirable behaviour.

The reliance on indirect methods of assessing student skills is also a major problem. It has been shown (Hinz, 1966) that how a student performs in reporting a history often bears little relationship to how well he or she actually relates to patients. Deficiencies in essential communication skills will, therefore, go unnoticed and allow teachers to preserve their belief that medical training succeeds in equipping students with these skills.

Since postgraduate training has generally relied on the same "apprenticeship method" it has suffered from the same deficiencies. Despite this most medical schools have been slow to change their training methods. Much of the resistance to training in communication skills has stemmed from the dominance of the bio-engineering ideology in medical care (Sanson-Fisher and Maguire, 1980). This approach stresses physical intervention to remedy underlying disease processes. It is established firmly in medical practice and is adhered to by the more powerful departments within medical schools. It usually ignores patients' emotional responses to illness and encourages doctors to maintain a distance from their patients, so as to strengthen their image as authority figures and increase their power to reassure patients.

Many doctors remain complacent about their communication skills because patients give them little feedback about any deficiencies. Yet, in independent surveys patients often express dissatisfaction about the way their doctors communicate with them. It is likely that doctors who accept the bio-engineering ideology convey to patients, albeit unwittingly, that their emotional needs are not the objective of the consultation. It has also been argued that doctors discourage feedback from patients so that they can maintain power over them (Waitzkin and Stoekle, 1972). Complaining directly about the care given may also conflict with the traditional passive sick role which patients are expected to adopt (Parsons, 1958). If patients do express dissatisfaction, doctors may interpret it as a consequence of the patients' worry about their illness rather than a reflection of how poorly they have communicated with them.

In the absence of patient feedback and direct observation of doctors' interactions with patients, it is easy to understand why many doctors refuse to accept that there is any need to change traditional training methods. Even if they accept that some doctors may be deficient in communication skills, they tend to argue that such skills cannot be taught ("you have the gift or you do not"), or that they have little impact on the delivery and outcome of care. This ignores the evidence reviewed already about hidden morbidity and other consequences of defective communication, as well as studies of newer approaches to training in these skills (Maguire *et al.*, 1978b, Carroll and Monroe, 1979).

RELUCTANCE TO COVER PSYCHOLOGICAL AND SOCIAL ASPECTS

Doctors appear especially reluctant to cover the possibility that patients have psychological and social problems in their own right, or as a consequence of established physical illness and its treatment. Recent studies have focused on the reasons for this.

When general practitioners who had been looking after cancer patients were interviewed in depth about their interactions with the patients, they suggested that several factors accounted for their avoidance of psychosocial aspects (Rosser and Maguire, 1982). First they assumed that any patients who developed problems would come to the surgery and tell the doctor about these difficulties. When faced with evidence that only a small proportion of patients did this, few accepted that they ought to ask questions routinely to elicit such problems, such as "How have you been feeling in yourself since the operation?" They felt that they did not have the time. Doctors were also concerned that if they did ask such questions they might "open Pandora's box". They might then be faced with problems they could not deal with. These included being asked questions about diagnosis, aetiology, treatment and prognosis which they found hard to answer. For example, how do you respond if a patient with advanced cancer asks "Should I continue this drug treatment?" when you know it is making her feel wretched and she may not live long anyway. It is better to manage the consultation so that patients have little chance to ask such questions, especially as the doctor may feel he or she has not been able to keep pace with the latest advances in treatment.

Probing patients' and relatives' emotional responses to serious illness, particularly depression, anxiety and sexual problems, is also avoided, because it brings doctors close to suffering and the real impact of illness and treatment. This may exhaust them emotionally and intensify feelings of guilt that they have failed the patient. This seems especially true when it is a child who is suffering from serious illness. Doctors may then find that they can no longer "switch off", and avoid taking their problems home. Active enquiry about psychological and social aspects is, therefore, better avoided.

While this need to maintain emotional distance may explain some of the deficiencies in communicating with cancer patients, it does not explain why similar deficiencies are evident when dealing with patients who present with less serious illnesses. Even when patients succeed in getting a message through that they are "depressed" or "very anxious" the doctor is likely to respond by saying "Of course you are. So would I be in your position. But you will find it gets easier over time". This tendency of doctors to dismiss as "understandable" symptoms of morbid anxiety and depression, because they are "reactive" to an established stress, is a general one within clinical practice (Derogatis et al., 1976; Maguire et al., 1980b). Doctors commonly believe that they can best help ill patients by jollying them along and encouraging them to look on the positive side rather than by focusing on possible areas of difficulty. In this view, questioning might cause patients to worry more than they would otherwise have done. Doctors, therefore, put the onus on patients and relatives to disclose any psychological and social problems which they are experiencing. However, a substantial proportion of patients fail to do so and the reasons for this non-disclosure warrant consideration.

RELUCTANCE TO DISCLOSE PROBLEMS AND ASK QUESTIONS

When patients or relatives are asked why they are reluctant to disclose any psychological and social problems or ask for advice and information, their reasons match closely the findings from the observations of doctor–patient interactions (Maguire et al., 1980b; Cartwright et al., 1973).

Patients correctly perceive doctors as busy and involved in the care of many others, and are loath to burden them any more. They also believe that doctors are primarily concerned with their physical well-being and are not sure that it will be acceptable if social or psychological concerns are mentioned. This uncertainty is usually based on past experience. When such concerns were previously hinted at, the doctor may have ignored them, changed the subject or enquired in an uninterested way. Little time may have been given to explain these problems. Instead, doctors are more likely to reach for a prescription pad to give a course of tranquillisers or sleeping tablets. Alternatively, patients may be told that this was how most people felt in the same situation, that it was "understandable" and did not merit any intervention. Such experiences often confirm patients' own beliefs that emotional problems are an inevitable consequence of their situation and that nothing can be done. There is, therefore, no point in mentioning them further.

When patients with serious physical illness become anxious or depressed they tend to feel that they are the only ones who are not coping. They may feel guilty and ashamed at their "inadequacy" or "weakness", and be afraid to mention that they are finding it difficult to cope. Disclosure might detract from the care given for their physical illness and lead to their being regarded as "neurotic", "uncooperative" and "ungrateful". It might also mean that they could be asked to see a psychiatrist; this is to be avoided, because of the stigma involved, and fears that they will be considered "mad", put on "tranquillisers" or have their liberty removed. They therefore try to put on a "brave face", or "pull themselves together". Only when it becomes impossible to do this any longer are they likely to reconsider mentioning their difficulties.

Another major reason for non-disclosure concerns the questions asked by doctors. Only rarely do the patients recall any doctor spontaneously asking how they have been feeling about their illness or treatment, their own view of it and the impact on their daily lives. Consequently, they interpret a general enquiry like "how are you today?" as aimed solely at their physical health. Patients' expectations of a doctor's interest can work in an opposite way. Those who are used to seeing psychiatrists may be reluctant to mention physical symptoms, believing that they are only concerned with psychological problems and being uncertain that they are "proper doctors". Other reasons commonly given for not asking and pursuing questions include: the lack of time, forgetting what they wanted to ask because they were worried, expecting to be fobbed off and being afraid of the answer. When patients have persisted in asking a question the doctor has often become brusque, irritated or ended the consultation.

It is widely assumed that most patients with serious illness, and their relatives, will turn to their general practitioners if they develop any further problems. However, this may not happen very often if the patient is being followed up at hospital regularly by a team who are expert in the management of their physical disease. Patients and their relatives tend to devalue their practitioner's care because he or she has had much less experience of the illness (Comaroff and Maguire, 1981). As a result, they fall between the two potential sources of help, since they do not disclose their problems either to the hospital team or practitioner. These barriers to effective communication between doctors, patients and relatives are formidable, but attempts must be made to overcome them if medical care is to become more effective.

THE NEED FOR CHANGES IN TRAINING METHODS

One obvious solution to the problems that have been outlined would be to change existing methods of medical education, so that medical students and doctors are much more likely to acquire the essential skills in communication during their undergraduate and postgraduate training. Over the last decade, there has been a growing number of attempts to teach communication skills more effectively (Carroll and Monroe, 1979). These have mainly been introduced by departments of psychiatry, psychology or general practice, and most attention has focused on teaching medical students and doctors to obtain accurate histories of patients' presenting problems. There has been little systematic attempt to teach doctors how to give information, break bad news, give reassurance or talk with the dying or bereaved (Meadow and Hewitt, 1972; Anderson, 1982).

Analysis of existing methods and deficiencies in skill has suggested that if training is to be superior to traditional approaches it must include certain components. The student or doctor must be given a model of interviewing which is appropriate for the tasks to be performed. Thus, it must include details about the areas to be covered as well as explicit guidance about the techniques that they will find helpful. Usually, this is given in the form of a handout or programmed text, but teachers are increasingly using videotape recordings to show the skills in action (Maguire et al., 1977).

Once the students or doctors have grasped the skills to be learned and data to be obtained, they need to practise under carefully controlled conditions. The task expected of the student should be made explicit by giving instructions such as the following example: "We want you to concentrate on finding out what the patient's presenting problems are. You must establish these first before you ask about any previous difficulties". The length of time allowed to complete the task should also be made clear and an indication given as to whose responsibility it will be to end the interview within that time. Moreover, the task given should be appropriate to the student's or doctor's level of training and experience. This also involves the careful selection of real patients who will be cooperative or present the required degree of difficulty. Alternatively, people may be trained to simulate problems of a given complexity and nature (Meadows and Hewitt, 1972; Maguire et al., 1977; Meier et al., 1982). This is a valid way of assessing the acquisition of skills since there is little difference between students' performances with real versus simulated patients (Sanson–Fisher and Poole, 1980).

The provision of feedback of performance by an experienced tutor using audiotape or videotape replay is a further crucial element. Such feedback should focus both on the data obtained and the skills used to obtain it. To be fully effective in giving feedback, teachers should realize how exposing and threatening seeing and hearing oneself is, especially when conducted amongst one's peers. Teachers should avoid the "hot seat" approach, where the student or doctor whose interview is being replayed is "grilled" and criticized. Strengths should be focused upon before weaknesses, and the recipient's feelings about the patient and interview conditions taken into account before any feedback is offered. There should also be a clear explanation of why certain behaviours are "desirable" or "undesirable" and discussion should be encouraged (Pendleton, 1982; Maguire, 1982).

Feedback is likely to be more effective if both teachers and students are given a rating scale which allows them to measure reliably how well they have performed and so determine how well they are progressing. Some techniques, such as doctors explaining who they are and what they want to do, are easily measurable in terms of present or absent (Maguire et al., 1978b). Other skills like "control" (the ability to keep patients to the point without upsetting or alienating them) may be measured on a visual analogue scale (from no control to excellent control) (Maguire et al., 1978b; Verby et al., 1979). An alternative method is to indicate if and when certain desired and undesired behaviours occur. It is then possible to provide students or trainees with profiles of their behaviours (Morrison and Cameron Jones, 1972).

Many courses have been described which include some if not all of these components, for example, Jason et al. (1971) and Cline and Garrard (1973). While there has been less effort to evaluate their effectiveness, the attempts made have generally been encouraging. In one study, 48 medical students were randomly allocated to one of four training conditions: training by the traditional apprenticeship method; or practice under controlled conditions and feedback, by television, by audiotape replay or by an instructor who had previously watched a videotape replay. Students taught by the traditional methods failed to show any significant improvement (Maguire et al.,

1978b). Only those who were given an audiotape or television feedback showed improvements, both in the data they could obtain and the techniques they used. In this study, students were given feedback individually on three practice interviews at weekly intervals. It was later found (Maguire *et al.*, unpublished) that this feedback was just as effective when carried out in small groups. Feedback training has also been shown to be effective with general practitioners (Verby *et al.*, 1979), even when those who are especially deficient in history-taking skills are selected (Goldberg *et al.*, 1980). Training has also beeen beneficial when given to physicians during their postgraduate training, especially in terms of their ability to empathize, respond to patients' feelings and cover psychosocial aspects (Robbins *et al.*, 1979). Other studies have been limited to the learning of specific skills such as empathy, and have demonstrated that these can also be taught (Sanson-Fisher and Poole, 1978). It seems reasonable to conclude that at least the skills involved in taking histories and being emphatic can be taught using appropriate methods. Methods of teaching other communication skills have yet to be properly evaluated. However, providing the skills are made explicit and the same components of training included, it is probable that they will be as successful.

Despite the superiority of feedback methods over traditional training in teaching some of the key skills, several questions need to be answered. Do the skills last and are they generalized to the student's or doctor's work with different types of patients? There have been few follow-up studies, but the preliminary evidence has been encouraging (Poole and Sanson-Fisher, 1981; Kauss *et al.*, 1980). Those who had received training in specific skills were still superior to those who had not, although they showed some decay when compared with the level of skills immediately after training. Another important question concerns the relationship between communication skills and specific outcome measures, such as diagnostic accuracy, patient satisfaction, compliance and adaptation. The demonstration of strong correlations between specific skills and outcome would enable training to focus on those skills. Some progress has been made in respect of the skills required to identify psychiatric problems. Those doctors who establish good eye contact at the outset, pick up verbal leads, clarify key complaints and are able to exercise appropriate control, are much more likely to identify problems than doctors who do not use these skills (Goldberg *et al.*, 1980). It is also heartening that patients have expressed clear preferences for being interviewed by students who have been rated highly on certain key skills, including response to verbal leads, precision and control (Thompson and Anderson, 1982).

It is also possible that these feedback methods would be even more effective in the short and longer term if they:

(i)   included the "bug in the ear" technique (Hunt, 1980), where students can be advised as they interview;

(ii) used a third person to review in detail what the patient and doctor were thinking and feeling at different points of the interview (*interpersonal process recall*, Kagan et al., 1969);

(iii) focused on practising only one skill at a time (*microcounselling*, Moreland et al., 1973);

(iv) allowed trainees to look at their own performances by themselves until ready to show them to someone else (Pendleton, 1982);

(v)   included feedback from the patient (Kent et al., 1981), or actual experience as a patient (Markham et al., 1979).

Nor is it clear when such skills-training should be given, or how it could best be integrated into the curriculum. Should it be the concern of a special department of medical communication, or could most teachers be taught to do it?

It will take some time before the need to teach these skills is widely accepted and these questions are answered. A much quicker solution, which has been adopted by some centres, is to rely on specialist workers to perform some of these key tasks. Specialist nurses or social workers have been employed to help deal with patients who suffer from serious life-threatening illnesses and/or need help to adapt to particular treatments. Stoma nurses or therapists are notable examples of this development. It is assumed that they will be able to help patients adapt to their stomas and provide any information, advice and support that is needed before and after surgery. In particular, such nurses seek to ensure that the patient can manage the stoma from day to day and has an adequate bag. There is little doubt that stoma nurses are well trained for such technical aspects of their work, but no reason to believe that they have been adequately trained in the relevant communication skills. Similar criticisms can be made of other specialists, including "chemotherapy", diabetic" and "mastectomy" nurses. For this reason, a study was conducted to see if a nurse who was first trained in the relevant skills was effective in helping women who underwent mastectomy for cancer of the breast.

The nurse was taught how to take a history, to give information and advice, provide reassurance and identify problems which needed help. One hundred and fifty two women were randomly allocated to routine care alone, or to such care plus regular visits by this nurse (Maguire et al., 1980c). The provision of advice, information and support failed to prevent problems. However, these skills allowed the nurse to recognize and refer those who needed help, and since this help was effective, those who received visits fared much better. This group of patients had significantly less anxiety, depression or sexual problems when assessed 12 to 18 months later. They were also much more satisfied with the care given. This confirms the expectation that communication skills can have a positive and important effect on the outcome of patient care, and highlights the importance of ensuring that such specialist nurses have been properly trained.

REFERENCES

Anderson, J. L. (1982). Evaluation of a practical approach to teaching about communication with terminal cancer patients. *Med. Educ.* **16**, 202–7.

Barbee, R. A. and Feldman, S. E. (1970). A three year longitudinal study of the medical interview and its relationship to student performance in clinical medicine. *J. Med. Educ.* **45**, 770–76.

Bennett, A., Knox, J. D. E. and Morrison, A. T. (1978). Difficulties in consultations reported by doctors in general practice. *J. R. Coll. Gen. Pract.* **28**, 646–651.

Bishop, J. M., Fleetwood-Walker, P., Wishart, E., Swire, H., Wright, A. D. and Green, I. D. (1981). Competence of medical students in history-taking during the clinical course. *Med. Educ.* **15**, 368–372.

Brody, D. S. (1980). Physician recognition of behavioural, psychological and social aspects of medical care. *Arch. Intern. Med.* **140**, 1286–1289.

Byrne, P. S. and Long, B. E. L. (1976). "Doctors Talking to Patients." HMSO, London.

Carroll, J. G. and Monroe, J. (1979). Teaching medical interviewing: a critique of educational research and practice. *J. Med. Educ.* **54**, 498–500.

Cartwright, A., Hockey, L. and Anderson, J. L. (1973). "Life before Death." Routledge and Kegan Paul, London.

Cline, D. W. and Garrard, J. N. (1973). A medical interviewing course: objectives, techniques and assessment. *Am. J. Psychiat.* **180**, 575–578.

Comaroff, J. and Maguire, P. (1981). Ambiguity and the search for meaning: childhood leukaemia in the modern clinical context. *Soc. Sci. Med.* **158**, 115–123.

Derogatis, L. R., Abeloff, M. D. and McBeth, C. D. (1976). Cancer patients and their physicians in the perception of psychological symptoms. *Psychosomatics* **17**, 197–201.

Devlin, H. B., Plant, J. A. and Griffen, M. (1971). Aftermath of surgery for anorectal cancer. *Br. Med. J.* **3**, 413–418.

Duffy, D. L., Hammerman, L. and Cohen, A. (1980). Communication skills of house officers: A study in a medical clinic. *Ann. Intern. Med.* **93**, 353–357.

Goldberg, D. P. and Blackwell, B. (1970). Psychiatric illness in general practice: a detailed study using new method of case identification. *Br. Med. J.* **2**, 439–441.

Goldberg, D. P., Smith, C., Steele, J. J. and Spivey, L. (1980). Training family doctors to recognise psychiatric illness with increased accuracy. *Lancet* **ii**, 521–523.

Helfer, R. E. and Ealy, K. F. (1972). Observations of paediatric interviewing skills. *Am. J. Dis. Childh.* **123**, 556–560.

Helfer, R. E. (1970). An objective comparison of the paediatric interviewing skills of freshmen and senior medical students. *Paediatrics* **45**, 623–627.

Hinz, C. F. (1966). Direct observation as a means of teaching and evaluating clinical skills. *J. Med. Educ.* **41**, 150–161.

Hunt, D. D. (1980). 'Bug in the ear' technique for teaching interview skills. *J. Med. Educ.* **55**, 964–6.

Janek, W., Burra, P. and Leichner, P. (1979). Teaching interviewing skills by encountering patients. *J. Med. Educ.* **54**, 401–407.

Jason, H., Kagan, N., Werner, A., Elstein, A. S. and Thomas, J. B. (1971). New approaches to teaching basic interviewing skills to medical students. *Am. J. Psychiat.* **127**, 1404–1407.

Kagan, N., Schauble, P., Regnikoff, A., Danish, S. J. and Krathwohl, D. R. (1969). Interpersonal process recall. *J. Nerv. Ment. Dis.* **148**, 365–374.

Kauss, D. R., Robbins, A. S., Abrass, I., Bakaitis, R. F. and Anderson, L. A. (1980). The long-term effectiveness of interpersonal skills training in medical school. *J. Med. Educ.* **55**, 595–601.

Kent, G. G., Clarke, P. and Dalrymple Smith, D. (1981). The patient is the expert: a technique for teaching interviewing skills. *Med. Educ.* **15**, 38–42.

Korsch, B. M., Gozzi, E. K. and Francis, V. (1968). Gaps in doctor–patient communication 1. Doctor–patient interaction and patient satisfaction. *Paediatrics* **42**, 855–871.

Ley, P. (1982). Satisfaction, compliance and communication. *Br. J. Clin. Psychol.* **21**, 241–254.

MacNamara, M. (1974). Talking with patients: some problems met by medical students. *Br. J. Med. Educ.* **8**, 17–23.

Maguire, P. (1976). The psychological and social sequelae of mastectomy. In "Modern Perspectives in the Psychiatric Aspects of Surgery" (J. G. Howells, ed.), pp. 390–420. Brunner Mazel, New York.

Maguire, G. P. and Granville-Grossman, K. L. (1968). Physical illness in psychiatric patients. *Br. J. Psychiat.* **114**, 1365–1369.

Maguire, P. and Rutter, D. (1976). Training medical students to communicate. In "Communication between Doctors and Patients" (A. E. Bennett, ed.), pp. 45–74. Oxford University Press, London.

Maguire, G. P., Julier, D. L., Hawton, K. E. and Bancroft, J. H. J. (1974). Psychiatric morbidity and referral on two general medical wards. *Br. Med. J.* **1**, 266–268.

Maguire, G. P., Clarke, D. and Jolly, B. (1977). An experimental comparison of 3 courses in history-taking skills for medical students. *Med. Educ.* **11**, 175–182.

Maguire, G. P., Lee, E. G., Bevington, D. J., Kuchemann, C. S., Crabtree, R. J. and Cornell, C. E. (1978a). Psychiatric morbidity in the first year after mastectomy. *Br. Med. J.* **1**, 963–965.

Maguire, P., Roe, P., Goldberg, D., Jones, S., Hyde, C. and O'Dowd, T. (1978b). The value of feedback in teaching interviewing skills to medical students. *Psychol. Med.* **8**, 695–704.

Maguire, P., Roe, P., Goldberg, D., Jones, S., Hyde, C. and O'Dowd, T. (1978b). The value of feedback in teaching interviewing skills to medical students. *Psychol. Med.* **8**, 695–704.

Maguire, P., Comaroff, J., Ramsell, P. J. and Morris Jones, P. H. (1979). Psychological and social problems in families of children with leukaemia. In "Topics in Paediatrics 1: Haematology and Oncology" (P. H. Morris Jones, ed.), pp. 141–149. Pitman Medical, London.

Maguire, G. P., Tait, A., Brooke, M., Thomas, C., Howat, J. M. T. and Sellwood,

R. A. (1980a). Psychiatric morbidity and physical toxicity associated with adjuvant chemotherapy after mastectomy. *Br. Med. J.* **281**, 1179–1180.

Maguire, P., Tait, A. and Brooke, M. (1980b). Mastectomy: a conspiracy of pretence. *Nursing Mirror* January 10, 17–19.

Maguire, P., Tait, A., Brooke, M., Thomas, C. and Sellwood, R. (1980c). The effect of counselling on the psychiatric morbidity associated with mastectomy. *Br. Med. J.* **281**, 1454–1456.

Maguire, P., Roe, P., Goldberg, D. and O'Dowd, T. (unpublished). The role of supervision and small groups in teaching interviewing skills.

Markham, B., Gessmer, M., Warburton, S. W. and Sadler, G. (1979). Medical students become patients: a new teaching strategy. *J. Med. Educ.* **54**, 416–418.

Marks, J. N., Goldberg, D. P. and Hillier, V. (1979). Determinants of the ability of general practitioners to detect psychiatric illness. *Psychol. Med.* **9**, 337–353.

Meadow, R. and Hewitt, C. (1972). Teaching communication skills with the help of actresses and videotape simulation. *Br. J. Med. Educ.* **6**, 317–322.

Meier, R. S., Perkowski, L. C. and Wynne, C. S. (1982). A method for training simulated patients. *J. Med. Educ.* **57**, 535–540.

Moreland, J. R., Ivey, A. E. and Phillips, J. S. (1973). An evaluation of microcounselling as an interviewer training tool. *J. Counsel. Clin. Psychol.* **2**, 294–300.

Morrison, A. and Cameron-Jones, M. (1972). A procedure for training for general practice. *Br. J. Med. Educ.* **6**, 125–132.

Muss, H. B., White, D. R., Michielutte, R., Richards, F., Cooper, M. R., Williams, S., Stuart, J. J. and Spurr, C. L. (1979). Written informed consent in patients with breast cancer. *Cancer* **43**, 1549–1556.

Palmer, B. V., Walsh, G. A., McKinna, J. A. and Greening, W. P. (1980). Adjuvant chemotherapy for breast cancer: side effects and quality of life. *Br. Med. J.* **281**, 1594–1597.

Parsons, T. (1958). Definitions of health and illness in the light of American values and social structure. *In* "Patients, Physicians and Illness" (E. Jaco, ed.). Free Press, Glencoe.

Pendelton, D. (1982). Doctor–patient communication. Gift or skill. *Gen. Pract. Vocat. Training* **4**, 24–30.

Platt, F. W. and McMath, J. C. (1979). Clinical hypocompetence: the interview. *Ann. Intern. Med.* **91**, 898–902.

Pollack, S. and Manning, P. R. (1967). An experience in teaching the doctor–patient relationship to first year medical students. *J. Med. Educ.* **42**, 770–774.

Poole, D. A. and Sanson-Fisher, R. W. (1980). Long-term effects of empathy training on the interview skills of medical students. *J. Patient Counsel. Health Educ.* **2**, 125–129.

Querido, A. (1963). "The Efficacy of Medical Care." Stenfert Kroese, Leiden.

Reynolds, P. M., Sanson-Fisher, R. W., Poole, A. D., Harker, J. (1982). Cancer and communication; information giving in an oncology clinic. *Br. Med. J.* **282**, 1449–1451.

Robbins, A. S., Kauss, D. R., Heinrich, R., Abrass, I., Dreyer, J. and Clyman, B. (1979). Interpersonal skills training: evaluation in an internal medicine residency. *J. Med. Educ.* **54**, 835–891.

Rosser, J. E. and Maguire, P. (1982). Dilemmas in general practice: the care of the cancer patient. *Soc. Sci. Med.* **16**, 315–322.

Sanson-Fisher, R. and Maguire, P. (1980). Should skills in communications be taught in medical schools? *Lancet* **ii**, 523–526.

Sanson-Fisher, R. W. and Poole, A. D. (1978). Training medical students to empathize—an experimental study. *Med. J. Aust.* **1**, 473–476.

Sanson-Fisher, R. W. and Poole, A. D. (1980). Simulated patients and the assessment of medical students' interpersonal skills. *Med. Educ.* **14**, 249–253.

Scott, N. C., Donnelly, M. B. and Hess, J. W. (1975). Changes in interviewing styles of medical students. *J. Med. Educ.* **50**, 1124–1126.

Thompson, J. A. and Anderson, J. L. (1982). Patient preferences and the bedside manner. *Med. Educ.* **16**, 17–21.

Verby, J. E., Holden, P. and Davis, R. H. (1979). Peer review of consultations in primary care: the use of audio-visual recordings. *Br. Med. J.* **1**, 1686–1688.

Verby, J., Davis, R. H. and Holden, P. (1980). A study of the interviewing skills of trainee assistants in general practice. *J. Patient Counsel. Health Educ.* **2**, 68–71.

Waitzkin, H. and Stoeckle, J. D. (1972). The communication of information about illness. *Adv. Psychosom. Med.* **8**, 180–215.

Weiner, S. and Nathanson, M. (1976). Physical examination: frequently observed errors. *J. Am. Med. Ass.* **236**, 852–855.

Weissman, M. M. and Klerman, G. L. (1977). The chronic depressive in the community: unrecognised and poorly treated. *Compr. Psychiat.* **18**, 523–531.

Wolf, S., Almy, T. P., Flynn, J. T. and Kern, F. (1952). Instruction in medical history-taking. *J. Med. Educ.* **27**, 244–252.

Wright, A. D., Green, I. D., Fleetwood-Walker, P. M., Bishop, J. M., Wishart, E. H. and Wire, H. (1980). Patterns of acquisition of interview skills by medical students. *Lancet* **ii,** 364–366.

6
Compliance with Medical Advice

MARSHALL H. BECKER and
IRWIN M. ROSENSTOCK

Many of the diseases that currently plague the human species are thought to be preventable and/or treatable. However, the success of preventive and therapeutic efforts depends not only on the efficacy of the suggested course of action, but also on the client's "compliance"—i.e. "the extent to which a person's behavior . . . coincides with medical or health advice" (Haynes *et al.*, 1979).

It seems only sensible that individuals would readily undertake public health and medical care recommendations so that they might avoid, or obtain relief from, illness; yet it is evident that substantial non-compliance occurs wherever some form of self-administration or discretionary action is involved. One reviewer of the compliance literature (Podell, 1975) calculates that, on average, only one-third of patients correctly follow physicians' directions. Sackett (1976) summarizes a good deal of the literature on the magnitude of the problem and points out that scheduled appointments for treatment are missed 20 to 50% of the time, while about 50 per cent of patients do not take prescribed medications in accordance with instructions. Recommended changes in habitual behaviours are even less frequently adhered to: smoking cessation programs are considered to be unusually effective if more than one-third of the entrants have reduced their smoking by the end of six months. Dietary restrictions are often not observed, and large percentages drop out of weight control programmes.

In light of these statistics, one might be tempted to assume a popular uninterest in, or even an aversion to, health-related activity, but such misinterpretation is quickly dispelled by the enormous market for over-the-counter medications, medical appliances, books about "wellness" and "self care," special foods, and the like. As Sir William Osler observed, "The desire to take medicine is perhaps the greatest feature which distinguishes

HEALTH CARE AND HUMAN BEHAVIOUR
ISBN 0–12–666460–9

175

man from animals" (Cushing, 1925). Clearly, the difficulty lies neither with arousing public interest in health matters nor with overcoming some widespread reluctance to acknowledge illness or attempt cure, but rather, in persuading individuals to adopt those regimens specified by health professionals.

A RATIONAL BASIS FOR NON-COMPLIANCE

The existence of these poor compliance levels often surprises health workers, to whom such behaviour appears counter-intuitive. Physicians overestimate the degree of co-operation achieved in their practices, and are unable to predict the likelihood of an individual patient's adherence to therapy (see Caron and Roth, 1968; Mushlin and Appel, 1977). Clinicians tend to blame non-compliance on the patient's personality, and express little desire to understand or little sympathy for the unco-operative patient (Davis, 1966), although their own compliance-related attitudes and performance are not unlike those of patients in general (Blackwell et al., 1978; Shangold, 1979).

A brief historical digression will help place the non-compliance phenomenon in better perspective. The era just preceding and following the turn of the nineteenth century witnessed the transition of medicine from an arcane and relatively powerless art to the beginnings of an effective science. Discovery of the germ theory of disease stimulated identification of specific causes of disease states, which in turn, led to development of equally specific environmental or personal interventions for the prevention or treatment of those diseases. By the middle of the twentieth century, the development and widespread diffusion of immunizations and antibiotics had brought the control of infectious disease to a point where mankind's expectations of medical science were raised well beyond what could, in reality, be accomplished.

A part of this reality was what we now know to be the multicausal nature of disease. Pre-twentieth-century approaches to disease aetiology lacked a clear distinction between necessary and sufficient conditions for the existence of disease states or even a clear definition of a disease state. It has only recently been realized that diseases rarely, if ever, result from single causes, and that any given disease may reflect the simultaneous occurrence of, and highly complex interactions among, physical, psychological, social and environmental events.

Consideration of treatments for the most prevalent conditions that presently afflict western society yields a picture of at least equal intricacy. Therapeutic regimens have become increasingly complex. The patient may be requested to ingest and/or apply a variety of medications at different intervals over varying time periods; to modify a number of life style practices, such as patterns of smoking, eating and drinking; to engage in stress-reduction activities and/or exercise programmes; and to alter aspects of his physical environment. Furthermore, none of these recommendations is guaranteed to prevent or cure the disease, or even to reduce severity of symptoms.

When health, disease, prevention and control are viewed in the light of these complexities, it is not surprising that the general public is often disturbed, confused, unrealistically hopeful, and unjustifiably disappointed with medical science. Having been educated to expect a single powerful preventive or treatment, the public often confronts a complex combination of prescriptions of uncertain effectiveness, and their unmet expectations exert an adverse effect on subsequent compliance with medical advice. By the time the average person has reached adulthood he has likely experienced many successes and many failures relative to health and medical recommendations.

Various effects on prevention or recovery of different levels of regimen co-operation can be elucidated with the aid of the paradigm presented in Fig.1. When health professionals think about patient compliance, they typically imagine cases which fall in cells "A" and "D", that is, achievement of the preventive or treatment goal is simply dependent upon whether or not the individual follows advice sufficiently.

	Illness prevented or patient gets well	Illness not prevented or patient does not get well
Adequate compliance	A	B
Inadequate compliance	C	D

Fig. 1 Some possible relationships between degree of patient compliance and health outcomes (after Sackett, 1976).

They, thereby, tend to forget that a great many therapeutic incidents occur which fall in the "deviant case" cells of the figure. For example, one commonly encounters (and experiences) circumstances wherein faithful adherence to a regimen does *not* yield the desired outcome (i.e. cell "B"):

the diagnosis may have been incorrect; the prescribed therapy may have been incorrect (or inadequate, or inefficacious); the patient may not have responded to a particular treatment; the preventive measure may not have been sufficient; and so forth. The "lesson" learned (or attitude developed) by the individual is, "Sometimes, even if you do everything the health professionals tell you to do, you still get sick/don't get well." Similar, but opposite, learning experiences are encountered in cell "C". Here, despite poor compliance, the patient nonetheless recovers (or does not become ill). Again, the wrong diagnosis may have been made and/or the host's natural defences may prove sufficient (much acute illness disappears without treatment, and symptoms of chronic disease may abate for long periods of time even in the absence of medical intervention). Moreover, high risk behaviours (e.g. cigarette smoking, over-eating, diets high in saturated fats and cholesterol) do not usually result in readily-observable illness in the short run (nor does *every* risk taker become ill even in the long run). Here, the "lesson" learned (and concomitant attitude developed) is, "Sometimes, even if you *don't* do everything the health professionals tell you to do, you still get well/don't get sick."

Furthermore, many persons have experienced (or heard about) the potential adverse consequences of different medications and therapies. Individuals are continually exposed by the mass media to controversies, contradictions, and often reversals with regard to public health and medical care recommendations (e.g. the recent debates about the merits and/or dangers of obtaining various influenza immunizations, sharply altering dietary patterns, achieving "ideal" body weight, and others). One is impressed by the contemporary relevance of Chapin's comment, made in 1915 that "The opprobrium of our art is that preventive medicine, like its other branches, has taught much that has had to be unlearned. We ought not to be surprised that people do not believe all we say, and often fail to take us seriously. If their memories were better, they would trust us even less" (Chapin 1915).

To provide a framework for discussion of the conditions under which people will or will not follow health recommendations, this chapter will utilize a classification scheme developed by Kasl and Cobb (1966), which distinguishes three classifications of health-related behaviour:

(i) *health behaviour*, activity undertaken by individuals who believe themselves to be healthy for the purpose of preventing disease or detecting disease in an asymptomatic state;

(ii) *illness behaviour*, activity undertaken by individuals who feel ill for the purpose of defining the state of their health and of discovering suitable remedy; and

(iii) *sick role behaviour*, activity undertaken by those who consider themselves ill for the purpose of getting well (including compliance with
prescribed therapeutic regimes).

PREVENTIVE HEALTH BEHAVIOUR

An understanding of preventive health behaviour requires initial consideration of several underlying issues. First, there is the question of whether the
concept of "health" (as distinct from illness) has any coherent meaning for
most people, or whether it is merely an analytic construct. Can preventive
behaviour be better explained by reference to a general concept of health, or
by considering particular kinds of health-related matters that may or may
not be related to each other? This matter has not been well studied. We do
not know, with any assurance, if people are guided by a dimension of
health. Becker *et al.* (1972) showed that a tendency to be aroused by
health-related stimuli and a general concern for health helps in explaining
mothers' decisions to adhere to a ten-day penicillin regimen prescribed for
their children. But, in another setting (Becker *et al.*, 1975), general concern
with health did not account for people's decisions to participate in a
programme to detect the Tay–Sachs trait. It should be noted that the first of
these studies concerned behaviour under conditions of diagnosed illness,
whereas the second concerned behaviour to be initiated by a healthy target
audience. Perhaps health consciousness helps to explain illness or sickness
(compliance) behaviour, but is less valuable in explaining preventive
behaviour. Haefner *et al.* (1967) showed that while correlations among four
preventive health actions studied (chest x-rays, medical and dental visits in
the absence of symptoms and toothbrushing after meals) were positive,
they were quite modest, and other investigators have been unable to
demonstrate the existence of a uni-dimensional preventive health orientation (Williams and Wechsler, 1972; Langlie, 1977).

A second issue concerns behaviours that may affect one's state of health,
but which are undertaken or avoided for motives other than the achievement of "health". For example, adults who habitually brush their teeth
shortly after arising each day and have done so since childhood probably
learned this behaviour early in life, for reasons unrelated to dental health (at
least in so far as they were concerned). In the adult, the behaviour is often
triggered by the various stimuli associated with the toothbrushing response:
awakening, experiencing an undesirable taste, and the like. A great many of
our behaviours that have implications for health (e.g. patterns of eating,
exercising, smoking) are of this sort, that is, responsive to social, environmental and other influences, and possessing large habitual components.

Whether our immediate response to a physical sign is to interpret it as a symptom or not is almost certainly habitual. These considerations have important implications for understanding, predicting and modifying behaviour. Attempts to get children to adopt specific, healthful behaviour patterns should not be restricted to health-related issues, but rather, should appeal to the entire panoply of relevant motives and incentives (within proper ethical bounds).

A third issue relates to the variety of ways in which people seek to satisfy a dominant motive. An important dimension in choice of health action is that of self care versus professional care. Parents who are motivated to prevent a particular disease in their children (e.g. influenza or poliomyelitis) may do so by obtaining professional help (e.g. immunization), or by initiating their own actions (e.g. prayer, keeping their children away from public places during the disease's peak season, and the like). Many policy makers believe that strains on the health care system could be reduced if people were encouraged to handle "minor" problems by themselves. However, the rationale underlying encouragement for more self care includes an implicit assumption that the way people handle these non-emergency conditions will be in accord with what health professionals would do if they were given responsibility. Advocates of self care may or may not be in accord with modern medical wisdom.

Over the past few decades, a variety of models have been constructed to help explain public response to preventive programmes, and as will be discussed later, patient compliance decisions (Cummings *et al.*, 1980). Although these formulations offer a number of different orientations and variables, they all contain elements of a particular model intially developed to predict compliance with such preventive health recommendations as obtaining immunizations, screening tests, and annual checkups (Becker, 1974a). This "Health Belief Model" contains the following elements (Fig. 2):

(i)   the individual's subjective state of readiness to take action, which is determined by both the person's perceived *susceptibility* to the particular illness and by his or her perceptions of the probable *severity* of the physical and social consequences of contracting the disease;

(ii) the individual's evaluation of the advocated health behaviour, in terms of its feasibility and efficaciousness (i.e. an estimate of the action's potential *benefits* in reducing susceptibility and/or severity), weighed against perceptions of physical, psychological, financial, and other costs or *barriers* involved in the proposed action; and

(iii) a *cue to action* must occur to trigger the appropriate health behaviour; this stimulus can be either internal (e.g. the perception of symptoms)

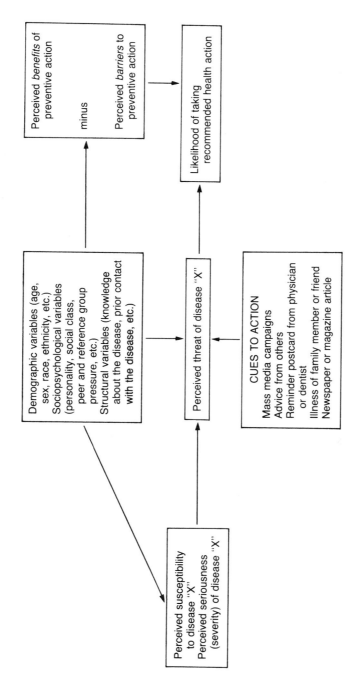

Fig. 2 The Health Belief Model.

or external (e.g. interpersonal interactions, mass media communications).

Although it is assumed that diverse demographic, personal, structural, and social factors can, in any given instance, influence an individual's health-related perceptions, these variables are not considered to be direct causes of health action.

The Health Belief Model has now been applied successfully in a large number of research efforts to explain and predict individual's health-related behaviours in preventive situations, including: screening for cervical, breast, or other cancers; screening for tuberculosis, heart disease, Tay-Sachs disease, and for dental problems; immunizations against various illnesses; adoption of an accident-preventive device; risk-reduction actions to prevent coronary heart disease; a postpartum programme of contraception; and well-child (preventive) clinic visits. The major results of these studies are summarized in Table 1.

To illustrate how the Health Belief Model (HBM) has been employed in studying preventive health behaviour, we describe a recent report of health beliefs and inoculation behaviour in reference to swine influenza, which in 1976, was widely believed by public health officials to threaten the population of the United States (Cummings et al., 1979).

Predictor variables included HBM dimensions, measures of behavioural

TABLE 1 Summary of studies using one or more Health Belief Model variables to predict compliance with preventive health recommendations

Investigator	Behaviour	Susceptibility	Severity	Benefit	Barrier
Hochbaum (1956; 1958)	TB X-ray screening	+	+	+	NM
Rosenstock et al. (1959)	Polio vaccination	+	+	+	+
Flach (1960)	Pap test	+	NM	+	NM
Leventhal et al. (1960)	Flu vaccination	+	+	NM	NM
Kegeles (1963a)	Dental visit	+	+	+	+
Kegeles (1963b)	Dental visit follow-up	+	0	+	+
Kirscht et al. (1966)	Dental, TB X-ray, cancer	0	0	+	NM
Suchman (1967)	Safety glove	+	+	+	0
Kegeles (1969)	Pap test	+	NM	+	NM
Tash et al. (1969)	Dental visit	−/+	+	+	+
Haefner and Kirsch (1970)	Preventive examinations: TB, cancer, heart	+	+	+	NM
Heinzelmann and Bagley (1970)	Physical activity programmes	+	+	+	NM
Campbell (1971)	Actions to prevent CHD	+	+	+	NM
Fink et al. (1972)	Breast cancer screening	+	+	+	NM
D'Onofrio (1973)	Acceptance of post partum contraception programme	+	+	+	+
Ogionwo (1973)	Cholera immunization	+	NM	+	NM
Becker et al. (1975)	Screening for Tay-Sachs	+	−	+	NM
Becker et al. (1977b)	Well-child (preventive visits)	+	+	+	NM
Cummings et al. (1979)	Influenza vaccination	+	+	+	+

+ = positive findings; − = negative findings; 0 = no association found; NM = not measured.

intention, physicians' advice and other variables hypothesized to have some potential impact on the decision to accept an inoculation. The research design consisted of a telephone survey one week prior to the start of a mass campaign and a follow-up survey on a random half of the sample immediately after the campaign and the other half two months later. One adult respondent was randomly chosen from each household selected into the sample. The subject group comprised 374 adults in the initial survey and 286 adults in the follow-up survey.

The following questions were addressed: (i) what is the relative importance of the social psychological attributes posited by the HBM in explaining inoculation behaviour? (ii) what are the interrelationships among HBM variables, behavioural intention, and non-attitudinal factors? and (iii) what is the relationship between intention to receive inoculation and subsequent behaviour?

Each of the four main HBM variables, perceived susceptibility, severity, efficacy and barriers, yielded a significant correlation with inoculation behaviour. Socio-economic status, a composite score of income and education, was the only demographic variable to have a significant relationship with vaccination behaviour. The other traditional demographic indicators (age, sex, marital status) demonstrated weak correlations with the dependent variable. It should also be noted that for those individuals who sought the advice of a physician, the physician's recommendation had a powerful influence on their subsequent behaviour. Finally, behavioural intention was significantly associated with behavioural outcome.

Additional analyses further illuminated these findings: path analysis supported a particular causal model, wherein the HBM variables were strong predictors of behavioural intention, which in turn, was a strong predictor of inoculation behaviour. The HBM influence on this behaviour is thus thought to be mediated through "behavioural intention".

ILLNESS BEHAVIOUR

Under what conditions will people seek professional help in the presence of symptoms? Before initiation of professional treatment, many activities may be undertaken in the effort to cope with episodes of health disturbance. Some episodes will result in a decision to do nothing or to self-medicate, even though, from a medical point of view, the condition requires professional attention. The timing of decisions to seek care is a further aspect of illness behaviour (Zola, 1973), and there is some evidence that certain people will typically wait longer than will others before acting on a disturbance (Becker et al., 1972). The behaviour that takes place in trying to define the state of one's illness is critical in the process leading to treatment, particularly because so many of the decisions are self-initiated. Illness behaviour is, therefore, closely related to decisions leading to either seeking professional help or delay in seeking care, and the use of non-prescribed medications and nostrums.

Most research on delay in seeking diagnosis has involved cancer (Kalmer, 1974; Green and Roberts, 1974). Clements and Wakefield (1972) have noted that non-delay in initiating diagnosis for cancer symptoms is similar to care-seeking for any type of symptom, thus suggesting that patterns of delay may be typical of particular individuals, unlike the patterns of health behaviour discussed earlier. In an extensive review of the literature concerning delay, Antonovsky and Hartman (1974) have noted that the findings are not entirely consistent or clear. In general, lower socio-economic status and lower educational levels are frequently (but not always) associated with delay. However, it is difficult to know whether socio-economic status or education is the more powerful factor, since the two are highly interrelated. No other socio-demographic characteristic has pro-vided a basis for firm generalizations about delay.

Antonovsky and Hartman (1974) further conclude that knowledge interacts with emotional factors. Thus, knowledge about cancer symptoms in combination with anxiety arising from beliefs that cancer cannot be prevented or cured, leads to greater delay, whereas such knowledge unaccompanied by severe doubts about preventability or curability is associated with less delay (see Rogers and Mewborn, 1976). These beliefs would appear to be closely related to the Health Belief Model variable "perceived benefits of action." The authors report a variety of studies on the role of various emotional reactions (for example, fear, guilt, fatalism, shame) on delay, with somewhat equivocal results. Reinterpretation of these findings in terms of Health Belief Model components might yield more comprehensive explanations (see Kelly, 1979). According to Anto-novsky and Hartman, personality, IQ, and measures of neuroticism have generally not been useful in accounting for delay (hypochondria, however, has been implicated in a tendency not to delay). Studies of coping styles have also not proved useful in distinguishing delayers from non-delayers. It appears that delayers more often believe in divine healing, whereas non-delayers have acquired habits of paying attention to symptoms and have faith in the medical profession. Antonovsky and Hartman were unable to find research on the effects of social influence on delay, though they correctly point out that such influences have been found to be important in other areas of preventive health behaviour. Finally, they conclude that a comfortable relationship between patient and doctor at the very least removes a barrier and facilitates non-delay or participation in preventive examinations.

EXPLANATIONS OF ILLNESS BEHAVIOUR

Two main types of explanation that seem appropriate to illness behaviour may be outlined briefly. One approach that has achieved some popularity represents a situational or structural perspective. The writings of Aday and Andersen (1974) illustrate this approach in their discussion of factors affecting access to health care; such access is, for a variety of reasons, unevenly distributed throughout the population. The model includes predisposing, enabling, and need factors as determinants of response to a health disturbance. Differential access to care is principally a function of the enabling factors, which include the resources available to the person for health care (e.g. money, a regular source of care, transportation and health insurance). To the extent that enabling factors are not present, likelihood of seeking care is diminished. By extension, it can be said that, in the face of a health threat, people will use those services that their resources permit them to obtain.

A second class of explanation relates to the cultural background of the individual. Differences among cultural groups are believed to result in variations in the interpretation of symptoms, in the manner in which symptoms are expressed, and in differential readiness to act on symptoms (Zola, 1973; Jenkins, 1966; Mechanic, 1968). For example, Zola found cultural differences in interpretation and response to symptoms between Americans of Irish and Italian descent. One could similarly use a cultural interpretation in explaining sex differences in illness behaviour (Mechanic, 1972); differences between male and female responses to symptoms are known to become socialized at a relatively early age.

Since culture generally operates on individual behaviour by influencing motivations and perceptions, it is entirely possible that the effects of culture can be specified by a socio-psychological perspective, for example, as illustrated by the Health Belief Model described earlier. Applications of the Health Belief Model to the area of illness behaviour have been reviewed by Kirscht (1974). Kirscht begins by pointing out that, since the Health Belief Model has been rarely utilized as a focus for research on illness behaviour, its applicability must be viewed largely by inference.

Andersen, for example, presents a model in which health beliefs are part of the set of predispositions to use health services, physicians and health insurance, and knowledge of disease (1968). In Health Belief Model terms, these seem to represent a general perception of the value of medical care. Other aspects of the model appear to include something like threat under the concept of "need".

A study of physician ultilization was conducted by Bice and White (1969) using data from interviews in the United States, England and Yugoslavia, and focusing on a two-week period of time. Empirical combination of a set of variables yielded "perceived morbidity", perhaps reflecting threat of a disease, as the best predictor of physician use. Second best was a measure of "tendency to use services", a composite of three items concerning what people said they would do if experiencing a health problem, which appears to measure the perceived value of medical care.

Suchman's work on health orientation (1966) represents a systematic attempt to bring together social-cultural factors and individual beliefs. In Suchman's scheme, the social structure in which a person lives is related to beliefs about medical care. Social structure is classified along a "parochial-cosmopolitan" dimension while health orientation is represented by the dimension of "popular–scientific" point of view. These dimensions are mutually reinforcing. Persons involved in more parochial groups hold more folk beliefs about health, delay in symptom recognition, and tend to attempt self-treatment. Suchman tested this formulation among persons who had experienced a recent serious illness. There was substantial confirmation of Suchman's hypotheses: a "scientific" view of medical care was associated with more concern about symptoms; parochialism appeared to induce more discussion of symptoms with lay persons; and those with popular health beliefs delayed longer before seeking care.

The approach outlined fits rather well with the Health Belief Model, where social factors are seen as affecting beliefs about seriousness and about the value of medical care. Suchman's measure of health orientation includes such dimensions as scepticism regarding medical care and knowledge of disease. Included in the measure of social organization are ethnic exclusivity and traditional family authority, both of which should be related to paths of action that are known and available to the individual.

SICK ROLE BEHAVIOUR

Efforts to describe and explain sick role behaviour have been summarized in a number of works (Becker, 1974b; Sackett and Haynes, 1976; Haynes et al., 1979; Kirscht and Rosenstock, 1979; Becker and Maiman, 1981). Most research aimed at understanding sick role behaviour has yielded an unsystematic multiplicity of findings. Part of the problem can be attributed to reliance on a medical model of patient behaviour that focuses on certain enduring (usually demographic) characteristics of the patient, on the nature of the illness as defined medically, and on characteristics of the regimen.

More generally, sick role behaviour has been viewed in the context of social roles originally set forth by Parsons (1951, 1972), who posited the "sick role" as a construct to account for the rights and obligations of the sick person in the context of American values. Parsons' discussion begins with the notion that the sick person suffers a disturbance of capacity. Once the incapacity is recognized, the individual moves into the sick role; occupants of this role are not held to be responsible for the incapacity since it is viewed as beyond their control, and they are, therefore, exempted from normal social role obligations. However, continued legitimation of the sick role requires that the occupant take every reasonable action toward achieving recovery, including (where appropriate) an obligation to seek technically competent help and to co-operate in the process of getting well.

In a review, Segall (1976) shows that, while Parsons' concept has been widely (and often, uncritically) accepted among medical sociologists, empirical work with the concept has uncovered many difficulties. For example, the model does not appear to account for psychiatric disorders. Also, the chronically-ill patient does not appear to be encompassed well by the sick role; indeed, by definition, chronic illnesses are not "curable" and the requirement on the patient would, therefore, be more one of adjusting to the condition than of trying to get well. Nonetheless, despite these problems, the concept seems to have some self-evident validity..

What are the relationships to sick role behaviours of personal, social, and situational variables? Historically, the search for correlates of adherence has been descriptive rather than explanatory. In many studies, a common aim was to identify groups of non-adherers, often with the hope that identification would solve the problem. For that reason, much of the research was essentially atheoretical.

Haynes' (1976a) review of "determinants" of compliance with medical regimens covered some 185 original research reports on a variety of factors: demographic characteristics of patients; features of the disease, the regimen, and the therapeutic source; aspects of patient–physician interaction; and socio-behavioural characteristics of patients. He concluded that only a few variables have demonstrated consistent relationships with patient adherence. Among these factors (all associated with lower rates of compliance) are: a "psychiatric" diagnosis; the complexity, duration, and amount of change involved in the regimen itself; inconveniences associated with operation of clinics; inadequate supervision by professionals; patient dissatisfaction; "inappropriate health beliefs"; non-compliance with other regimens; and family instability. This summary is noteworthy for what it does not include, that is, the many variables studied that have not yielded consistent relationships with adherence across different situations and regimens, such as demographic factors, personality characteristics, level of knowledge, health status and social norms. Other reviewers have also noted that few associations are found between compliance and ordinary social characteristics of patients, such as age, sex, and education (Becker and

Maiman, 1975; Kasl, 1975). It would appear that a "defaulting" personality does not exist, because personality measures have had little success in predicting compliance, and because measures of different aspects of compliance have, in general, shown relatively low levels of association. Kasl (1975) notes that characteristics of the regimen and the nature of the patient–provider relationship have yielded associations with compliance, although socio-demographic characteristics of patients are not reliable predictors.

Application of the Health Belief Model to sick role behaviour has often yielded positive results. Where an illness has been diagnosed and a course of therapy recommended, the individual's perception of the threat represented by symptoms or by the future course of the condition becomes central. It is in relation to this threat that possible actions and their costs can be evaluated when decisions are made. A recommendation by a health professional becomes one possibility, to be judged by its perceived value for dealing with the threat, and in light of possible barriers to acting.

Becker and Maiman (1975) have reviewed much of the literature on patient adherence from the point of view of the HBM. In examining the relationship between perceived susceptibility and following medical advice, researchers have employed the concepts of "resusceptibility" and "belief in diagnosis," as some diagnosis of illness has already been made. For example, one investigator reported that compliance with a regimen of long-term penicillin prophylaxis by college students with a history of rheumatic fever was greater for those with higher subjective estimates of the likelihood of having another attack (Heinzelman, 1962). Similarly, other researchers have found significant positive associations between a mother's belief in the possibility of her child's contracting rheumatic fever again and compliance, both in administering the penicillin and in clinic attendance (Elling et al., 1960). One study obtained substantial correlations between a mother's compliance with a regimen (penicillin and clinic appointment-keeping) prescribed for the child's acute illness (otitis media) and her feeling that the child was resusceptible to the present illness, her belief in the accuracy of the diagnosis, and her perception that her child was "easily susceptible to disease" (Becker et al., 1972). Similar measures of the susceptibility construct have been shown to be related to compliance with anti-hypertensive regimens (Kirscht and Rosenstock, 1977), a diet regimen for obese children (Becker et al., 1977a), a drug regimen to prevent or control asthma attacks in children (Becker et al., 1978), dietary intake restrictions and medications for patients with end-stage renal disease who are receiving regular hemodialysis (Hartman and Becker, 1978), and mothers' use of over-the-counter medications for their symptomatic children (Maiman et al., 1982).

Although *physicians'* estimates of the severity of an illness are not usually predictive of patient co-operation, the concept of patient-perceived severity has yielded results that are positive and consistent: the level of perceived severity of the condition (either for one's self or one's child) regularly predicts adherence to the regimen (Becker *et al.*, 1972, 1977a, 1978; Charney *et al.*, 1967; Gordis *et al.*, 1969; Hartman and Becker, 1978; Kirscht and Rosenstock, 1977). Unke the situation applying to preventive health actions, a prescribed regimen suggests that a diagnosis of illness has been made, and the patient is either experiencing symptoms or, as in the case of rheumatic fever prophylaxis, has experienced them before. It may, therefore, be that the presence of physical symptoms produces an elevating or "realistic" effect on perceived severity, motivating the patient to follow the physician's instructions as long as indications of illness persist (or to avoid their recurrence). Indeed, patients often state that they stop taking their medicine as soon as they feel better.

As is the case for preventive behaviour, perception of benefits is often shown to be related to patient compliance with medication and other therapies. Several investigators have found belief in the ability of penicillin to prevent recurrence of rheumatic fever to be predictive of adherence to the regimen (Elling *et al.*, 1960; Heinzelmann, 1962). In one study, "belief in the efficacy of clinic medications" predicted regular administration of the prescribed penicillin (Becker *et al.*, 1972); others have shown that subjects with stronger positive beliefs about the value of adherence to their doctor's instructions (in terms of feeling healthier and reducing the chance of future strokes, heart attacks, and kidney problems) were more likely to report medication compliance and to have filled and refilled their prescriptions (Kirscht and Rosenstock, 1977). Finally, several studies obtained significant associations between the patient's faith in the benefits of medical intervention and degree of co-operation with diet and medication therapies (Becker *et al.*, 1977a, 1978; Hartman and Becker, 1978).

Certain perceptions of characteristics of the regimen are fairly consistent predictors of compliance with prescribed therapies. Cost and side effects are usually associated with poor compliance, and the greater the duration of the therapy, the more compliance decreases over time. The degree of behavioural change required is also negatively correlated with patient co-operation, and the general rule is that prescribed actions are easier to obtain than eliminations of proscribed behaviours (Haynes, 1976b). Findings from research employing part or all of the HBM to study sick role behaviours are summarized in Table 2.

Finally, while all of the studies mentioned have assessed (and sometimes tried to alter) the attitudes and beliefs of health care consumers, quite encouraging results are available from research which employed HBM

TABLE 2   Summary of studies using one or more Health Belief Model variables to predict compliance with prescribed medical regimens

Investigator	Behaviour	Susceptibility	Severity	Benefit	Barrier
Elling et al. (1960)	Penicillin	+	NM	+	NM
Heinzelmann (1962)	Penicillin	+	+	+	NM
Bergman and Werner (1963)	Penicillin	NM	NM	NM	0
Charney et al. (1967)	Penicillin	NM	+	NM	NM
Gabrielson et al. (1967)	Follow-up care	NM	+	+	+
Gordis et al. (1969)	Penicillin	−	+	0	NM
Becker et al. (1972)	Penicillin	+	+	+	NM
Kirscht and Rosenstock (1977)	Anti-hypertensive regimens	+	+	+	+
Becker et al. (1977a)	Weight-loss diet	+	+	+	+
Becker et al. (1978)	Asthma medication	+	+	+	+
Hartman and Becker (1978)	Dietary restrictions and medications (hemodialysis patients)	+	+	+	+
Maiman et al. (1982)	Mother-initiated medications for their children	+	NM	+	+

+ = positive findings; − = negative findings; 0 = no association found; NM = not measured.

concepts in an attempt to modify the attitudes and behaviours of *physicians*, in order to achieve improvements in the compliance levels of their patients. In a controlled clinical trial, Inui and associates (Inui et al., 1976) assigned one of two groups of physicians to receive special tutorials (about one to two hours in length), whose content emphasized both compliance difficulties experienced by patients with hypertension and possible strategies (based on the HBM) for altering patient beliefs and behaviours. After only a single session, physicians in the experimental group were observed to spend a greater proportion of clinic visit time on patient teaching, and their patients later exhibited higher levels of knowledge and appropriate beliefs about hypertension and its treatment. Moreover, the patients of tutored physicians were subsequently more compliant with the treatment regimen and demonstrated better blood pressure control.

DROPPING OUT OF TREATMENT

The drop-out phenomenon has not been well studied except in the psychiatric area. Nevertheless, premature withdrawal from treatment is a significant problem in disease control. For example, it is reported that 37 per cent to 50 per cent of tuberculosis patients cease treatment against medical advice (Drolet and Porter, 1949; Wilmer, 1956); with regard to anti-hypertensive therapy, as many as 50% of patients drop out during the first year, most of them during the first two months of treatment (Armstrong et al., 1962; Caldwell et al., 1970).

Why do people discontinue treatment? To begin with, the picture may not be as bleak as the drop-out rates suggest. Baekeland and Lundwall (1975) conclude (in a review of psychiatric literature) that not all drop-outs are lost to treatment, since many of them seek care elsewhere; moreover, some persons may drop out because their health has improved. These reviewers conclude that likelihood of dropping out is also positively related to: social isolation or lack of affiliation; negative therapist attitudes and behaviour; low personal motivation; long waiting time for treatment; low socio-economic status; young age; female sex; and social instability.

It should be emphasized that features of the treatment setting and system of care are clearly involved in the problem of drop-out. Relatively simple changes in the system, such as reminders and provider continuity, have demonstrated notable effects on keeping patients in treatment for alcoholism (Baekeland and Lundwall, 1975). Similarly, modification of clinic procedures toward more personalized, convenient care has proved valuable in reducing drop-out among hypertensive patients (Finnerty et al., 1973a; Steckel and Swain, 1977). Finally, in a review of the drop-out and broken-appointment problem in general adult clinics, Deyo and Inui (1980) conclude that most successful interventions have concentrated on features of clinic organization (e.g. individual time appointment systems, specific physician assignment, mailed prospective reminders, access to physician by telephone, elimination of pharmacy delays) and on interactions between patient and provider (e.g. educational efforts aimed at conveying knowledge of disease, its therapy and the importance of continuing care; modifying health beliefs; eliciting and discussing reasons for previously missed appointments).

It has long been known that many clients referred by one agency for care at another never complete these referrals. For example, Levine et al., (1969) have shown that most children referred to child guidance clinics for service fail to obtain service at those clinics. Cauffman and others (1974) have probed this problem and emerged with some surprising findings. The overall aim of their project was to develop and implement an on-line computer system for making referrals for health care throughout the Los Angeles area, using a comprehensive health service data bank to which health workers in various agencies would be linked by terminal devices. Thirteen diverse agencies in the East Los Angeles Health District participated in a feasibility study of the system. Over the study period, data were collected on a total of 471 consumers, each with a single referral. It was found that over 40 per cent of consumers referred for care did not receive care; some of these appeared for care but did not receive it, perhaps for good medical reasons, but 34 per cent of the total group did not even appear at the care facility.

Only two factors studied showed significant relationships to referral follow-through: whether the consumer was given a specific appointment with a provider, and whether the consumer was given the name of a person to see at the provider's office. Those consumers given specific appointments and/or a named person to contact were more likely to show than were other consumers.

These findings are reasonable, and the action implications seem obvious. Of greater theoretical importance are those factors that did not distinguish shows from no-shows. These included sex, age, type of health problem, convenience problems (including transportation, language, child care, parking), financial difficulties, time interval between referral and appointment, distance from care, and type of provider. Some of the "non-findings" are surprising, especially those concerning convenience problems in obtaining care. It is clear that referral failures are widespread, and it it likely that the rate of no-shows could be reduced by giving clients specific appointments with named providers.

PROVIDING INFORMATION AND MODIFYING BELIEFS

It was noted earlier that the relationship of knowledge to adherence is not clear because the concept of knowledge has been used to cover too broad a range of information. On the one hand, provision of information about the nature of illness and its treatment, at a fairly abstract level, has generally not increased compliance with medical recommendations. Sackett et al. (1975) and Kirscht and Rosenstock (1979) informed hypertensive patients about their condition, both studies utilizing control groups that did not receive the information. While there was increased knowledge among those who were informed, there was no subsequent effect either on compliance or on blood pressure levels. Tagliacozzo et al. (1974) looked at the effects of special nurse instruction on patients with chronic diseases attending an out-patient clinic (a control group received the regular care procedures). The intervention was formally structured to cover specific information about diseases and treatment. In terms of *main* effects on staying in treatment, following medical advice, or even changing attitudes, there was little impact. However, some *interaction* effects occurred: compliance was increased among those with more knowledge of illness, multiple illnesses, high anxiety, favourable attitudes toward the clinic and those who felt their illness was serious.

Under some conditions, then, provision of information may influence compliance. In a well-controlled experiment with randomly assigned experimental and control groups, Haefner and Kirscht (1970) were able to increase perceived threat of illness (susceptibility and severity), as well as perception of benefits of following professional health advice; such belief changes led to a statistically significant increase in the number of subsequent visits to the doctor for check-ups, in the absence of symptoms. To take another example, Becker and others (1977b) studied the effects of communications on obese children attending a weight control clinic. Mothers of these patients were randomly assigned to one of three groups: a high-threat communication condition, a low-threat communication, and a non-communication control. Following an initial visit to the clinic, the messages were delivered orally in a standardized format, followed by receipt of a reinforcing booklet. Each patient then received dietary counselling and reappointments to the clinic. The groups receiving either of the communications lost significantly more weight than did the controls, through four follow-up visits, and the group receiving the high-threat message lost more weight than did the one receiving the low-threat version. Initial health beliefs regarding health threats, the child's susceptibility to illness, and the benefits of weight loss were predictive of subsequent success in reducing weight. In this instance, providing "persuasive" information resulted in better adherence to the diet.

Information intended specifically to inform patients about their regimen can also increase compliance. McKenney and associates (1973) selected fifty hypertensive patients of whom half met monthly with the pharmacist while the other half continued with the usual level of care. The pharmacist meetings included discussion of medications and counselling regarding treatment. Members of the intervention group significantly increased their knowledge and subsequent regimen compliance, and exhibited better blood pressure control.

The foregoing examples support the view that, if patients know more about their disease and its treatment, they will sometimes comply more readily with drug dosage (Sackett et al., 1978) and scheduling regimens (Hulka et al., 1975). Variability in the effects of patients' knowledge on compliance may be attributed to several factors: (i) knowledge about particular details of the prescribed therapy is essential for correct compliance; (ii) patients frequently do not possess all the information they need to follow the regimen; but (iii), as indicated earlier, providing the necessary information to the patient does not, in itself, ensure subsequent co-operation.

The first two factors were studied (Svarstad, 1976) in clients of a health centre serving a low-income population. About 50% of these patients could not correctly report how long they were supposed to continue taking their medications, 26% did not know the dosage prescribed, 17% could not report the prescribed frequency for taking their medications, 16% thought that their drugs marked "p.r.n." were to be taken regularly, and 23% could not identify the purpose of each drug they were taking. When these conditions were examined in relation to compliance, it was found that about 70% of those who correctly understood their physician's instructions were adhering to their regimens, but only about 15% of patients complied if they made one or more mistakes in reporting facts about the regimen. In this study, the investigator also rated each doctor–patient encounter for clarity of oral or written instructions about the regimen. Of those patients receiving clear instructions, 62% understood and 54% complied. Of those patients who received confusing instructions, 40% understood and only about 30% complied. Clearly, it is important for physician instructions about a drug regimen to go beyond exposition and achieve communication.

Other studies have shown that the aspect of medical care about which patients express the greatest dissatisfaction is the amount and form of information they receive from their physicians (McKinlay, 1972). Medical terms are often misunderstood by the patient. One study (Francis et al., 1969) found that patients thought "lumbar puncture" meant draining the lungs, "incubation period" was interpreted as an instruction to the patient to stay in bed, and terms such as "work-up" and "history" were found to have no medical meaning to many patients.

The third factor mentioned above is addressed in a study (Johannsen et al., 1966) of patients with chronic conditions who were treated at a large urban hospital out-patient clinic. For patients with considerable disease experience, there was no association between knowledge and compliance with appointments to return to the clinic; however, such association was substantially significant for patients with little prior disease experience and for those whose clinic visits were hampered by social factors. Thus, for individuals who are motivated to comply, but who are ignorant of the correct procedures, the provision of information should be beneficial; however, for already-knowledgeable, but insufficiently-motivated patients, additional information about the regimen is unlikely to enhance compliance.

A good start toward acceptable compliance is physician instructions based on these points: (i) patients remember best the first instructions presented; (ii) instructions that are emphasized are also better recalled; (iii) the fewer the instructions given, the greater will be the proportion remembered (Podell, 1975). When new or complex information is offered, the physician may wish to evaluate comprehension by requesting the patient to repeat essential elements of the message, particularly the specific actions required by the treatment plan. As many as one-half of the physician's statements are forgotten by the patient almost immediately; therefore, written instructions should be provided whenever possible in order to reinforce the oral communication.

IMPROVING WAYS OF PROVIDING CARE

Changes introduced into the system of care may enhance compliance, if they provide increased support and clearer expectations for a patient. Finnerty and others (1973b) modified clinic procedures, including definite appointments, better monitoring and more sensitivity to patients' needs, that led to dramatic reduction in drop-out. Wilber and Barrow's (1972) utilization of home visits by a nurse resulted in greater compliance and better management of blood pressure.

Two experimental tests of the benefits of continuity of care, both conducted in paediatric settings, yielded different conclusions. Gordis and Markowitz (1971) studied a continuous care system set up for a randomly assigned group of children who received penicillin prophylaxis for rheumatic fever. Continuous care was provided by two paediatricians who handled all medical problems of the children. Children in a control group were given the usual clinic care, being seen by different physicians at each visit. When compliance with the penicillin regimen was assessed over 15 months (through collection of periodic urine samples taken on a random schedule), no differences between the groups were found. The second study (Becker et al., 1974) involved setting up two areas in a large paediatric care centre: one featured assignment of families to particular physicians, the other comprised the usual clinic arrangement with rotating staff and sub-clinics. Families were randomly assigned to the continuous or the discontinuous system. After a year, the continuous care system was shown to yield significantly greater appointment-keeping compliance and satisfaction on the part of patients, as well as greater staff satisfaction with both work situation and with patients.

As indicated earlier, compliance is reduced when the regimen requires an alteration of the patient's life-style, or is (i) complex, (ii) of long duration, (iii) inconvenient, or (iv) expensive (Haynes, 1976b; Johannsen et al., 1966; Podell, 1975; Kirscht and Rosenstock, 1977). Regimens can be made simpler by minimizing the number of different medications, the number of doses, and variations in scheduling. Ways to do this include using preparations that combine several drugs or drug actions, giving larger and less frequent doses, and prescribing drugs or preparations with more sustained action. However, Weintraub (1976) cautions that these methods are not without danger, especially for the patient who is capriciously compliant. Large-dose tablets may increase the frequency of accidental and suicidal overdoses, and serious therapeutic consequences may result from missing a single dose if the one omitted during a day is the only one prescribed. The physician may also work toward synchronizing the taking of several medications and avoid routine prescription of additional non-essential medicines (such as vitamins and tranquilizers) that may add considerably to the overall complexity of the total regimen.

Shorter term therapy, or at least the perception of it, can be accomplished by scheduling follow-up visits in quick succession when progress can be demonstrated, thus providing the patient with a feeling of accomplishment and a sense of the treatment's importance. If life-style must be altered (e.g. because of diet, exercise, or abstinence from smoking), these changes should be introduced over the course of several or many visits, taking the behaviours one at a time, reinforcing whatever compliance is achieved, and only then adding the next objective. (Matthews and Hingson, 1977.) Inconvenience can be minimized by matching the medication schedule to the patient's regular daily activities; this will also make pill-taking easier to remember (Sackett *et al.*, 1978).

IMPROVING THE DOCTOR–PATIENT RELATIONSHIP

It is in the crucial communication between doctor and patient that the patient develops an understanding of the disease and its treatment (Stiles *et al.*, 1979); patient satisfaction and compliance are two outcomes with clearly-documented relationships to this verbal exchange (Francis *et al.*, 1969).

Coe and Wessen (1965) have suggested that numerous aspects of the physician–patient interaction, such as impersonality and brevity of encounter, negatively affect patient behaviour, and more-recent reviews support their conclusion (Becker and Maiman, 1975). Lack of communication, particularly communication of an emotional nature, is usually seen as the problem. Davis (1968) found that particular communication patterns are associated wth patients' failure to comply with doctors' advice. Such patterns include circumstances in which tension in the interaction is not released and in which the physician is formal, rejecting, or controlling, disagrees completely with the patient, or interviews the patient at length without later providing feedback. Francis and others (1969) report that a mother's compliance with a regimen prescribed for her child is better when she is satisfied with the initial contact, regards the physician as friendly, and feels that the doctor understood the complaint. Further, they found that key factors in non-compliance included the extent to which patients' expectations from the medical visit were left unmet, lack of warmth in the doctor–patient relationship, and failure to receive an explanation of diagnosis and cause of the child's illness.

Many other investigations have also shown positive correlations between compliance and patient satisfaction with the visit, the therapist, or the clinic, including perceptions of convenience and of waiting times before and during appointments (Becker and Maiman, 1975). Compliance is greater when patients feel their expectations have been fulfilled, when the physician elicits and respects patients' concerns and provides responsive information about their condition and progress, and when sincere concern and sympathy are shown.

A relatively recent development, that attempts to capitalize on (and in some ways improve) the relationship between provider and patient, is the "therapeutic contract". Both parties set forth a treatment goal, the specific obligations of each part in attempting that goal, and a time limit for its achievement. Lewis and Michnich (1977) argue that, as a compliance-enhancing intervention, the contract is supposed to work by clarifying and making explicit relative responsibilities of both provider and consumer in achieving an agreed-upon goal and by transferring some power from provider to consumer. Available data support the provider–client contract as a tool for increasing the likelihood of patient compliance (Steckel and Swain, 1977; Cummings *et al.*, 1981).

SUPERVISION AND SOCIAL SUPPORT

Hospitalized patients exhibit better compliance than day-patients, who, in turn, are more compliant than out-patients. A variety of before-and-after studies have demonstrated increased patient co-operation when frequency of out-patient visits is increased, home visits are added, patients receive negative feedback about non-compliance, and there is continuity of care (Haynes, 1976b). There are ways to extend supervision beyond the time the patient spends at the office or health facility; these include reminder calls about the regimen and/or the follow-up visit, and instructions that the patient keep a record of which pills were taken each day and at what time.

Social support seems to be important in long-term treatment plans that require continuous action on the part of the patient (Davis, 1968; Caplan *et al.*, 1976). For example, studies of weight control have shown that those persons who received assistance from another family member in cueing or in reinforcement of proper eating behaviour were more likely to lose weight and to maintain their weight loss (Stuart and Davis, 1972). Similar outcomes have been described for the family's influence on compliance in taking medications (Willcox *et al.*, 1965). A family's own health beliefs and its evaluation of the patient's illness and treatment may influence adherence, and compliance may also be altered if the family assumes responsibility for the sick member's care and provides sympathy, support, and encouragement. Success is greatest when the family's normal roles and patterns are compatible with the illness of the patient, or when the family members are willing to make accommodating changes in their lives and in the family environment (Becker and Green, 1975).

MEASURING COMPLIANCE

Compliance is far from being a uni-dimensional concept; it generally includes a wide array of different behaviours. Health recommendations may range from such relatively simple, one-time actions as obtaining an immunization to permanent modifications in life-long habits. The differences in behavioural complexity among different regimens must be considered in attempting to understand and explain compliance. Consider the range and diversity of behaviours that are often prescribed for the newly-diagnosed hypertensive: taking medication daily; losing weight and maintaining that weight loss; reducing sodium intake; smoking cessation; reducing alcohol consumption; initiating an exercise programme; returning regularly to the physician; and so forth. These are very diverse behaviours, with different determinants, requiring different sets of knowledge, motivations, and skills. It has been shown that an individual's compliance with different elements of a regimen may vary considerably (see Hartman and Becker, 1978; Kirscht *et al.*, 1981).

Patient non-compliance can be manifested in a variety of behaviour patterns; for example: not undertaking recommended diagnostic actions or habits (e.g. not obtaining regular check-ups or having blood pressure assessed annually, not learning or performing self-examination procedures); delay in seeking care for symptoms of illness; failure to keep follow-up appointments or to complete a recommended referral to another provider or to a laboratory for diagnostic work; not filling a prescription; not taking prescribed medication (at all, or as instructed).

ASSESSMENT PROBLEMS

An important issue in the study of compliance with professional recommendations is measuring the behaviours involved. Relatively simple to measure are those behaviours which are formally recorded; thus, assessment of appointment keeping or of immunizations obtained is fairly straightforward (although these visits and services are not always recorded). However, the many behaviours (usually private) that are not subject to regular entry in medical records pose measurement problems of greater magnitude.

There is a considerable literature on assessment of medication behaviour (Gordis, 1976). Measures vary in their apparent validity and directness. Ideally, we would like to observe directly the extent to which patients consume prescribed drugs; because that is generally not possible, investigators have utilized pill counts or looked for traces of drugs in blood or urine tests. Pill counts are not easy to perform, and pose a series of problems. For example, medications are not always kept in their original containers, supplies are divided up and containers are not returned on request. Moreover, frankly-acknowledged pill counting may cause patients to dissemble. Physiological assessments have advantages, but they are often costly, and may also alter behaviour if patients know they are being tested. In addition, because of individual differences, variation occurs in blood level of a drug even under conditions of perfect compliance, and there may be problems relative to how long an indicator will be present.

Many investigators rely on the patient's own description of his/her compliance behaviours. Although self-report may yield over-estimates of adherence to recommendations (Gordis et al., 1969), many studies of medication adherence which have compared self-report with other methods of assessment have yielded high intercorrelations (Feinstein et al., 1959; Francis et al., 1969; Becker et al., 1972; Becker et al., 1978). Sackett and his colleagues found that a non-threatening clinical interview was 90 per cent predictive of non-compliance in a group of hypertensive patients (1978). Many types of behaviour related to health recommendations are quite difficult to measure except through asking questions; for example, eating behaviour, physical activity, occurrence of symptoms, alcohol consumption and smoking.

Yet another difficulty is introduced by the fact that investigators employ widely-differing definitions of "compliance". In studies initiated by clinicians, non-compliance is often established as the point below which the desired preventive or therapeutic results are likely to be achieved. At the other end of the scale, behavioural scientists (who are seeking to understand why a patient is not following advice) are apt to view as non-compliance any notable deviation from the prescribed course of therapy, even if such deviation has no clinical effect. Some researchers have divided their study populations into "compliers" and "non-compliers" on purely statistical bases (e.g. persons falling above and below median or mean levels of adherence in that group), thereby ignoring both biological *and* behavioural considerations; and others have selected arbitrary cut-points (e.g. because some level of non-compliance seemed "intolerable" or "significant" to the investigator, or because that level was employed in previous research).

With such enormous possibility for variation in non-compliance behaviour and its assessment, it is hardly surprising that seemingly conflicting findings abound. These problems also point up the dangers inherent in attempting to summarize the vast compliance literature in order to derive general "principles" of compliance determinants and strategies across studies of different illnesses, regimens, compliance measures, and patient populations.

THE CONSUMER'S "RIGHT" TO NON-COMPLIANCE

"Intelligent non-compliance" describes the situation wherein a prescribed mediation is purposely not taken and the patient's reason for non-compliance appears valid when analysed dispassionately (Weintraub, 1976). Some examples of circumstances in which the non-compliant patient is better off include: (i) mis-diagnosis or inappropriate prescribing; (ii) the patient experiences substantial adverse reactions or side-effects; and (iii) when patients with long-term conditions become aware that they or their disease has changed in such a way as to obviate the need for continuance of the prescribed therapy. Physicians rarely attempt to monitor their patients' compliance behaviour and often do not re-evaluate the need for continued therapy (particularly for chronic conditions).

Related to the concept of intelligent non-compliance are the many current efforts to alter the traditional view of the doctor–patient relationship (in which the obedient patient is the passive recipient of prescribed instructions) to one in which "patients have expectations of the doctor, evaluate the doctor's actions, and are able to make their own treatment decisions" (Stimson, 1974). Researchers supporting this approach contend that such terms as "failure to co-operate," "doctor's orders," "instructions," "defaulting," "disobedience" and even the widely used term "compliance" help to perpetuate an atmosphere of expectation in which the dictatorial physician gives orders to the submissive patient. Frequently-proposed alternative language includes "adherence", "drug omissions" and "therapeutic alliance". The patient-provider contracts described earlier are a step in the direction of achieving consensual regimens.

Education about health may be regarded as having two components: information necessary to make appropriate decisions, and behavioural skills necessary to act on that information. Health professionals have not only the right, but also the obligation to provide information to an uninformed client or public and to make a responsible effort to provide it in a manner that assures it will be received and understood. Then, for the motivated clients or population who wish to act on the knowledge, the professional would seem to have the further obligation to give instruction in those behavioural skills necessary to satisfy those motives. To illustrate, the coronary patient (or general public) may not be fully aware of the relationship between cigarette smoking and heart disease. It becomes an obligation of the health sciences to educate both patients and the public on that matter. Then, for cigarette smokers who wish to cut down smoking or give it up entirely, it is a further responsibility of the professional to assist them in doing so, using whatever ethical means the state of the art offers.

SUMMARY AND CONCLUSIONS

It has been observed that the number of reviews of the compliance literature now exceeds the number of original studies done on this topic; and the number of original studies is considerable. With the plethora of papers and books summarizing new research and reviewing old, it is not surprising to discover a diversity of findings. Moreover, when one looks at preventive health behaviour in contrast with sick role behaviour, somewhat different relationships emerge between adherence and psychosocial factors. Among the strongest associations with both preventive and curative recommendations are certain psychological dispositons, particularly components of the Health Belief Model. Generally speaking, beliefs about threat to health (perceived susceptibility to, and severity of, illness) and about the efficacy or benefits of recommended preventive or curative actions are strongly associated with following professional health recommendations. Similarly, knowledge of nature and rationale of the specific recommendations that are made are associated with increased co-operation. Persons who receive meaningful social support and who demonstrate substantial stability of their primary social groups are also more likely than their opposite numbers to undertake suggested health practices.

The associations described generally apply across both treatment and preventive actions. If we look at preventive health behaviours alone, several additional associations are generally observed. Females are more likely than males to participate in preventive health actions, as are persons of higher education and income.

Returning to compliance with therapeutic regimens, having a personal, continuous source of care and supportive interactions with a provider are associated with adherence to treatment recommendations. The occurrence of disabling symptoms is a strong predictor of seeking and following medical advice. Various aspects of the recommended action are associated with compliance. The more complex the recommended action, the longer the duration of time required for treatment and the more the regimen interferes with other personal behaviours, the less complete will be compliance with the regimen.

While there is interest in factors that are positively associated with adherence, it is equally important to review those variables which generally (and perhaps surprisingly) show little or no consistent relationship with following health recommendations for the treatment of disease. For example, socio-demographic characteristics, such as age, sex, education, and income, evidence no consistent relationships with adherence to treatment. General knowledge about health and illness, intelligence, locus of control, and general satisfaction with the health system are also not consistently related to compliance.

Research on intervention strategies to modify health-related behaviour, particularly complex behaviour, is at a fairly early stage of development. However, the provision of relevant and appropriate information about the particulars and logic of the regimen does appear to increase compliance. Moreover, there is evidence that increasing the perceived threat of illness, as well as the perceived benefits of the suggested course of action, also increases compliance, both with preventive and treatment recommendations. There is also evidence that improving ways of providing care will enhance compliance; this includes setting definite appointments, maintaining better continuity of monitoring for adherence (as well as providing continuity in general) and using home visits by a nurse. Modifications in the ways of providing care that will simplify procedures are likely to increase compliance, including minimizing the number of different medications and doses, introducing complex changes a little at a time, and matching regimen schedules to the patient's regular daily activities.

The use of the therapeutic contract is gaining increasing support as a procedure for increasing compliance. Whether this is effective because it provides for reinforcement of a series of achievable goals or because it transfers some power from the provider to the client, what is important for the practitioner is that such contracts appear to work. Finally, the use of social support from significant others, usually family members, has been shown to improve compliance with medical regimens.

There is now available a great deal of descriptive and explanatory material concerning the correlates of non-compliance, both with preventive and treatment regimens. Work on strategies for enhancing compliance is of much more recent origin, but has yielded promising results. We strongly recommend the launching of demonstrations based on sound theoretical considerations that will provide further confirmation of the effectiveness of various change strategies across a variety of health conditions, recommended health actions, and client populations.

REFERENCES

Aday, L. A. and Andersen, R. (1974). A framework for the study of access to medical care. *Health Services Res.* **9**, 208–220.

Andersen, R. (1968). "A behavioural model of families' use of health services". Research series No. 25. Center for Health Administration Studies, University of Chicago, Chicago.

Antonovsky, A. and Hartman, H. (1974). Delay in the detection of cancer: a review of the literature. *Health Educ. Monogr.* **2**, 98–125.

Armstrong, M. L., Bakke, J. L., Dodge, H., Conrad, L. L., Freis, E. D., Fremont, R. E., Kirkendall, W. M., Pilz, C. G., Ramirez, E. A., Richardson, D. W. and Williams, J. H., Jr, (1962). Double blind control study of hypertensive agents. *Arch. Int. Med.* **110**, 222–237.

Baekeland, F. and Lundwall, L. (1975). Dropping out of treatment: a critical review. *Psychol. Bull.* **82**, 738–783.

Becker, M. H. (ed.), (1974a). The health belief model and personal health behavior. *Health Educ. Monogr.* 2(4), 324–508.

Becker, M. H. (1974b). The Health Belief Model and sick role behavior. *Health Educ. Monogr.* 2(4), 409–419.

Becker, M. H. and Green, L. W. (1975). A family approach to compliance with medical treatment: a selective review of the literature. *Int. J. Health Educ.* **18**, 173–182.

Becker, M. H. and Maiman, L. A. (1975). Sociobehavioral determinants of compliance with health and medical care recommendations. *Med. Care* 13(1), 10–24.

Becker, M. H. and Maiman, L. A. (1980). Strategies for enhancing patient compliance. *J. Comm. Health.* 6(2), 113–135.

Becker, M. H. and Maiman, L. A. (1981). Patient compliance. *In* "Drug Therapeutics: Concepts for Physicians" (K. L. Melmon, ed.) pp. 65–79. Elsevier, New York.

Becker, M. H., Drachman, R. H. and Kirscht, J. P. (1972). Predicting mothers' compliance with pediatric medical regimens. *J. Pediatri.* 81(4), 843–854.

Becker, M. H., Drachman, R. H. and Kirscht, J. P. (1974). A field experiment to evaluate various outcomes of continuity of physician care. *Am. J. Pub. Health* 64(11), 1062–1070.

Becker, M. H., Kaback, M., Rosenstock, I. M. and Ruth, M. (1975). Some influences of public participation in a genetic screening program. *J. Comm. Health* **1**, 3–14.

Becker, M. H., Maiman, L. A., Kirscht, J. P., Haefner, D. P. and Drachman, R. H. (1977a). The health belief model and dietary compliance: a field experiment. *J. Health Soc. Behav.* 18, 348–366.

Becker, M. H., Nathanson, C. A., Drachman, R. H. and Kirscht, J. P. (1977b). Mothers' health beliefs and children's clinic visits: a prospective study. *J. Comm. Health* 3, 125–135.

Becker, M. H., Radius, S. M., Rosenstock, I. M., Drachman, R. H., Schuberth, K. C. and Teets, K. C. (1978). Compliance with a medical regimen for asthma: a test of the health belief model. *Pub. Health Rep.* **93**, 268–277.

Bergman, A. B. and Werner, R. J. (1963). Failure of children to receive penicillin by mouth. *New Engl. J. Med.* **268**, 1334–1338.

Bice, T. W. and White, K. L. (1969). Factors related to the use of health services: an international comparative study. *Med. Care* **7**, 124–133.

Blackwell, B., Griffin, B., Magill, M. and Bencze, R. (1978). Teaching medical students about treatment compliance. *J. Med. Educ.* **53**, 672–675.

Caldwell, J., Cobb, S., Dowling, M. D. and Jongh, D. D. (1970). The dropout problem in antihypertensive therapy. *J. Chron. Dis.* **22**, 579–592.

Campbell, D. A. (1971). A study of the preventive health behaviour of a group of men with increased risk for the development of coronary heart disease. Ph. D. dissertation, Ohio State University.

Caplan, R., Robinson, E. A. R., French, J. R. P., Jr., Caldwell, J. R. and Shinn, M. (1976). "Adhering to medical regimens". Ann Arbor, Institute for Social Research, University of Michigan.

Caron, H. W. and Roth, H. P. (1968). Patients' cooperation with a medical regimen. *J. Am. Med. Assoc.* **203**, 922–926.

Cauffman, J. G., Lloyd, J. S., Lyons, M. L., Cortese, P. A., Beckwith, R. L., Petit, D. W., Wehrle, P. F., McBroom, E. and McIntire, J. R. (1974). A study of health referral patterns. *Am. J. Pub. Health* **64**, 331–356.

Chapin, C. V. (1915). Truth in publicity. *Am. J. Pub. Health* **5**(6), 493–502.

Charney, E., Bynum, R., Eldredge, D., MacWhinney, J. B., McNabb, N., Scheiner, A., Sumpter, E. A. and Iker, H. (1967). How well do patients take oral penicillin? A collaborative study in private practice. *Pediatrics* **40**, 188–195.

Clements, J. and Wakefield, J. (1972). Symptoms and uncertainty. *Int. J. Health Educ.* **15**(2), 113–122.

Coe, R. M. and Wessen, A. (1965). Social-psychological factors influencing the use of community health resources. *Am. J. Pub. Health* **55**, 1024–1031.

Cummings, K. M., Jette, R. P. T., Brock, B. M. and Haefner, D. P. (1979). Psychosocial determinants of immunization behavior in a swine influenza campaign. *Med. Care* **17**, 639–649.

Cummings, K. M., Becker, M. H. and Maile, M. C. (1980). Bringing the models together: an empirical approach to combining variables used to explain health actions. *J. Behav. Med.* **3**, 123–145.

Cummings, K. M., Becker, M. H., Kirscht, J. P. and Levin, N. (1981). Intervention strategies to improve compliance with medical regimens by ambulatory hemodialysis patients. *J. Behav. Med.* **4**, 111–127.

Cushing, H. (1925). "Life of Sir William Osler" Vol. 1, The Clarendon Press, Oxford, p. 616.

Davis, M. S. (1966). Variations in patients compliance with doctors' orders: analysis of congruence between survey responses and results of empirical investigations. *J. Med. Educ.* **41**, 1037–1048.

Davis, M. S. (1968). Variations in patients' compliance with doctors' advice: an empirical analysis of patterns of communication. *Am. J. Pub. Health* **58**, 274–288.

Deyo, R. A. and Inui, S. (1980). Dropouts and broken appointments: a literature review and agenda for future research. *Med. Care* **18**, 1146–1157.

D'Onofrio, C. A. (1973). Motivational and promotional factors associated with acceptance of a contraceptive method in the postpartum period. Ph. D. dissertation, University of California, Berkeley.

Drolet, G. and Porter, D. (1949). "Why Patients in Tuberculosis Hospitals Leave Against Medical Advice." New York Tuberculosis and Health Association, New York.

Elling, R., Whittemore, R. and Green, M. (1960). Patient participation in a pediatric program. *J. Health Hum. Behav.* **1,** 183–191.

Feinstein, A., Wood, H. F., Epstein, J. A., Taranta, A., Simpson, R. and Tursky, E. (1959). A controlled study of three methods of prophylaxis against streptococcal infection in a population of rheumatic children: II. Results of the first three years of the study, including methods for evaluating the maintenance of oral prophylaxis. *New Eng. J. Med.* **260,** 697–702.

Fink, R., Shapiro, S. and Roeser, R. (1972). Impacts of efforts to increase participation in repetitive screenings for early breast cancer detection. *Am. J. Pub. Health* **62,** 328–336.

Finnerty, F. A., Jr., Mattie, E. and Finnerty, F. A., III (1973a). Hypertension in the inner city: I. Analysis of clinic dropouts. *Circulation* **47,** 73–75.

Finnerty, F. A., Jr., Shaw, L. and Himmelsbach, C. (1973b). Hypertension in the inner city: II. Detection and follow-up. *Circulation* **47,** 76–78.

Flach, B. (1960). "Participation in Case Finding Programs for Cervical Cancer" Administrative Report, Cancer Control Program, United States Public Health Service. Government Printing Office, Washington, D.C.

Francis, W., Korsch, B. M. and Morris, M. J. (1969). Gaps in doctor–patient communication: patient's response to medical advice. *New Engl. J. Med.* **280,** 535–540.

Gabrielson, I. W., Levin, L. A. and Ellinson, M. D. (1967). Factors affecting school health follow-up. *Am. J. Pub. Health* **57,** 48–59.

Gordis, L. (1976). Methodologic issues in the measurement of patient compliance. *In* "Compliance with Therapeutic Regimens" (D. L. Sackett and R. B. Haynes, eds), pp. 51–66. Johns Hopkins University Press, Baltimore.

Gordis, L. and Markowitz, M. (1971). Evaluation of the effectiveness of comprehensive and continuous pediatric care. *Pediatrics* **48,** 766–776.

Gordis, L., Markowitz, M. and Lilienfeld, A. (1969). The inaccuracy of using interviews to estimate patient reliability in taking medications at home. *Med. Care* **7,** 49–54.

Green, L. W. and Roberts, B. J. (1974). The research literature on why women delay in seeking medical care for breast symptoms. *Health Educ. Monogr.* **2,** 129–177.

Haefner, D. and Kirscht, J. P. (1970). Motivational and behavioral effects of modifying health beliefs. *Pub. Health Rep.* **85,** 478–484.

Haefner, D., Kegeles, S. S., Kirscht, J. P. and Rosenstock, I. M. (1967). Preventive actions concerning dental disease, tuberculosis, and cancer. *Pub. Health. Rep.* **82,** 451–459.

Hartman, P. E. and Becker, M. H. (1978). Noncompliance with prescribed regimen among chronic hemodialysis patients: a method of prediction and educational diagnosis. *Dialysis and Transplantation* **7,** 978–989.

Haynes, R. B. (1976a). A critical review of the "determinants" of patient compliance with therapeutic regimens. *In* "Compliance with Therapeutic Regimens" (D. L. Sackett and R. B. Haynes, eds), pp. 26–39. Johns Hopkins Unversity Press, Baltimore.

Haynes, R. B. (1976b). Strategies for improving compliance: a methodologic analysis and review. In "Compliance with Therapeutic Regimens" (D. L. Sackett and R. B. Haynes, eds), pp. 69–82. Johns Hopkins University Press, Baltimore.

Haynes, R. B., Taylor, D. W. and Sackett, D. L. (eds), (1979). "Compliance in Health Care." Johns Hopkins University Press, Baltimore.

Heinzelmann, F. (1962). Determinants of prophylaxis behavior with respect to rheumatic fever. J. Health Hum. Behav. **3**, 73–81.

Heinzelmann, F. and Bagley, R. W. (1970). Response to physical activity programs and their effects on health behavior. Pub. Health Rep. **85**, 905–911.

Hochbaum, G. M. (1956). Why people seek diagnostic x-rays. Pub. Health Rep. **71**, 377–380.

Hochbaum, G. M. (1958). "Public Participation in Medical Screening Programs: A Socio-Psychological Study", Public Health Service Publication 572. Government Printing Office, Washington, D.C.

Hulka, B. S., Kupper, L. L., Cassel, J. C. and Efird, R. L. (1975). Medication use and misuse: physician-patient discrepancies. J. Chron. Dis. **38**, 7–21.

Inui, T. S., Yourtee, E. L. and Williamson, J. W. (1976). Improved outcomes in hypertension after physician tutorials: a controlled trial. Ann. Intern. Med. **84**, 646–651.

Jenkins, C. D. (1966). Group differences in perception: a study of community beliefs and feelings about tuberculosis. Am. J. Soc. **71**, 417–429.

Johannsen, W., Helimuth, G. and Sorauf, T. (1966). On accepting medical recommendations. Arch. Environ. Health **12**, 63–69.

Kalmer, H. (ed.), (1974). Reviews of research and studies related to delay in seeking diagnosis of cancer. Health Educ. Mongr. **2** (whole No. 2).

Kasl, S. V. (1975). Social-psychological characteristics associated with behaviors which reduce cardiovascular risk. In "Applying Behavioral Science to Cardiovascular Risk" (A. J. Enelow and J. B. Henderson, eds). American Heart Association, New York.

Kasl, S. V. and Cobb, S. (1966). Health behavior, illness behavior, and sick role behavior. Arch. Environ. Health **12**, 246–266 and 531–541.

Kegeles, S. S. (1963a). Some motives for seeking preventive dental care. J. Am. Dent. Ass. **67**, 90–98.

Kegeles, S. S. (1963b). Why people seek dental care: a test of a conceptual formulation. J. Health Hum. Behav. **4**, 166–173.

Kegeles, S. S. (1969). A field experiment attempt to change beliefs and behavior of women in an urban ghetto. J. Health Soc. Behav. **10**, 115–124.

Kelly, P. T. (1979). Breast self-examinations: who does them and why. J. Behav. Med. **2**, 31–38.

Kirscht, J. P. (1974). The health belief model and illness behavior. Health Educ. Monogr. **2**(4), 387–408.

Kirscht, J. P. and Rosenstock, I. M. (1977). Patient adherence to antihypertensive medical regimens. J. Comm. Health **3**, 115–124.

Kirscht, J. P. and Rosenstock, I. M. (1979). Patients' problems in following recommendations of health experts. In "Health Psychology" (G. Stone, F. Cohen and N. E. Adler, eds), pp. 189–215. Jossey-Bass, San Francisco.

Kirscht, J. P., Haefner, D. P., Kegeles, S. and Rosenstock, I. M. (1966). A national study of health beliefs. J. Health Hum. Behav. **7**, 248–254.

Kirscht, J. P., Kirscht, J. L. and Rosenstock, I. M. (1981). A test of interventions to increase adherence to hypertensive medical regimens. Health Educ. Q. **8**(3), 261–272.

Langlie, J. (1977). Social networks, health beliefs, and preventive health behavior. *J. Health Soc. Behav.* **18**, 244–260.

Leventhal, H. Hochbaum, G. and Rosenstock, I. (1960). Epidemic impact on the general population in two cities. *In* "The Impact of Asian Influenza on Community Life: A study in Five Cities" DHEW, PHS, Publication No. 766. U.S. Government Printing Office, Washington D.C.

Levine, S., Scotch, N. A. and Vlasak, G. J. (1969). Unraveling technology and culture in public health. *Am. J. Pub. Health* **59**, 237–244.

Lewis, C. E. and Michnich, M. (1977). Contracts as a means of improving patient compliance. *In* "Medication Compliance: A Behavioral Management Approach" (I. Barofsky, ed.), pp. 69–75. Charles B. Slack, Thorofare, N.J.

McKenney, J. M., Slining, J. M., Henderson, H. R., Devins, D., Barr, M., Stern, M. P., Farquhar, J. W., Maccoby, N. and Russell, S. H. (1973). The effect of clinical pharmacy services on patients with essential hypertension. *Circulation* **48**, 1104–1111.

McKinlay, J. B. (1972). Some approaches and problems in the study of the use of services: an overview. *J. Health Soc. Behav.* **13**, 115–152.

Maiman, L. A., Becker, M. H., Cummings, K. M., Drachman, R. H. and O'Connor, P. A. (1982). Effects of sociodemographic and attitudinal factors on mother-initiated medication behavior for children. *Pub. Health Rep.* **97**, 140–148.

Matthews, D. and Hingson, R. (1977). Improving patient compliance: a guide for physicians. *Med. Clin. N. Am.* **61**, 879–889.

Mechanic, D. (1968). "Medical Sociology." Free Press, New York.

Mechanic, D. (1972). Social psychologic factors affecting the presentation of bodily complaints. *New Engl. J. Med.* **286**, 1132–1139.

Mushlin, A. I. and Appel, F. A. (1977). Diagnosing patient noncompliance. *Arch. Intern. Med.* **137**, 318–321.

Ogionwo, W. (1973). Socio-psychological factors in health behavior: an experimental study on method and attitude change. *Int. J. Health Educ.* **16**, 1–32.

Parsons, T. (1951). "The Social System", Free Press, New York.

Parsons, T. (1972). Definitions of health and illness in the light of American values and social structure. *In* "Patients, Physicians, and Illness" 2nd Ed, (E. G. Jaco, ed.), 107–127. Free Press, New York.

Podell, R. N. (1975). "Physician's Guide to Compliance in Hypertension." Merck, Rahway, N.J.

Rogers, R. W. and Mewborn, C. (1976). Fear appeals and attitude change: effects on a threat's noxiousness, probability of occurrence, and the efficacy of coping responses. *J. Personality Soc. Psychol.* **34**, 54–61.

Rosenstock, I. M., Derryberry, M. and Carriger, B. K. (1959). Why people fail to seek poliomyelitis vaccination. *Pub. Health Re.* **74**, 98–103.

Roth, H., Caron, H. and Hsi, B. (1971). Estimating patient's cooperation with his regimen. *Am. J. Med. Sci.* **262**, 269–273.

Sackett, D. L. (1976). The magnitude of compliance and non-compliance. *In* "Compliance with Therapeutic Regimens" (D. L. Sackett and R. B. Haynes, eds), pp. 9–25. Johns Hopkins University Press, Baltimore.

Sackett, D. L. and Haynes, R. B. (1976). "Compliance with Therapeutic Regimens." Johns Hopkins Universty Press, Baltimore.

Sackett, D. L., Haynes, R. B., Gibson, E. S., Hackett, B. C., Taylor, D. W., Roberts, R. S. and Johnson, A. L. (1975). Randomized clinical trial of strategies for improving medication compliance in primary hypertension. *Lancet* **i**, 1205–1207.

Sackett, D. L., Haynes, R. B., Gibson, E. S., Taylor, D. W., Roberts, R. S. and Johnson, A. L. (1978). Patient compliance with antihypertensive regimens. *Patient Counsel Health Educ.* **1**, 18–21.

Segall, A. (1976). The sick-role concept: understanding illness behavior. *J. Health Soc. Behav.* **17**, 162–169.

Shangold, M. M. (1979). The health care of physicians: do as I say and not as I do. *J. Med. Educ.* **54**, 668.

Steckel, S. B. and Swain, M. A. (1977). Contracting with patients to improve compliance. *J. Am. Hosp. Ass.* **51**, 81–84.

Stiles, W. B., Putnam, S. M., Wolf, M. H. and James, S. A. (1979). Interaction exchange structure and patient satisfaction with medical interviews. *Med. Care* **17**, 667–681.

Stimson, G. V. (1974). Obeying doctor's orders: a view from the other side. *Soc. Sci. Med.* **8**, 97–104.

Stuart, R. B. and Davis, B. (1972). "Slim Chance in a Fat World." Research Press, Chicago.

Suchman, E. A. (1966). Health orientation and medical care. *Am. J. Pub. Health* **56**, 97–105.

Suchman, E. A. (1967). Health behavior: a model for research on community health campaigns. *J. Health Soc. Behav.* **8**, 197–209.

Svarstad, B. L. (1976). Physician–patient communication and patient conformity with medical advice. *In* "The Growth of Bureaucratic Medicine: An Inquiry into the Dynamics of Patient Behavior and the Organization of Medical Care" (D. Mechanic, ed.) pp. 220–238. Wiley, New York.

Tagliacozzo, D., Luskin, D. B., Lashof, J. C. and Ima, K. (1974). Nurse intervention and patient behavior: an experimental study. *Am. J. Pub. Health* **64**, 596–603.

Tash, R. H., O'Shea, R. M. and Cohen, L. K. (1969). Testing a preventive-symptomatic theory of dental health behavior. *Am. J. Pub. Health* **59**, 514–521.

Weintraub, M. (1976). Intelligent noncompliance and capricious compliance. *In* "Patient Compliance" (L. Lasagna, ed.), p. 39–47. Futura Publishing Company, New York.

Wilber, J. and Barrow, J. (1972). Hypertension—a community problem. *Am. J. Med.* **52**, 653–663.

Willcox, D. R. C., Gillan, R. and Hare, E. H. (1965). Do psychiatric outpatients take their drugs? *Br. Med. J.* **2**, 790–792.

Williams, A. and Wechsler, H. (1972). Interrelationship of preventive actions in health and other areas. *Health Serv. Rep.* **87**, 969–976.

Wilmer, H. (1956). The relationship of the physician to the self-discharge behavior of tuberculosis patients. *In* "Personality, Stress, and Tuberculosis" (P. Sparer, ed.), 248–265. International Universities Press, New York.

Zola, I. K. (1973). Pathways to the doctor – from person to patient. *Soc. Sci. Med.* **7**, 677–689.

7

Psychological Care of Acute Coronary Patients

RUE L. CROMWELL and JEFFREY C. LEVENKRON

All of us can point to attitudes and actions which we feel are psychologically good for sick people. Lacking controlled research evidence we can nevertheless base these attitudes upon a background of personal experience and clinical observation. There are differences in opinion, however, as to whether these attitudes and actions directly affect physical recovery and well-being.

The effects of psychological interventions after admission to the coronary care unit (CCU) may be limited to offering comfort to acutely ill patients. Alternatively, these early psychological interventions may influence the course of physical recovery from coronary disease (see Chapter 3 for a discussion of possible mechanisms). Some feel that there is no special need for professional understanding or psychological training in order to deliver "good psychological care". Others, however, take the view that such psychological care cannot be so intuitive, that what is good for one patient is not necessarily good for another, and that one cannot just naively generalize from one's own experience—even professional experience—to the entire population of acute coronary patients. It is possible that good psychological care can be attained only when personality differences, environmental stresses, and the interactions among them are separately understood. For example, what may be reassurance to one person may provoke anxiety in another (see Chapter 6 for discussion of similar issues in relation to surgery).

The purpose of this chapter will be to review selected investigations which bear upon these issues. However, a major part of the work to be presented here will be based upon a programme of investigation conducted

HEALTH CARE AND HUMAN BEHAVIOUR
ISBN 0–12–666460–9

by the senior author and others (Cromwell *et al.*, 1977), although other relevant subsequent work will also be reviewed.

THE VANDERBILT/HOLY CROSS PROJECT

How much should a patient with a heart attack be told about the nature and severity of his condition? How much should he be allowed to do in the way of diversional stimulation? Should he be allowed to participate in his own care? Or, on the other hand, should he be given a highly limited stimulus environment and limited activity? Will psychological interventions have an effect only upon the patient's comfort, on his degree of compliance with the nurses' and with doctors' advice, or will they have a direct effect upon survival and recovery? Does the acute myocardial infarction (MI) patient react to stress in a way different from other patients? Independently of the psychological interventions, can outcome be predicted—not only the patient's sense of comfort and degree of co-operation, but, more important-ly, the potential outcome of another myocardial infarction or death? Finally, can factors be identified which differentiate the MI patient in personality and constitution from other patients, including those in a coronary unit who do not have myocardial infarction?

The National Institute of Mental Health (USA) asked that a project be set up as a collaboration between the Vanderbilt University Department of Psychiatry and the Coronary Care Unit of Holy Cross Hospital, Silver Spring, Maryland, to address these questions. It is not to be expected that a single research project will answer all questions, or that it will answer any one question definitely. The intent of the project was to make whatever inroads that were possible into these questions.

SUBJECTS OF THE STUDY

Of the 309 patients studied, 229 had been admitted to the coronary care unit with suspected acute myocardial infarction. The remaining 80 were compa-rably ill patients elsewhere in the hospital and without cardiovascular involvement. Of the 229 coronary care unit patients, 80% were given complete study and 20% were discharged too soon for complete study. The 229 represented 66% of the 347 patients under 60 who were admitted to the coronary care unit during that period. The major reasons for not being in the study were that (i) the length of coronary unit stay was too short; (ii) the physician or patient failed to give informed consent; or (iii) the patient was judged by us to be too seriously ill to participate in the study. Patients above 60 were not studied because of possible complications beyond acute myocardial infarction. Since those discharged early from the coronary care unit could not be studied and those judged too severely ill were not studied, the sample may be described as intermediate in range of severity. Failure to give informed consent tended to occur with physicians who wanted none of their patients in the study; therefore, this did not appear to be an important selective factor. The mortality rate on the coronary unit during the period of study was 18%, but since there was zero mortality among those participating in the study, the 18% originate completely from those over 60 and those rejected for study because of severity. As will be described later, eight in our group died during the 12-week follow-up period, and 12 were rehospitalized with a recurrent infarction during that time. Of the patients admitted to the coronary care unit during this period, 49% met the strict retrospective criteria for acute myocardial infarction (by USPHS cardiologists not involved with or knowledgeable of our procedures) and 51% were disconfirmed for acute myocardial infarction. This circumstance presented the opportunity for an on-ward non-MI control group which was not discriminable by our research group until after our procedures were completed. Final diagnoses among these on-ward non-MI patients included cardiac exhaustion, congestive heart disorder, pancreatitis and duodenal ulcer.

THE INTERVENTION (NURSING CARE) STUDY

Each of the 183 patients who underwent complete study was assigned to one of eight psychological treatment groups in a $2 \times 2 \times 2$ factorial design. This assignment was pre-arranged, before the individual arrived onto the coronary care unit and with only the knowledge that he/she was a potential candidate for study. The three dimensions along which the psychological treatments differed were:

(i)   high vs low amount of information given to the patient about the nature and severity of his condition;

(ii) high vs low amount of diversional stimulation and activity allowed the patient; and

(iii) high vs low amount of participation in self treatment and care.

Each patient was assigned as "high" or "low" on each of these conditions. A given patient, for example, may have an assignment in the high information/low diversion/high participation group.

Information Conditions

The "high information" condition included:

(i) a tape recording with extensive information about heart attacks, their causes, and treatments;

(ii) a shorter tape focusing upon support, reassurance, and a description of the coronary unit environment;

(iii) an option to hear these tapes again as requested;

(iv) extensive literature from the American Heart Association and other sources explaining heart attacks, how the heart works, and coronary treatment;

(v) a house physician assigned to explain extensively this same information;

(vi) agreement by the private physicians to be as informative as possible with these patients; and

(vii) participation by the nurses in giving full explanations about heart disease and the coronary unit.

The "low information" condition included:

(i) only the support-and-reassurance tape;

(ii) no literature;

(iii) house physicians assigned to limit comments to support, reassurance, and generalities;

(iv) agreement by the personal physicians to do likewise and to give a minimum of factual detail; and

(v) the nurses' declining to answer factual questions but instead referring such questions to the physicians.

Diversion Conditions

The "high diversion" condition included:

(i) a bed area with a large window and television set;

(ii) a mobile art object suspended outside the window;

(iii) a position near the entrance to the unit so that the traffic pattern offered additional stimulation;

(iv) full access to magazines, books, and newspapers;

(v) expanded visiting privileges (unless the patient himself chose otherwise because of fatigue, illness, or other reason);

(vi) agreement by the nurses and the coronary unit staff to engage these patients in friendly conversation; and

(vii) unlimited time of visitation by the clergy.

The "low diversion" conditions included:

(i) no television;
(ii) no window;
(iii) limited visual stimulation from the bed;
(iv) no books, magazines, or newspapers allowed;
(v) visitation only by the immediate family for limited time periods; and
(vi) visits by nurses and coronary unit staff only for purposes of carrying out assigned duties.

Participation Conditions

The "high participation" condition included:

(i) instructions to activate the ECG tape of the cardiac monitor whenever the patient felt a symptom;
(ii) a daily regime of mild isometric exercises designed to prevent embolism;
(iii) a foot pedalling exercise to be done while being monitored for heart rate, blood pressure, and ECG; and
(iv) a general attitude that the patient is to participate in his own recovery effort.

These ECG tapes were appropriately identified and given to the private physician during his next visit.

The "low participation" condition included complete bed rest, except for self feeding. Patients were told to lie quitely and their needs would be taken care of by the coronary nursing staff. Emphasis was placed upon reduced physical movement.

Patients in the "low" conditions were not stimulus-deprived; instead, their experience was much like that of the usual care received on a regular hospital ward without a television set. With the high staff/patient ratio on the coronary care unit a moderate level of stimulation was unavoidable and high quality medical care was insured.

Parallel to these three psychological intervention variables were three personality variables of particular interest: repression–sensitization (Ullmann, 1962), scanning (Silverman, 1964; Davis et al., 1967), and locus of control (Rotter, 1966). The repression–sensitization variable, also called "inhibiting vs facilitating anxiety", refers to the tendency of individuals to fail to process (or to repress) versus to be more sensitized to and more efficiently process information as a consequence of an increased level of anxiety. Scanning refers to the rate in which an individual processes information in his environment. It is measured not through questionnaire or inventory but through visual size estimation. Size over-estimators process information at a low rate. Size under-estimators process information at a high rate. Locus of control refers to the degree to which individuals view the outcome of life events as under internal vs external control.

The dependent variables of the intervention (nursing care) study were various indices of recovery (vs recurrence of MI and/or death), comfort and co-operation.

INTERACTING HYPOTHESES

Having described the major independent and dependent variables, a word is now appropriate about the a priori hypotheses. The authors initially questioned the earlier simplistic notion of "coronary prone personality", i.e. that specific diseases should be associated with specific personalities. Likewise, we questioned whether specific stresses, objectively defined, were related to specific diseases. Instead, we proposed that a personality-stress interaction would be the most sophisticated and useful way by which to understand how health can become affected by psychological factors. In other words, neither high nor low information about the nature of one's heart condition, for example, is inherently stressful or debilitating. Likewise, we felt, a given personality characteristic, such as being a represser or a sensitizer, would not be associated with a specified disease or, in itself, debilitative to health. On the other hand, repressers given a high amount of information about what is wrong with them may be distressed and their health may be negatively affected by this circumstance. Also, sensitizers, we felt, would be distressed and negatively affected in health if they did *not* receive information about their condition. Thus, the notion of personality-stress interaction was formulated. This interactionist view is, of course, highly consistent with the more current and empirically based descriptions of the coronary prone personality (Glass, 1977).

Regarding diversion, it was hypothesized that a high (or extensive) scanner would be distressed (and debilitated in health accordingly) if he were deprived of diversional activity; whereas the low scanner would be distressed and debilitated if given a high amount of diversional activity.

Regarding participation in treatment, the personality variable, locus of control, was hypothesized to play a similar role. Those who tend to see the outcome of events to be under their own control should be comforted by the opportunity to participate in self care. On the other hand, they should be distressed by the idea of complete bed rest and letting other people take care of them. Likewise, those who see the outcome of events as resulting from chance or from control by others should be pleased by the low participation conditions, where others take complete responsibility for their treatment. If, on the other hand, they were to be given responsibility for self care and treatment, then this should prove stressful.

In this way, the intervention study pursued questions which physicians and nurses have frequently asked themselves and each other: "How much should the patient be told?" "What should I let him do?" "To what extent should he be made inactive and his own needs be taken care of by others?"

RESULTS OVERVIEW

Before reviewing specific results, an overview of results of the entire project is important. Otherwise, the reader could become bogged down among the numerous individual results, even though only a limited number are abstracted in this chapter.

First, the results for the MI patients tended, by and large, to be different from those for the non-MI comparison groups. This was only partly the result of their earlier discharge. Numerous other variables were fundamentally different. In spite of some similarities, the MI patients tend to represent a distinctly different population from other patients. Second, our preconceived notion about the interaction between personality and environmental events leading to stress and debilitation was not strongly borne out by the data. While some findings indeed emerged, the more striking findings concerned the separate roles of the psychological interventions and of the personality variables, not the interactions between them. Third, the psychological (nursing care) interventions showed no appreciable impact upon the long term indices of recovery (such as death within 12 weeks, recurrence of acute MI within 12 weeks), but a remarkable impact was shown upon the length of coronary unit and hospital stay. Fourth, and contrarily, the personality variables had their greatest impact upon predicting outcome and the biological consequences of illness. These results will be reported in a later section which describes the "Prediction Study".

INTERVENTION RESULTS

The most salient cluster of converging findings from the intervention study concerned how extensive information to the patient about the nature of his condition was coupled with other intervention variables. If the high information was coupled with high participation in self treatment or with high diversion (but not both), then the outcome was favourable. If the high information was coupled with neither high participation nor high diversion, then the outcome was unfavourable. Specifically, a significant triple interaction ($P = 0.01$) occurred in predicting length of coronary unit stay as a function of information, diversion and participation. A similar triple interaction ($P = 0.02$) occurred among these variables as they affected length of stay in the hospital after leaving the coronary care unit. Patients with high information, low diversion and low participation had a mean stay in the coronary unit of 7.8 days and in the hospital of 28.0 days. Patients with high information, low diversion, and high participation had a mean stay in the coronary unit of 5.5 days and mean hospital stays of 20.9 days. If the high information was combined with high diversion rather than high participation, then the mean stay was still relatively low: 5.7 days in the coronary unit and 19.5 days in the hospital. The other intervention conditions fell in between these extremes, which accounted for the triple interactions.

These results brought a humbling message to the investigators. First, there is no simple answer to the question "How much should the patient be told?" The effect of the information depends upon what is coupled with it. Second, our sophisticated hypotheses appeared to be superseded by a commonsense everyday notion: If you are going to give an individual serious and important information, you should also provide a means for them to do something about it or else divert their minds from it. Specifically, if you are going to tell an acute MI patient about the severity of his condition, you should give him options to participate in self-care or else ample diversion to aid coping.

Other findings also supported this information-coupling notion. When information and participation were both high (or both low), then the number of cardiac monitor alarms for deviant heart rate were relatively few. If one condition was high and the other low, then the number of alarms was greater.

It is notable that these intervention effects carried over to hospital stay (where the psychological interventions were not carried out), but that they did not carry over to the follow-up period of 12 weeks (where rehospitalization with recurrent MI and death from MI were recorded). It is not surprising that the non-MIs showed no effect, since they were given the news of disconfirmation of MI and were discharged as quickly as possible.

When the study was designed it was assumed that stress would be the mediating variable to account for these differences in patient status and outcome. Indeed, as described in the information-coupling hypothesis, this may be the case. With results at hand, however, other alternative interpretations also present themselves. One interpretation concerns the learning to be sensitive to relevant symptoms. It has long been known from psychological research that learning is enhanced when learning material is presented with minimal proactive and retroactive interfering activity. Thus, the high information/low diversion/low participation patient would have the optimal conditions by which to learn and report relevant symptoms to his physician. While this could not account for the beneficial effect of coupling with high participation or the cardiac monitor alarm results, it would indeed suggest a scenario in which this "high/low/low" group would have the longest stay in both coronary unit and hospital. The patient learns, becomes sensitized to, and reports relevant symptoms; the physician becomes concerned about these reports and, out of caution, keeps the patient in the hospital longer.

A third interpretation concerns which patients protest and complain. As with the previous interpretation, it is assumed that the discharge of a patient by a physician is determined by social psychological variables in addition to the health status of the patient. For example, it is assumed that normatively patients will be discharged sooner when they or family members complain about the length of stay in the hospital. If such is the case, a particular effect may occur for the patient who is given information about the seriousness of his condition but who is then left to think about it with little diversion or participation in self-treatment. Such a patient may decide the hospital is the place to be. With selectively less complaining, such patients may have longer coronary unit and hospital stays.

It is unlikely that chance factors or group differences in sampling could account for these results. Also, the findings on length of stay cannot be attributed to the habits of individual physicians. Over 30 different private physicians were responsible for making the discharge decision for their respective patients.

As will be discussed later, the lengths of coronary unit and hospital stays were not reliably related to MI recurrence or death during the follow up period. Therefore, it is not possible to conclude whether these findings were a function of health status, social psychological variables, or both. In any case the economic implications are substantial. The cost of these additional days of specialized care are considerable.

As mentioned earlier, very few findings emerged to support the hypotheses that interactions between personality and environment affected coronary treatment outcome. Perhaps the most striking of these findings was one which did not lend itself to ordinary statistical evaluation. Every single patient who died or who had a recurrent MI during the 12-week follow-up period had the hypothesized incongruence between locus of control and the participation condition. That is, they were either internal locus of control with low participation in self treatment or external locus of control with high participation in self treatment. None of the patients in the two congruent conditions died or had recurrent MIs during the follow-up period. Statistical significance was not possible; however, this observation should be kept in mind for future investigation. If valid, an interpretation should account for the fact that the patients were no longer in the coronary unit or hospital when the negative consequences occurred. For example, if a patient found the treatment experience of the coronary unit incompatible with his personality, he might be prone to resist seeking treatment once the crucial symptoms of another MI appeared. Consequently, a more fully developed MI or death would be more likely to occur.

Also in line with the hypothesized interaction was the finding that the number of monitor alarms for high heart rate was a function of the interaction of information and repression–sensitization ($P = 0.05$). Sensitizers who received low information and repressers (the less anxious) who received high information had the greater number of alarms per day. The congruent combinations (sensitizers with high information and repressers with low information) had significantly fewer alarms.

It should be noted here that during the course of this study no evidence was found that the repression–sensitization scale actually measured repression. Instead, the scale essentially measured high vs low anxiety and was highly correlated with other anxiety scales. Consequently, the results concerning repression–sensitization will be interpreted in terms of anxiety.

Also, in line with the above finding and the hypothesized interaction was the finding that the co-operation with nurses on the coronary care unit was significantly different for the congruent vs incongruent combinations of information and repression–sensitization ($P = 0.02$). Sensitizers (the more anxious) with high information and repressers (the less anxious) with low information were more co-operative than those with the alternate combinations. Among the non-MI patients, those with the congruent combinations were transferred out of the coronary unit sooner than those with the incongruent combinations (means, 2.7 and 3.3 days for the congruent combinations; 4.2 and 4.3 days for the incongruent combinations; $P = 0.001$).

For the personality-treatment combinations of scanning and diversion the results were opposite to prediction. The number of monitor alarms for high heart rate was greater for minimal scanners with low diversion (3.5/day) and extensive scanners with high diversion (2.4/day) than for extensive scanners with low diversion (1.6/day) and minimal scanners with high diversion (1.9/day) ($P = 0.002$). Also, an unpredicted effect occurred for the diversion conditions alone. Those who later died in the follow-up period tended to be more often in the high diversion condition. If valid and interpretable, this would suggest that the availability of high diversion may have led some patients not to take their cardiac illness seriously and, therefore, may not have taken necessary precautions against recurrence.

THE PREDICTION STUDY

Both the potential aetiological factors of myocardial infarction and the psychosocial factors involved in treatment may be better understood when the predictive value of each variable is examined. As with the intervention study, the dependent variables toward which predictions were attempted are recovery, comfort and co-operation indices. It should be noted that this is not a retrospective prediction of the initial MI but a prospective study of recurrent MI and other variables related to health status. In order to reduce the reporting of spurious results from the examination of many predictor variables, the correlations had to be significant at the 0.05 level in each of two split samples of the data. Once this criterion was achieved, the total sample was then used to calculate the correlation and P values reported here. The only exceptions to this rule are in the case of death and rehospitalization from a recurrent MI. As mentioned earlier, the number of positive instances is so small that statistical analysis even without split samples is problematic. Consequently, in these latter cases the alpha level is reduced to 0.025 for the point biserial correlations. Even with this precaution, the findings on death and recurrence are of importance, not for conclusions but for exploration by future investigators.

Subsequent *death* during the follow-up period was predicted by two kinds of variables. A low score for social affection on the Nowlis Mood Adjective Checklist at the *end* of the coronary unit stay predicted a higher probability of death ($P = 0.005$). Although unpredicted in this study, the finding is in accord with the proposed psychosocial syndrome of "giving up" (Schmale, 1964). The other variables predicting death were all measures of plasma non-esterized fatty acids (NEFA). As will be noted later in the psychological stress study, plasma NEFA was measured on several occasions on the coronary unit. Six of these measures, not necessarily subsequent to a known stressful experience, were significant predictors of death within 12 weeks (r, 0.38 to 0.63; P, 0.025 to 0.005).

Rehospitalization with another MI was predicted by four psychological variables and three biological ones. Extensive scanning (as measured by degree of visual size underestimation) ($r = 0.39$; $P = 0.0005$), number of cards guessed during the solvable card guessing task (also interpretable as a scanning measure) ($r = 0.36$; $P = 0.005$), level of depression (MMPI) at the beginning of the coronary unit stay ($r = 0.30$; $P = 0.005$), and repression–sensitization (high anxiety) ($r = 0.31$; $P = 0.005$) were the significant psycho-

logical predictors. The three biological variables predicting rehospitalization with MI within 12 weeks were sedimentation rate ($r=0.30$; $P=0.005$),
17-hydroxycorticosteroid level at 3.30 p.m. following an unsolved task
between 10.45 and 11.00 a.m. ($r=0.40$; $P=0.005$), and highest recorded
systolic blood pressure while on the coronary unit ($r=-0.30$; $P=0.025$).

Several aspects of these findings are worthy of note. This was the first
time in which psychological and biological variables had been compared in
a prospective study of recurrence of MI, and it is remarkable that the
psychological variables were stronger predictors than the biological ones.
Second, scanning, the inferred rate at which an individual processes
information, appears very worthy of further examination. In this respect, it
should also be noted that these findings, in the view of the authors, seem to
support the concept of "coronary prone personality" (Rosenman *et al.* 1970;
Freedman and Rosenman, 1974), a view of which the investigators were
originally sceptical as opposed to the interaction hypothesis. Third, sedimentation rate has not typically been one of the strong predictors with
respect to coronary outcome studies. On the other hand, cholesterol, often
mentioned in other studies, fell short of the strict criteria which were used
for significance here. Fourth, the corticosteroid results will become more
clear in the following section on response to stress, when the prolonged
elevation of steroids in MI patients is discussed. Fifth, the blood pressure
finding, it should be noted, is in the inverse direction: the lower the peak
blood pressure, the higher the likelihood of rehospitalization.

The length of stay in the coronary care unit was analysed as another index
of recovery of MI patients. Although intervention variables, as reported in
the previous section, were important determinants of transfer from the
coronary unit, we find here that personality variables were not. Instead,
only biological predictors were significant: severity of symptoms during the
first 24 hours on the unit ($r=43$; $P=0.005$), number of days delay before
psychological testing was begun (obviously based upon the severity level;
$r=0.43$; $P=0.005$), serum glutamic oxylacetic transaminase (SGOT;
$r=0.41$; $P=0.0005$), most severe symptoms while on the coronary unit
($r=0.41$; $P=0.0005$), number of days with temperature over 99° F ($r=0.38$;
$P=0.0005$), LDH ($r=0.36$; $P=0.0005$), number of alarms for high heart
rate ($r=0.33$; $P=0.005$), highest temperature while on the coronary unit
($r=0.32$; $P=0.0005$), and level of severity of symptoms after the first 24
hours ($r=0.30$; $P=0.005$).

For the on-ward non-MI controls three predictors of length of coronary
unit stay were significant: severity of symptoms after the first 24 hours
($r=0.52$; $P=0.005$), LDH ($r=0.46$; $P=0.0005$), and number of days delay
before psychological testing began ($r=0.25$; $P=0.01$).

The over-riding predictor of length of hospital stay for MI patients was the length of coronary unit stay (and the variables which predicted this stay). In addition, only one 17-OH-CS measure and the relatives' (usually spouses') estimation that the patient had an internal locus of control personality were significant.

Number of days before return to work was analysed as a recovery index. In line with what is often observed in other studies, none of the variables in this project significantly predicted this variable. It would seem that the amount of time before returning to work has to do with factors other than the patient's biological health status, the personality variables studied here, or the psychological interventions studied here.

Co-operation with the coronary nurses was unrelated to the attitude toward co-operating with doctors' orders. Co-operation with nurses was predicted by moods of aggression and egotism upon entering the coronary unit ($r = -0.29$; -0.22; $P = 0.005$, 0.01). The greater the moods of aggression and egotism, the less the co-operation. Attitude of co-operation with doctors' orders was predicted only by one of the NEFA measures, and this was probably a spurious relationship.

Level of comfort on the coronary unit was predicted solely by drop in temperature ($r = 0.29$; $P = 0.005$). The greater the drop in temperature, the greater the comfort.

THE RESPONSE TO PSYCHOLOGICAL STRESS

Numerous opportunities for stress occur in the natural environment of the acute coronary patient. Learning of or wondering about decisions made in the workplace in his/her absence; budgetary matters or child discipline in the home during the patient's absence; telephone calls confronting the patient with problems to solve by people who do not perceive the severity of the illness; impatience with nurses, doctors, and other coronary staff when the coronary victim is forced unwillingly into the role of an ill person—all of these are frequently reported by acute coronary and other patients.

Whether these day-to-day stressful situations have a lasting debilitative effect upon the patient's health is a reasonable question. Also, it is reasonable to ask if the response of the acute MI patient to such stress is different from that of other patients. A simple card-guessing task was devised which would produce slightly less autonomic stress response than an exciting television programme or card game. The task simply consisted of observing a series of cards, each having an X or O on it, and predicting which of the two letters would appear on the next card. The task was divided into two parts. On one day, the cards were in a pre-arranged order so that a repeating series was quickly anticipated and solved. On the next day the cards were in random order so that the task could not be solved. The difference between the two tasks was the psychological experience of success or failure.

Heart rate and the finer plethysmographic responses of blood volume and pulse amplitude were measured before, during and after the tasks, which were given between 10.45 and 11.00 a.m. on consecutive days. Blood samples were drawn at 7.30 a.m., 10.45 a.m., 11.00 a.m., 12.10 p.m., 3.30 p.m., and 11.30 p.m., on the two days when the tasks were administered. For a day-to-day scan, blood samples were also drawn at 10.45 a.m. on all other days on the coronary unit. These blood samples were used for assays of plasma 17-hydroxycorticosteroids (17-OH-CS) and plasma non-esterized (free) fatty acids (NEFA). Besides the immediate pre- and post-measures from blood at 10.45 a.m. and 11.00 a.m. on task days, a second post-task measure was done at 12.10 p.m. This time was chosen because the half life of 17-OH-CS is normatively 70 min. The 7.30 a.m., 3.30 p.m., and 11.30 p.m. measures were done in order to track the circadian rhythm of 17-OH-CS. Also, the later measures allowed the examination of delayed deviations in plasma level subsequent to the stress task. Only selected salient findings from the full report (Cromwell et al., 1977) are summarized here.

Changes occurred in blood volume from the task to post-task periods, thus reflecting changes associated with the discovery that the task had been solved or failed. A significant interaction occurred among groups, periods (task, post-task), and days (solvable vs unsolvable task) ($F = 10.84$, $df = 1/12$, $P = 0.006$). This interaction resulted from the fact that blood volume of MI patients increased while blood volume of the non-MI patients decreased following the failure experience.

Both groups increased in pulse amplitude once the unsolvable task was underway (i.e. from pre-task to task). Then, once failure was realized (once the unsolvable task was over) the MI patients sharply decreased and the non-MI patients sharply increased in pulse amplitude. This yielded another significant triple interaction ($F = 10.82$, $df = 1/12$, $P = 0.007$). When the groups were analysed separately, only the increase in the non-MI patients was significant ($F = 5.90$, $df = 1/12$, $P = 0.03$). However, since most MI patients showed the downward trend, nonparametric tests of the MI change were significant.

The disruptions in the circadian rhythm of 17-hydroxycorticosteroid level on the days of the task administrations were analysed by comparing the MI and non-MI groups across time periods of 10.45 a.m., 11.00 a.m., and 12.10 p.m. A significant interaction occurred between groups and time points ($P = 0.05$). Regardless of solvability of the task the MI and non-MI groups reacted to the task in very different ways. The non-MI controls showed an immediate but slight elevation in response to the stress task, but 70 min later they were fully restored to the level of the circadian rhythm. The MI patients, by contrast, showed only a minimal immediate elevation, but 70 min later had a markedly high elevation. The latter difference was statistically significant ($P = 0.005$).

This pattern of response in the MI patients is similar to that found in hospitalized depressed patients, in that the latter, tend to accumulate rather than dissipate 17-OH-CS in response to stress (Wehmer, 1966). It is as if both the depressed and MI patients ruminate about a failure experience after it has occurred.

The NEFA assay seemed to be highly sensitive to the stress of attaching electrodes and drawing blood, but not to the stress of failure. Moreover, the second post-measure at 12.10 p.m. showed that a NEFA response was still taking place in both groups (either to stress or caloric intake). Potentially most important, however, was the predictive value of NEFA after the failed task with respect to survival during the follow-up period. Finally, heart rate seemed to be the most sensitive to the actual activity during the tasks.

After the results of the Vanderbilt/Holy Cross project were analysed, a frequent question was raised as to whether the differences between the MI and non-MI patients, if replicable, should be linked to the MI personality. That is, are the differences present specifically at the time of the infarct, or are they present before and after the infarct as well? To answer a part of this question a later study was carried out by Klorman (1977). She examined acute hospitalized MI patients, post cardiac (three months or more dis-charged) MI patients, and non-MI controls on the finger plethysmographic responses to solvable and unsolvable tasks. In general, the differences among groups supported the notion that the post-cardiac group was more similar to the acute hospitalized MI group in contrast to the non-MI controls. A more detailed examination of time points during tasks and rest periods was conducted, and the results were not identical to the original study. For blood volume all groups had marked decrease in blood volume on the unsolvable as opposed to the solvable task, with subsequent fluctuations following the unsolvable task. For pulse amplitude all groups showed an initial constriction followed by a steady increase in amplitude during the unsolvable task. For the acute MI group, however, this change consisted of a large rapid decrement followed by a gradual increase; whereas the non-MI group showed only a small decrement followed by a sharp and strong increase. The post-MI group showed an intermediate trend, similar to the acute MI group but less marked. These results support the notion that certain response characteristics of the MI cannot be attributed solely to the presence of an active acute lesion. Whether subject sampling or method accounted for the differences which occurred between these results and the original study cannot be determined.

THE COMPARISON STUDY

In order to understand the mechanisms underlying intervention with the acute myocardial infarction patient, it is first necessary to understand in what ways the MI patient differs from the non-MI control. This has already been discussed in the previous section on response to stress. In this section, other variables of the Vanderbilt/Holy Cross project will be reported, which distinguish the two groups. It will be recognized that this analysis, which shows group differences, is different from the analyses which predict outcome (with or without given interventions).

Of the 37 variables in which differences were shown, 17 could be viewed as potential (although not confirmed) predictive or vulnerability variables. The other 20 differences are the inevitable result of the cardiac lesion itself. Unless otherwise indicated, differences reported here will be between the MI patients and the on-ward non-MI controls.

Examination of the potential vulnerability variables indicated that the acute MI patients are older (compared to off-ward non-MI controls, $P=0.0001$) and more likely to be male (compared to on-ward controls, $P=0.06$; off-ward controls, $P=0.0003$). The MI patients are more likely to have positive histories of heart disease in themselves ($P=0.04$) and in their families ($P=0.0002$). According to both themselves and their relatives they bottle up tension (self-report $P=0.003$; relatives' $P=0.02$), have greater external locus of control (self report $P=0.003$; relatives $P=0.009$), and have very little exercise (self-report $P=0.09$; relatives' report $P=0.04$). In addition, the MI patients themselves reported greater denial of hostility (compared to off-ward non-MIs only, $P=0.01$), greater perfectionism (compared to off-ward non-MIs only, $P=0.005$), and greater control of self ($P=0.007$). Upon entering the coronary unit the MI patients had greater moods of sadness ($P=0.002$) and egotism ($P=0.03$). The MI patients scored higher on the total coronary proneness scale developed by the investigators (compared to on-ward controls $P=0.004$; compared to off-ward controls $P=0.0002$). This scale included dimensions of bottling up tension, scanning, perfectionism, exercise and over-eating. Two variables often reported for MI patients in other studies fell short of statistical significance: cholesterol ($P=0.08$) and depression ($P=0.09$).

An examination of these results together with the results for predicting outcome show that the patterns are not identical. The variables which separate the MI from the non-MI patient are not necessarily the same as those which predict outcome for the MI patients. Often investigators make the mistake of assuming that the variables on which a pathological or risk group is different from a control group are automatically the outcome (or vulnerability) predictors. The results here demonstrate that this is a hazardous assumption.

SUBSEQUENT INTERVENTION STUDIES

Since publication of the Vanderbilt/Holy Cross project, there has been a growing interest in behavioural methods for patients with coronary heart disease (CHD). Undoubtedly, this interest has been prompted by the mounting collection of confirming studies which identify CHD risk factors, as well as by a growing optimism for the expected course and recovery of patients with CHD. Indeed, one can find numerous papers that address the educational practices and psychological care procedures advocated for use with patients who have CHD (Farquhar, 1978; Pollock and Schmidt, 1979; Wenger and Hellerstein, 1978). These include: physical conditioning, risk factor education and modification, and supportive intervention. However, these almost exclusively describe care delivered after the patient has been transferred from the CCU, either to a general medical in-patient setting (e.g. to a "step-down" unit), or more typically, to an out-patient setting following discharge from hospital. By virtue of the time of these interventions, they represent not acute psychological care but cardiac rehabilitation. These are, therefore, more properly the concern of another chapter of this volume (see Chapter 11).

By comparison, there are precious few new studies of, or even clinical commentaries on, psychological care given to coronary patients in the acute state, as characterized by CCU admission. In light of the findings from the Vanderbilt/Holy Cross project, the compelling question is "Why hasn't more been done?" One answer may be found by considering the purpose and complexity of the CCU, as well as the reported clinical observations of patients who receive this special life-sustaining and time-limited care.

Admission to the CCU usually occurs during the most hyperacute phase of CHD, such as that precipitated by the crisis of an MI. Treatment in this early post-infarction phase (sometimes referred to as Phase I Rehabilitation) seeks to achieve physiologic stability. Priority is given to medical management, since coronary care facilities evolved in response to the need for sophisticated technology in caring for such patients. For this reason alone, the investigation of psychological and emotional factors may be relegated to secondary importance.

A second factor may have arisen from the clinical observations of psychological and emotional reactions often exhibited by acute coronary patients. It is now widely accepted that the crisis of MI often produces reactions of intense anxiety and depression (Lloyd and Cawley, 1978), in response to which some patients become hopeless (Engel, 1968) while others cope using denial (Hackett and Cassem, 1978). These emotional reactions of the patients are often thought to preclude any "rational" (or cognitive) understanding of the coronary event or active participation in the early recovery phase. Indeed, some clinicians have advised *delaying* the provision of information which seeks to clarify the MI and the recovery process: "The best time to clarify these misconceptions and impart the facts is just before the patient leaves the hospital. At this time, the doctor should discuss medications, activities, diet, and various restrictions, as well as the tendency of the family to overprotect and baby the patient" (Hackett and Cassem, 1978). Although some believe CCU patients are unable to process this information, the results of the Vanderbilt/Holy Cross project suggest that information presented in Phase I rehabilitation is indeed processed.

Related to these observed emotional reactions is the concern by professionals that acute coronary patients may be adversely affected by early interventions. In the anxious and/or depressed state that often accompanies MI, some believe that presenting detailed information or encouraging active self-participation in care will inevitably exacerbate these untoward emotional reactions and possibly jeopardize physiologic stability. Again, the data reported here do not bear out this speculation. It is worth reiterating that some patients achieve greater comfort from these interventions.

Finally, a fourth reason why further research has been limited may be related to the ways in which psychological care is conceptualized. For example, psychological care is often translated by the medical community as meaning "psychotherapy", which even in its brief or time-limited form, extends beyond the temporal limits of Phase I coronary care. Moreover, psychotherapy generally addresses behavioural and emotional reactions through ongoing contact with a specially trained therapist (see Gruen, 1975). Furthermore, it often focuses upon specific post-rehabilitation goals, such as resumption of sexual functioning (McLane *et al.*, 1980). Our view of psychological care has not been limited to psychotherapy. Instead, care is seen as changing the social and physical environment as experienced by the patient. Viewed in this way, psychological care can be fully integrated into the total structure of acute coronary care. Thus, "it makes a difference" in both immediate and longer-term patient outcomes.

In spite of the limited amount of research beyond the Vanderbilt/Holy Cross project, a few exceptions are worth noting. Pozen *et al.* (1977) exposed 102 acute MI patients to daily contact with a nurse-rehabilitator, from the day of their admission to the CCU. Patients were seen individually by the nurse, for 30 minutes daily, while in the CCU, then for 1 hour on alternate days following transfer to a convalescent area within the hospital. The content of contacts focused on: (i) imparting information on MI and its treatment; (ii) discussing plans for a return to normal functioning; and (iii) minimizing anxiety. In small group meetings following transfer from the CCU, diet, medication, prescribed activity, risk factors, and the recognizing of cardiac symptoms were further discussed. While the intervention method was neither standardized nor limited to the CCU, the result was quite promising. Intervention was found to increase significantly the return-to-work rate and to decrease cigarette smoking behaviour at a six-month follow-up. However, anxiety at discharge did not differ between treatment and control patients.

In a second paper, Johnston et al. (1976) report the clinical findings for 350 MI patients who were placed on an eight-step activity and exercise sequence. Upon admission to the CCU, patients gradually increased their participation in: (i) self-grooming, bathing and sitting behaviours; (ii) an hourly schedule of range-of-motion exercises; and (iii) recreational or diversional activities. Following transfer to a general medical ward, the extent of these self-care activities, exercises, and recreational pursuits broadened. At a one-year follow-up, more than 50% of the survivors were working, 66% adhered to fat-controlled diets, 77% continued to exercise, 91% of the prior hypertensives had controlled blood pressure, and 60% of the smokers were abstinent.

Although the results of this uncontrolled clinical investigation should be viewed with great caution, it provides some support for the belief that early behavioural intervention can be especially helpful in promoting risk factor reduction (Wenger and Mount, 1974).

SUMMARY AND CONCLUSIONS

In spite of increased interest in the psychological aspects of coronary heart disease the systematic investigation of psychological care of patients in the acute phase has been remarkably limited. Except for the extensive Vanderbilt/Holy Cross study, reported here, studies have focused primarily upon the effect of educative and self-participating activities upon back-to-work record and the changing of coronary-related habits. In spite of prevalent attitudes against intervening with the acute patients, all of these efforts, including the Vanderbilt/Holy Cross study, give clearly promising leads to relevant care procedures.

In the Vanderbilt/Holy Cross study, many findings emerged that need to be considered according to the separate criteria of (i) death, recurrence and physical status factors, (ii) length of stay in coronary unit and hospital, (iii) co-operation and comfort, and (iv) psychological well-being. Independent of intervention, psychological variables were more powerful than biological variables in predicting recurrent myocardial infarction (MI) with death or rehospitalization. Length of stay in both coronary unit and hospital were influenced by information, diversion and participation conditions on the coronary unit. If information about the patient's condition is coupled with self-participation in treatment or with diversion, the coronary unit and hospital stays are shortened. On the other hand, if information is not coupled with follow-up activity, the lengths of stay in treatment are lengthened. Co-operation with nurses proved to be quite independent of compliance with doctors' advice. Finally, the psychological and biological variables which differentiate the MI from the non-MI patient are not necessarily the same variables which predict outcome following an acute MI.

In conclusion, the importance of psychological factors in the treatment and outcome of acute myocardial infarction seems inescapable. On the other hand, much more explanation and replication is needed to understand the mechanisms by which these psychological factors have their biological effect.

REFERENCES

Cromwell, R. L., Butterfield, E. C., Brayfield, F. M. and Curry, J. J. (1977). "Acute Myocardial Infarction: Reaction and Recovery." Mosby, St. Louis, MO.

Davis, D. W., Cromwell, R. L. and Held, J. M. (1967). Size estimation in emotionally disturbed children and schizophrenic adults. *J. Abnorm. Psychol.* **72,** 395–401.

Engel, G. L. (1968). A life setting conducive to illness: the giving up—given up complex. *Ann. Intern. Med.* **69,** 293.

Farquhar, J. W. (1978). "The American way of Life need not be Hazardous to your Health." Norton, New York.

Freedman, M. and Rosenman, R. H. (1974). "Type A Behavior and your Heart." Fawcett Publications, Greenwich, Conn.

Glass, D. C. (1977). "Behavior Patterns, Stress, and Coronary Disease." Erlbaum, Hillsdale, N.J.

Gruen, W. (1975). Effects of brief psychotherapy during the hospitalisation period on the recovery process in heart attacks. *J. Consult. Clin. Psychol.* **43,** 223–232.

Hackett, T. P. and Cassem, N. H. (1978). Psychological aspects of rehabilitation after myocardial infarction. *In* "Rehabilitation of Coronary Patients" (N. K. Wenger and H. K. Hellerstein, eds). Wiley, New York.

Johnston, B. L., Cantwell, J. D. and Fletcher, G. F. (1976). Eight steps to inpatient cardiac rehabilitation: The team effort-methodology and preliminary results. *Heart Lung* **5,** 97–111.

Klorman, R. S. (1977). "Plethysmographic Responses to Experimental Stress in Acute and Recovered Myocardial Infarction Patients" Ph.D. dissertation, Indiana University. University Microfilms, Ann Arbor.

Lloyd, G. G. and Cawley, R. H. (1978). Psychiatric morbidity in men one week after first acute myocardial infarction. *Br. Med. J.* **2**, 1453–1454.

McLane, M., Krop, H. and Mehta, J. (1980). Psychosexual adjustment and counselling after myocardial infarction. *Ann. Intern. Med.* **92**, 415–519.

Pollock, M. L. and Schmidt, D. H. (1979). "Heart Disease and Rehabilitation." Houghton Mifflin, Boston, MA.

Pozen, M. W., Stechmiller, J. A., Harris, W., Smith, S., Fried, D. D. and Voigt, G. C. (1977). The nurse rehabilitator's impact on patients with myocardial infarction. *Med. Care.* **15**, 830–837.

Rotter, J. B. (1966). Generalised expectancies for internal vs external control of reinforcement. *Psychol. Monogr.* **80**, No. 609.

Rosenman, R. H., Freedman, M., Straus, R., Jenkins, C. D., Zyzanski, S. K. and Wurm, M. (1970). Coronary heart disease in the Western Collaborative Group Study. *J. Chron. Dis.* **23**, 173–190.

Schmale, A. (1964). Object loss, "giving up", and disease onset. *In* "Medical Aspects of Stress in the Military Climate" pp. 433–448. Walter Reed Army Institute of Research, Washington D.C.

Silverman, J. (1964). The problem of attention in research and theory in schizophrenia. *Psychol. Rev.* **71**, 352–379.

Ullmann, L. P. (1962). An empirically derived MMPI scale which measures facilitation–inhibition of recognition of threatening stimuli. *J. Clin. Psychol.* **18**, 127–132.

Wehmer, G. M. (1966). "The effects of a stressful movie on ratings of momentary mood, experienced anxiety and plasma 17-hydroxycorticosteroid level in three psychiatric groups." University Microfilms, Ann Arbor, Michigan.

Wenger, N. K. and Mount, F. (1974). An educational algorithm for myocardial infaction. *Cardiovasc. Nurs.* **10**, 11–15.

Wenger, N. K. and Hellerstein, H. K. (eds), (1978). "Rehabilitation of Coronary Patients." Wiley, New York.

8
Psychological Preparation for Surgery

ANDREW MATHEWS and
VALERIE RIDGEWAY

Is recovery from surgery significantly influenced by psychological factors?
Can we relate recovery to differences among individuals, such as personality traits, or to situationally determined cognitive and emotional processes?
If so, what mechanisms could underlie such effects? This chapter is an
attempt to address such questions by examining research evidence on the
effects of psychological preparation prior to surgery, or other invasive
medical procedures.

In an earlier review (Mathews and Ridgeway, 1981), we concluded that
there was reasonably convincing evidence that individuals high in neuroticism or trait anxiety were subject to more complications or slower recovery
from surgery than were those with low neuroticism or anxiety. Even if we
can accept such findings as valid, they are not easy to interpret. Perhaps
personality variables such as high neuroticism lead to slower recovery, or
perhaps physiologically vulnerable people tend to be both highly neurotic
and slower to recover from surgery, without any direct causal links
between them. Experimental evidence that recovery variables are modulated by psychological intervention would allow less equivocal conclusions, and it is with this evidence we are mainly concerned.

It is now quite widely accepted by hospital staff that patients should
understand what will happen to them during and after surgery. There is
much less agreement, however, concerning the type of information that
should be given, whether it should be tailored to individuals, and the nature
and extent of its consequences. Even if patients have a right to basic
information about their treatment, the content and effectiveness of such
information needs to be carefully reviewed. If relatively successful methods
emerge, they can be more widely implemented, while other methods may
prove to be either less influential or actually harmful in some cases. Such

HEALTH CARE AND HUMAN BEHAVIOUR
ISBN 0–12–666460–9

findings should carry direct benefits to both patients and staff, by helping to select the most effective and economical methods, and to determine the optimal means of delivery.

An important, if more distant objective, is the investigation of mechanisms that could underlie any link between psychological variables and physical recovery. Assuming that effects may extend beyond mere demand effects on self-report measures, a number of possibilities exist. Psychological preparation may act by providing reassurance, or by dispelling fearful ideas, so as to reduce pre-operative anxiety. Post-operatively, patients who are better informed about the significance of the procedures they undergo and the sensations they experience, may be less alarmed by them when they occur. Additionally, any instructions given may lead patients to behave differently, in ways that serve either to accelerate or impede physical recovery. These psychological mechanisms may clearly operate to a greater or lesser extent in different types of patients or medical procedures. For example, it has been suggested that patients who prefer to avoid thinking about surgery in advance may be made more rather than less anxious by unwanted information. At a physiological level, it seems that the stressful conditions associated with an operation can have quite far-reaching effects on inhibition or enhancement of pain, resistance to infection, rate of blood clotting, and other mechanisms likely to be involved in physical recovery from surgery (Mathews and Ridgeway, 1981). However, recent research goes against any simple equation between level of psychological reaction to "stress", and the various components of hormonal and autonomic response (see Chapter 3). For this reason, if preparation influences recovery via endocrine or immune system reactions, then we should not expect measures of emotional state to relate to recovery in any simple or linear fashion.

TYPES OF PREPARATION

Possibly the most common form of preparation is that of giving the patient information about the various procedures that the patient will experience before and after the operation, for example, skin preparation, aftermath of anaesthesia, intravenous feeding, and so forth. Most patients express a strong interest in such details, although a minority do not, either because they feel they already have sufficient knowledge or because they believe the information will be too upsetting. Preparation for other medical procedures such as invasive examinations, tend to focus on the actual event, during which the patient must actually cooperate. It is often not clearly stated in studies whether information of this type is given in order to reassure (e.g. to dispel alarming fantasies) or to forewarn the patient of upsetting events that

TABLE 1

Types of preparation	Example item
Procedural information	"After the operation, you will go to the recovery room, where specially trained nurses will care for you."
Sensation information	"It is normal to feel a sharp, burning sensation along the line of the incision."
Behavioural instructions	"You should try to cough four times each am and pm to keep your chest clear."
Modelling	"This film shows someone like you coping with the same procedures that you will experience."
Relaxation	"Try to concentrate on relaxing the muscles of your body whenever you feel tense."
Cognitive coping training	"You say you are worried about the anaesthesia. How could you make those thoughts more positive?"

require preparation (e.g. so as not to be taken by surprise and thus unable to cooperate at crucial moments). Such *procedural* information can be contrasted with *sensation* information when patients are advised about what they are likely to feel (see Table 1). In the work of Johnson *et al.* (1973, 1974, 1978a,b) a rationale has been consistently used to the effect that anxiety will be reduced by a close match between expectation and actuality. Unanticipated events, or more severe discomfort than expected may cause the patient to think things are not going according to plan, and thus increase anxiety.

Other information commonly included concerns actual *behavioural instructions*; telling patients what they should do after surgery or during a medical procedure. Since it is supposed that such behaviour will directly accelerate physical recovery, the effectiveness of instructions depends on the patient's compliance. Many studies have combined behavioural instructions and both types of information, so that it is difficult to know the relative contribution of each to any improvements in recovery.

Modelling may be seen as another distinct way of conveying information. With the use of a filmed model experiencing the procedure, information may be conveyed simultaneously about procedure, sensations (via the model's remarks) and appropriate behaviour. This method has more commonly been used with children than with adults (Melamed, 1977).

Other methods can be seen as more explicit attempts to reduce patients' anxiety, for example, via *relaxation*, hypnotic or otherwise. These efforts can also be directly linked to symptom reduction by suggesting that relaxation techniques should be used when pain occurs.

Reassurance is commonly provided in a very general way, by showing sympathy and concern, or more directly by encouraging the expression of fears that can then be set aside, or by emphasizing positive aspects of the experience. Although this is a non-specific component included in most good patient care, more specific training in *cognitive coping techniques* has also been used. In this method, patients are first encouraged to identify fears and worries and then to systematically counter them. This may be done by reinforcing the patient's own preferred coping technique (e.g. Kendall *et al.*, 1979) or by more standard training of patients to produce positive self-statements (Langer *et al.*, 1975).

It can be seen that many quite disparate methods may be included under the heading of psychological preparation and may have quite different effects. Before considering comparative effectiveness, however, we must first consider the various ways in which recovery has been assessed. We may then be in a position to determine whether specific types of preparation may act on different recovery variables.

MEASURES OF RECOVERY

Direct comparisons across studies are frequently complicated by the fact that different investigators use many different outcome measures. Some investigators use relatively few measures, whereas other researchers collect indices of numerous kinds of patient reaction, both psychological and physical. With the studies where one or only a few outcome measures are reported (number of medications but not length of stay, for example) it is obviously impossible to know whether the preparation intervention might have been found to be more influential if other types of data had been collected.

Different types of outcome data also have very different implications for possible mechanisms underlying any effects. If, for example, the consequences of preparation were to be confined to self-reported reductions in anxiety and increases in satisfaction, speculations about psychophysiological mechanisms would obviously be redundant. Even if some clinical indices of recovery were shown to be influenced by preparation, caution should be exercised when interpreting such results. Many of the recovery indices used, such as pain or nausea, are dependent on patient self-report and thus are likely to be influenced by mood state and expectations deriving from psychological interventions. Furthermore, apparently objective measures, such as analgesic use and discharge date, may also be heavily influenced by patients' subjective experience and behaviour, since staff must frequently rely on reports by the patient in arriving at medical decisions. Very few studies have included physiological measures and objective indices of medical recovery, although these would provide much clearer indications of the extent to which psychological factors may directly influence physical processes involved in recovery. Examination of the impact of preparation on subjective, behavioural and physiological indices may thus reveal which of several different possible processes are involved in the promotion of recovery.

For these reasons, we have attempted to classify outcome measures commonly used into standard groups or areas (i.e. behaviour, clinical ratings, length of stay, medication, mood, pain and physical: see Table 2). In evaluating the relative effectiveness of preparation, the number and type of areas sampled can be taken into account, as well as how many of them show significant effects.

TABLE 2 Measures commonly used to assess recovery

Behaviour	Specific observations of behaviour relevant to recovery (e.g. ambulation)
Clinical ratings	Rating systems used by staff to assess other aspects of recovery or adjustment (e.g. confusion)
Length of stay	Time from surgery to discharge
Medication	Counts of medication given (usually analgesics)
Mood	Self-reported mood (e.g. anxiety, depression) using standard scales
Pain	Self-reported pain measures on standard scales
Physical	Physiological indices (e.g. temperature, blood pressure) or medical complications (e.g. respiratory infection)

A few studies have used a composite recovery index, assigning an arbitrary point system to various items like pain, number of times the patient was nauseated, and so forth. While some overall view of recovery may be desirable, at this stage it seems of dubious theoretical value, and may serve to obscure specific effects attributable to particular types of preparation. Unfortunately, it seems impossible at present to construct any sort of hierarchy of patient recovery variables, with some factors being secondary to others, and some having more general implications. There may be more scope for useful scales within particular areas, such as the return to normal activities, and a preliminary attempt to construct a Guttman scale along these lines was reported by Williams *et al.* (1976).

Methods of preparation have also been categorized according to the use made of the various components identified earlier; for example, procedural or sensation information, behavioural instructions, and relaxation training. In some instances, investigators have clearly been interested in just one type of intervention. Often, however, an analysis of methods shows that other aspects of preparation are incorporated. For example, a patient might be told about medical procedures that are likely to happen in some detail (procedural information), but some exercises (coughing, deep breathing, etc.) may also be touched upon and encouraged. A combined approach could well turn out to be advantageous to patients, but again poses some difficulties for evaluating the psychological benefits of preparation in any simple way.

TYPES OF PATIENT AND PROCEDURE

Most studies have used mixed patient groups (for example, of different ages and sex) or have studied patients receiving a wide range of surgical procedures. This seems inadvisable, since pain tolerance and other relevant variables are known to differ according to such individual differences, while different operations can have widely varying impact on the recovery indices commonly used. In this chapter, we have chosen to focus mainly on major surgery with adult patients and have attempted to specify the degree of sample homogeneity with respect to surgery.

Work with children has been excluded as the child may have a limited understanding of surgery, and as a result, the procedures that may reduce anxiety in children are likely to differ from those appropriate to adults, and may well lead to different conclusions concerning mechanisms (see Melamed, 1977). Minor procedures, such as dental work, IUD insertions or child birth, have been studied (see Anderson and Masur, 1983, for a full review), but again may not clearly relate to major surgery and consequently have for the most part been excluded. Despite this, some studies dealing with invasive medical procedures that seem in our view to clarify issues relevant to surgery, are discussed in a later section. With the above exceptions, we have reviewed all studies of surgery that appear to be methodologically adequate. In practice, this meant excluding studies that did not include at least one randomly-assigned control group, that did not involve the systematic collection of post-operative measures relevant to recovery, or did not apply statistical analysis to this data. All studies meeting these criteria are summarized in Tables 3 and 4.

IS PREPARATION EFFECTIVE IN PROMOTING RECOVERY?

The question of whether preparation is effective can be approached in several different ways. One method (see Mumford et al., 1982) is to submit all studies to a meta-analysis; that is, to calculate mean effect sizes based on differences between experimental and control groups as a proportion of control group standard deviations. Such an exercise results in the finding of effect sizes averaging about half a standard deviation overall, so that Mumford et al. (1982) conclude that preparation can have significant effects, particularly on co-operation with treatment, duration of hospitalization and post-operative complications. Less information was extracted about type of intervention, although greater effect sizes tended to be associated with combinations of educational and psychotherapeutic approaches. Although the use of meta-analysis allows more precise quantification of overall effects, as used by Mumford et al. it does not differentially weight results in terms of methodological adequacy or theoretical significance.

An alternative to including all studies is to select only those judged methodologically capable of answering a particular theoretical question. In our view, the first, and possibly the most important, question is whether *any* of the specific forms of preparation that have been described produce effects over and above those that can be attributed to general reassurance and the special attention of a caring person. In answering this question, it is apparent that only studies including a randomly assigned attention–control group can be considered. Preparation studies which have control groups receiving no special attention beyond routine hospital care may suggest the clinical merits of preparation, but cannot eliminate rival hypotheses for the effects of preparation based on the often powerful effects of attention and its psychological implications. An adequate control group might involve talking with the investigator about plausibly relevant material, for example, health-related topics or general information about the hospital. Whenever possible, the information should be dispensed in similar mode, for example, on audiotape if the preparation message was presented in that way, and should be of similar duration. Ideally, a check should be made that patients expected similar benefit from both specific preparation techniques and the control conditions, although this has rarely, if ever, been done.

In reviewing the literature, surprisingly few studies were found to include an adequate control group matched for the additional attention paid to patients given systematic preparation. However, these few appear to show that preparation does produce significant benefits not attributable to attention alone. A summary of the relevant studies (indicated a) can be found in Table 3, together with others not including attention–control groups. At this stage, however, only those using attention controls will be discussed.

In the early study of Egbert et al. (1964) effects were found on both medication and time in hospital, and similar findings were reported by De

Long (1970), Hayward (1975), Flaherty and Fitzpatrick (1978), and Reading (1982). The differences observed in these studies concerned several areas of measurement, including pain report, use of analgesics, clinical observations and reduced length of stay. This might suggest a rather widespread effect of preparation on recovery variables, but it should be noted that the different studies used a wide range of measures, some of which failed to show significant results.

Furthermore, the studies concerned a range of different preparation methods, often used in combination, so that it is not clear which components have the most impact. However, since it seems to be established that some forms of preparation are linked to significantly improved recovery above and beyond that due to non-specific attention, we can now turn to a more detailed discussion of this second issue, namely, that of the relative efficacy of the different methods that have been evaluated.

WHICH PREPARATION METHODS ARE MOST EFFECTIVE?

Table 3 summarizes simple evaluative studies relevant to this question, all having randomly assigned control groups, although not necessarily matched for attention. More complex comparative studies, where different methods or components have been systematically contrasted are shown in Table 4, and will be considered in greater detail in a later section.

Only the first three studies have been classified as using information alone (Andrew, 1970; Vernon and Bigelow, 1974; Reading, 1982), unconfounded with behavioural instructions or discussion of worries. In these studies effects (if any) seemed rather modest, with only one significant finding out of a total of nine areas sampled across the three studies. Furthermore, the relevant study concerned laparoscopy (Reading, 1982), a very mildly traumatic procedure that could be classed as an invasive investigation rather than surgery. Thus, although the data on the usefulness of information alone is not extensive, it appears unexpectedly weak or even negative. Further consideration will be given to the reasons for this in the light of other studies, which specifically contrast the effects of information concerning sensations and procedure.

Behavioural instructions alone (to cough, breathe deeply, exercise, etc.) have been evaluated by several workers (e.g. Lindemann and Van Aernam, 1971), but only one study, that of Fortin and Kirouac (1977), used appropriate controls. Outcome was evaluated in four areas, clinical ratings, length of stay, medication, and mood, and group differences favouring the instructed group were found on ratings of physical function, analgesic injections and self-rated comfort. As with information, a full discussion of behavioural instructions will be deferred until after account has been taken of studies where it has been combined or contrasted with other methods. However, it can be noted that, on the basis of the present data, evidence in favour of instruction effects is rather more impressive than that for information.

Four investigations were classified as using a combination of information and instructions, starting with the frequently cited study of Egbert et al. (1964), and the time spent on each element is often difficult to assess. In the same way, the degree of active reassurance is difficult to gauge in many studies. However, all of these studies using mixed information/instruction had at least one significant result following their preparation intervention, and some found multiple effects (see Table 3). In view of the results noted in studies of information or instructions alone, it would seem likely that at least some of the power that has been attributed to information may thus reside in the specific behavioural instructions commonly incorporated.

Another group of three studies incorporated multiple components designed to reduce anxiety by dealing with worries expressed by patients, as well as providing some information and/or instructions. However, it is noteworthy that one report in this group did not show significant benefit for any outcome variable, and another found only weak effects. Dumas and Johnson (1972) failed to achieve any impact with a programme aimed at providing emotional support, although a previous study had suggested that it was associated with some minor beneficial consequences, such as reduced vomiting (Dumas and Leonard, 1963). Lindeman and Stetzer (1973) found some evidence of reduced palmar sweat activity following a similar procedure, but this applied only to a subgroup of patients having minor as opposed to major surgery, and no other outcome measure revealed any benefit. As with information alone, the evidence of clinical benefit attributable to emotional support and non-directive discussion of patients' worries is extremely weak. The one study showing strong effects (Schmitt and Woodridge, 1973) included behavioural instructions as well as information and group discussion, so that once again some of the observed impact may be due to the instructional component.

There is some evidence that relaxation can produce useful results (e.g. Flaherty and Fitzpatrick, 1978) despite other negative findings. Two of these negative studies (Surman et al., 1974; Field, 1974) used hypnotic relaxation, which may be less appropriate as a means of patient self-control, while another negative report (Aiken and Henrichs, 1971, not listed in Table 3) found that muscular relaxation failed to reduce delirium after cardiac surgery. To summarize the evidence reviewed so far, the beneficial effects of behavioural instructions, sometimes in combination with the provision of information or relaxation training, seem distinctly more

TABLE 3 Controlled evaluations of preparation for surgery

Study[a]	Surgery	Outcome measures[b]	Comments
(i) *Preparation based on information alone*			
Andrew (1970)	Mostly hernia	Behaviour Length of stay Medication	Pre-recorded preparation
Vernon and Biglow (1974)	Hernia	Clinical rating Mood	Pre-recorded preparation
Reading (1982)[a]	Laparoscopy	Behaviour Medication[b] Mood Pain	Attention control group. Informed patients had fewer analgesics
(ii) *Preparation based on behavioural instruction alone*			
Fortin and Kirouac (1976)	Diverse abdominal	Clinical rating[b] Length of stay Medication[b] Mood[b]	Composite ratings of physical function showed significant effect of preparation
(iii) *Preparation combining information and instructions*			
Egbert (1964)[a]	Diverse abdominal	Length of stay[b] Medication[b] Pain	Attention-control group
De Long (1970)[a]	Cholecystectomy and and hysterectomy	Length of stay[b] Recovery index[b]	Attention-control group Composite measure of recovery Pre-recorded preparation
Hayward (1975)[a]	Diverse mostly hysterectomy	Behaviour[b] Medication[b] Mood Pain[b]	Attention-control group[b]
Boore (1978)	Diverse abdominal	Behaviour	Prepared patients had

Pain
Physical[b]

(iv) Preparation combining discussion of worries with information/instruction

Study	Type	Measures	Notes
Dumas and Johnson (1972)	Diverse gynaecological	Length of stay Medication Mood Physical	Included some information/instruction. Earlier study found reduced vomiting
Lindeman and Stetzer (1973)	Diverse	Clinical rating Length of stay Physical[b]	Included information. Palmar sweat reduced following preparation, but only for minor surgery
Schmitt and Woodridge (1973)	Diverse	Behaviour[b] Length of stay[b] Medication[b] Mood[b] Physical[b]	Included both information and instruction. Significant effects included pulse and BP reductions

(v) Preparation involving muscular or hypnotic relaxation

Study	Type	Measures	Notes
Field (1974)	Orthopaedic	Clinical ratings Length of stay Mood Pain	Hypnotic relaxation plus some information
Surman (1974)	Cardiac	Clinical ratings Medication Mood Pain	Hypnotic relaxation plus some discussion of worries
Flaherty and Fitzpatrick (1978)[a]	Diverse	Medication[b] Pain[b] Physical[b]	Attention control group although allocation not strictly random

[a] Indicates studies including an attention control group.
[b] Indicates areas of measurement showing significant effects of preparation at 5% level of significance or better.

TABLE 4 Studies contrasting different preparation methods

Study	Surgery	Intervention group	Outcome measures	Comment
Chapman (1970)	Hernia (53)	(i) Procedural information (ii) Discussion of worries (iii) Routine care control	Length of stay[b] Medication[b] Mood	Both forms of preparation reduced analgesic use and stay
Langer et al. (1975)[a]	Mixed abdominal (60)	(i) Cognitive coping (ii) Information (iii) Combination (i) + (ii) (iv) Attention control	Clinical ratings[b] Length of stay Medication[b]	Significant main effect in favour of coping groups
Felton et al. (1976)	Diverse (62)	(i) Discussion and reassurance (ii) Information and instructions (iii) Routine care control	Mood[b] Physical	Poor analysis, but anxiety less in group (i)
Johnson et al. (1978a)	Cholecystectomy (81) Hernia (68)	Six-group factorial: Sensation ± instructions Procedure ± instructions No information ± instructions	Behaviour Length of stay[b] Medication[b] Mood Pain	Main effect of sensation on stay Main effect of instructions on drugs
Johnson et al. (1978b)	Cholecystectomy (58) Hernia (57)	Six-group factorial: Specific instructions ±	Behaviour Length of stay	Sensory information repeated (vs. once only)

	sensation No instructions ± repeat sensation		Pain	
Picket and Clum (1982)	Cholecystectomy (59)	(i) Cognitive distraction (ii) Relaxation training (iii) Relaxation information (iv) Routine care control	Medication[b] Mood[b] Pain[b]	Cognitive distraction most effective particularly with internal LOC
Ridgeway and Mathews (1982)[a]	Hysterectomy (60)	(i) Cognitive coping (ii) Information and instruction (iii) Attention control	Behaviour Clinical ratings[b] Medication[b] Mood[b] Pain[b] Physical	All significant effects favoured cognitive coping, but information also reduced worry
Wilson (1982)	Cholecystectomy (33) Hysterectomy (37)	(i) Information (ii) Relaxation training (iii) Combination (i) + (ii) (iv) Routine care control	Behaviour[b] Length of stay[b] Medication[b] Mood Pain[b]	Significant effects favoured relaxation, but all interventions decreased stay and relaxation increased adrenaline

[a] Indicates studies including an attention control group.
[b] Indicates areas of measurement showing significant effects of preparation at 5% level of significance or better.

impressive than do those of either information alone, or general reassurance based on discussing patients' worries.

Such an impression, however, is based only on simple evaluative studies employing one preparation and one control group. We now turn to more complex studies, which simultaneously contrast different methods of preparation, allowing more definitive conclusions. These studies are summarized in Table 4, with the types of intervention used and their outcome being indicated. The investigations reported by Chapman (1970) and Felton *et al*. (1976) suggest that, contrary to our earlier conclusion, discussion of worries and reassurance may reduce anxiety, medication use and recovery time. Both these studies utilized routine care controls, however, rather than matching for attention, and the measures and analysis used were limited. Reductions in anxiety are to be expected as a consequence of a pre-operative visit by a sympathetic person, irrespective of information content or specific discussion of worries, thus inflating the probability of differences from controls receiving only routine care. Hence, Leigh *et al*. (1977) found significant anxiety reductions in patients given the opportunity to discuss an information booklet, but not in those receiving the identical booklet without a visit. Nonetheless, the positive findings of Chapman (1970), in the absence of mood changes, do suggest that information and/or discussion can have more widespread effects, possibly in the context of low level routine care.

A possible explanation of the variable effects of preparation is provided by the experiments carried out by Johnson and her colleagues (1978a, 1978b), designed to test the importance of sensation (as opposed to procedural) information. The results of these experiments provide some, if inconclusive, support for the authors' hypothesis that only information about sensations is relevant. In the first study (1978a), six groups were randomly assigned to all possible combinations of behavioural instructions or no instructions, and sensation, procedural or no information. Ignoring interactions with level of pre-operative fear, only two significant effects emerged; patients given sensation information had shorter stays in hospital, but patients given behavioural instructions took fewer analgesics. In a second study (1978b) all patient groups were given sensation information, although this was repeated just before the operation in the case of half of them. These two groups were then sub-divided according to whether they were provided with specific behavioural instructions, non-specific instructions, (giving less details about actual exercises) or no instructions at all. Once again there were few unequivocal effects of preparation; analgesic use was reduced in those patients receiving sensation information on two occasions rather than one, and no other main effects were significant. Combined with the earlier result, this does suggest that sensation information has some impact, albeit rather a limited one, while procedural information does not necessarily have any role at all. The earlier conclusion about the role of behavioural instructions is also somewhat weakened by the finding that this manipulation reduced medication use in only one of the two studies.

Relaxation training was examined in two comparative studies, with somewhat contradictory results. Pickett and Clum (1982) found relaxation to be ineffective compared with an alternative cognitive method (see later) although their patients received only one tape-recorded relaxation session, the day before surgery. By contrast, Wilson (1982) found relaxation to be superior to information (both sensation and procedural) on a number of variables. In turn, the provision of information was superior to the routine care control condition, but only for one variable, length of stay. Like Pickett and Clum, Wilson taught patients to relax the day before surgery, but tapes were left for them to use during subsequent practice, which may account for the greater impact of relaxation in this study. Although one might assume that relaxation exerted its effect via greater reductions in anxiety, there was no direct evidence for this, and indeed relaxation was associated with higher levels of urinary adrenaline than other conditions. Such a finding suggests that the relevant mechanism may have more to do with the promotion of active coping behaviour than with simple anxiety reduction *per se*.

This suggestion finds more support from the three comparisons involving an explicit cognitive coping strategy. In one of them (Pickett and Clum, 1982) this took the form of an apparent distraction manoeuvre, in which patients were required to think first about their worries concerning surgery, and then re-direct their attention to alternative pleasant imagined scenes. This simple procedure produced both lower post-surgical anxiety than did relaxation and lower maximum pain scores than the routine care control conditions, particularly in patients with internal locus of control. Although the design used by Pickett and Clum was limited in a number of respects, the superiority of cognitive coping strategies is strongly supported by two further studies. Langer et al. (1975) used a related intervention method, but rather than simple distraction, patients were asked to replace worries concerning surgery by selective focusing on the positive aspects of hospitalization, and to rehearse these positive thoughts rather than any negative aspects of their experience. Ratings of anxiety and stress made by nurses indicated lower levels in patients trained using this technique, compared with patients given sensation and procedure information, and this superiority was also reflected in lower analgesic use. Ridgeway and Mathews (1982) used a somewhat stronger information condition which included some instructional components, but again found cognitive coping training to be superior on several measures. In this last study, the rationale of each condition was described in a booklet designed to equate patient expectancy, and the contents of each booklet was then amplified during individual bedside interviews. Although patients judged the information booklet to be the most useful, recovery in these patients did not differ from those in the attention control group, while the cognitive coping condition appeared to reduce reports of pain both in hospital and during the three-week post-discharge period. As in the study by Wilson, however, no differences in overall anxiety levels between groups emerged at any stage, other than differences in specific worries about the surgery itself.

Results of studies considered in this section allow us to expand somewhat on the simple conclusion that at least some forms of preparation are effective. Information and behavioural instruction can form an effective component of preparation, especially if information includes adequate descriptions of the sensations to be experienced. However, in most cases where information has been systematically contrasted with alternative methods, it has proved less powerful. Among the alternative methods, relaxation appears to have rather variable results; for example, it remains unclear why it had more effect in the hands of Wilson than in those of Pickett and Clum. More careful delineation of parameters of training, and the use of more powerful methods such as live rather than taped training (see Borkovec and Sides, 1979) might clarify this issue.

Studies using systematic training in cognitive strategies are few, but the three discussed here reveal remarkable unanimity in finding cognitive coping to be the most effective procceure among those examined. Given the limited data base, conclusions cannot be drawn with great confidence, but enough evidence exists to assert that cognitive coping methods are probably superior to information and/or instructions along in reducing subjective pain and the need for analgesics following surgery. It is not clear whether other indices of recover, particularly physiological parameters or medical complications, are similarly influenced, leaving the question open as to whether autonomic or immunological mechanisms are involved. In the absence of such evidence, it may be better to limit speculation to the possible mechanisms by which cognitive processes may influence recovery via emotional and behavioural consequences.

Despite finding some support for Johnson's view that sensation information is more helpful than procedural, the associated hypothesis concerning its mechanism was not so clearly supported. If sensation information acts by reducing the perceived mismatch between expected and actual sensation, then it should also be more effective in reducing post-surgical anxiety. This was not found to be true in Johnson's own experiments (1978a, 1978b), nor were general changes in mood found to be specific to the more effective techniques used in some other studies (Wilson, 1982; Ridgeway and Mathews, 1982). An alternative hypothesis, that we favour, is that overall level of anxiety may be less relevant to outcome than the specific significance attributed by patients to events experienced following surgery. Hence, a sensation (or procedure) will induce alarm only if it is interpreted as a sign that something has gone seriously wrong. Although this is more likely in the case of unexpected sensations, even expected sensations may induce alarm if they are perceived as threatening. The undue attention and concern about particular feelings or symptoms that may follow could then have a number of adverse consequences, including increased reports of pain and demand for analgesics, and reluctance to follow behavioural instructions involving exercise. Such consequences would seem to be sufficient to account for most, if not all, of the documented effects of preparation. Even such apparently objective medical indices as respiratory complications can be seen as the end result of a chain of events, beginning with excessive concern about the significance of pain or other post-operative sensations, leading to reluctance to breathe deeply or take exercise, and finally to physical symptoms such as respiratory problems. While emotional state may also have more direct effects on physical and medical variables, mediated by the autonomic nervous system (see Chapter 3), behavioural consequences, such as increased complaints and avoidance of self-help behaviour, provide a more parsimonious explanation.

Cognitive strategies should be relatively powerful in combating these maladaptive behavioural consequences (distress, complaints, avoidance, etc.), provided the patient can use the methods effectively in dealing with alarming thoughts arising from the prospect or consequences of surgery. Relaxation may or may not have similar results, depending on whether it is used by the patient as a effective strategy to deal with specific worries or related obstacles to recovery. The use of these strategies (reinterpretation of sensations, redirection of attention to positive ideas or relaxation) may lead directly to a reduction in symptom complaints, or such decreases may follow from the patient's *belief* that use of these methods affords some degree of control over his or her own condition. The case for this latter hypothesis has been argued strongly (see Langer *et al.*, 1975) on the basis of evidence from a variety of experiments where the perception of individual control has been shown to carry important psychological and physical benefits. In the case of surgery, one obvious beneficial consequence has already been cited; namely that a sense of control will lead to patients being more motivated to comply with behavioural instructions relevant to their own recovery. Another consequence having important implications is that patients may become less concerned about pain and other events that previously they felt unable to understand or influence (see Pennebaker *et al.*,

1977). The perception of personal control, whether it is a cause or perhaps also an effect of self-help behaviour, may thus lead to reduced reports or complaints of pain, and in turn to fewer analgesics being prescribed or to earlier discharge. The hypotheses outlined here will be further evaluated later in this chapter in the light of evidence from subsequent sections, including the possibility of interactions between personality and preparation for surgery, or for other medical procedures.

MEDICAL PROCEDURES OTHER THAN SURGERY

Some studies have examined threatening investigatory procedures such as cardiac catheterization (e.g. Finesilver, 1978), as an alternative to surgery. Although typically less damaging or traumatic, in common with surgery these procedures elicit anxiety, pain, a sense of loss of control and concern over outcome. In the case of surgery the patient normally receives a general anaesthetic and thus feels more loss of control, pain is more severe and prolonged, and fear about the outcome more intense. Medical procedures, by contrast, are relatively brief, and usually require only local anaesthetic or minor tranquillizers. The patient is conscious, may be an active participant and the requirements for rest and medication afterwards are slight. As a result, physical recovery variables are less relevant, and the main targets of psychological intervention are the reduction of anxiety during the procedure itself and facilitation of the patient's active cooperation. While the two types of events do vary in their demands, medical procedures can be used to study patients' reactions to events similar to surgery, in the same way that the study of volunteers with mild fears may shed light on the problems of more severe clinical phobias. For this reason, we have chosen to include studies of medical procedures other than surgery where they may be expected to relate to surgery in at least some aspects.

Despite the differences outlined above, results of experiments concerned with medical procedures reveal a rather similar pattern of effects to those arising from studies of surgical recovery. Johnson and her colleagues (Johnson et al., 1973; Johnson et al., 1974; Fuller et al., 1978) have performed a series of investigations comparing the effects of sensation information with other preparation methods prior to endoscopy, or pelvic examination. Information about the sensations to be expected was found to reduce behavioural signs of stress, such as arm movements or gagging, and the need for tranquillizers, during endoscopy. Other methods, such as procedural information and behavioural instructions (for example on breathing techniques to avoid gagging as a tube is passed down the throat) also have some effects although less consistently so. Findings were thus generally in the direction predicted by the accurate expectation hypothesis. However, since there were very few clearly significant differences between sensation information and alternative methods, support for the hypothesis is not overwhelmingly strong.

Cognitive coping procedures have also been examined, and found to be effective in two out of three studies. Kendall *et al.* (1979) contrasted training in cognitive coping strategies with an educational approach mostly concerned with procedural details about a forthcoming cardiac catheterization. Both interventions reduced self-rated anxiety during cateterization, although on physicians' ratings the cognitive technique was superior. Similar results were obtained for sigmoidoscopy by Kaplan *et al.* (1982) in that both cognitive coping and relaxation training proved independently effective in reducing anxiety, compared with an attention-control condition. Two types of cognitive coping condition were used in which patients were encouraged, through the use of a taped model, either to appraise their own coping ability positively or to focus on the doctor's expertise. Although trends favoured internal re-appraisal by the patient, there were no significant differences between the two strategies.

One discrepant result arose from a well controlled comparison of cognitive coping using stess-inoculation methods with an attention-control and a no treatment control group, for a mildly painful X-ray procedure, the knee arthogram (Tan and Poser, 1982). Unexpectedly, neither patients nor blind assessors' ratings of pain showed differences attributable to the preparation, despite the experimental group reporting a greater use of cognitive strategies during the X-ray procedure.

This last result prevents an unequivocal conclusion that as with surgery, cognitive coping methods are consistently effective in reducing anxiety and pain during medical procedures. Although the reason for the one discrepant result remains unclear, it involved a painful but relatively non-threatening procedure in comparison with the two studies previously cited. It is possible that cognitive coping techniques may have greatest effects where anxiety and uncertainty are high; that is, under circumstances where much of patients' discomfort arises from alarming ideas and idiosyncratic worries, rather than from acute pain alone. If so, then perhaps patients may be more appropriately prepared for the acute but transient pain of the knee arthogram with appropriate information about sensations, rather than the hour of stress inoculation used by Tan and Poser. On the other hand, procedures such as cardiac catheterization, where anxiety and uncertainty are almost certainly very high, may be more appropriately managed using cognitive coping methods.

In comparison with invasive medical procedures, major surgery would seem to be characterized both by greater intensity and chronicity of pain, *and* by greater worry and uncertainty. As a result it might be predicted that both sensation information and cognitive coping methods can produce measurable benefits in the case of surgery, albeit on different parameters. It seems likely that the patients' fears and worries about surgery may be the major factor interfering with behaviour relevant to recovery, so that, of the two methods, cognitive coping would generally be favoured.

PERSONALITY VARIABLES AND RESPONSE TO PREPARATION

It would be both theoretically important and clinically useful if it could be shown that variations in the effectiveness of psychological preparation for surgery depended on measurable cognitive or emotional differences among patients. Results often show that only a proportion of patients benefit from preparation, suggesting that it might be possible to select in advance those patients most likely to profit. From the theoretical point of view, identification of individual differences relevant to preparation effects might reveal something of the mechanisms underlying links between preparation and recovery.

In the review cited previously (Mathews and Ridgeway, 1981), we have already summarized evidence that high levels of trait anxiety or neuroticism are associated with more pain, medical complications, and slower recovery. Furthermore, and contrary to earlier views (e.g. Janis, 1958) that both high and low levels of pre-operative anxiety were detrimental, associations found between anxiety and recovery indicate a linear relationship: the greater the level of fear prior to surgery the poorer the recovery. This was illustrated in an experiment by Johnson *et al.* (1978a) in which patients were divided into two equal groups on the basis of pre-operative fear levels. The group characterized by high pre-operative fear reported more intense post-operative pain sensations, greater difficulty in walking, and more emotional distress following surgery. This last effect also interacted with that of information and instructions, however, to give a somewhat more complicated picture. Both behavioural instructions and sensation (as opposed to procedural) information unexpectedly worsened negative mood in low fear patients, and the expected improvement in mood followed such preparation only in high fear patients. Thus, although procedural information did not result in any detrimental consequences (or much benefit for that matter), it appears that other more powerful types of preparation can paradoxically worsen the mood of low fear patients. Presumably, the provision of instructions and sensation information may provoke such patients into making inappropriate cognitive or behavioural coping attempts, which run counter to their needs or preferences, and serve to increase rather than decrease emotional arousal.

The suggestion that preparation can be emotionally harmful if given to the wrong type of patient has been put forward frequently, although until recently the evidence has remained unconvincing. Early attempts in this direction utilized the inadequately validated dimension of repression–sensitization, contrasting those individuals said to avoid attending to or thinking about emotional stimuli and those whose preferred coping strategy is to remain vigilant and acquire information about possible threat. The study by Andrew (1970) is frequently quoted to the effect that avoidant (or repressing) patients did worse with preparation than without, although this only applied to one measure (analgesic medication), and the preparation used did not in fact benefit patients overall to any significant extent. In the related study by De Long (1970), which did find an overall effect of preparation, the patients said to use vigilant (or sensitizing) styles profited more from preparation than did those with avoidant (or repressing) styles. Since the measures used to assess repression–sensitization correlate very highly with anxiety (see Cohen and Lazarus, 1973), these findings may relate less to coping style *per se* than to pre-operative fear levels. As indicated earlier, low pre-operative fear predicts poor response to some forms of preparation in its own right (Johnson 1978a). Thus, patients who are said either to have low pre-operative fear or to show avoidant cognitive styles, may be inappropriate candidates for psychological preparation, other than routine procedural information.

Less support for the expected interaction between individual differences and a benefit derived from preparation comes from Wilson (1981). A new measure said to reflect denial (e.g. endorsement of items such as "it's best not to think about the future when something unpleasant is going to happen") did not relate to pre-operative fear, but high scores did predict smoother recovery. High fear patients recovered less well, as expected, but neither fear nor denial measures interacted with the effects of information. The only significant interactions found indicated that high fear patients derived less benefit from relaxation training, while information was more effective for patients rated as having aggressive tendencies.

Turning to other medical procedures, the repression–sensitization distinction has also been shown to modulate the effect of a modelling video tape shown prior to endoscopy (Shipley et al., 1978, 1979). Patients viewed the video tape not at all, once or three times. Heart rate was found to be reduced in proportion to the number of times the tapes were viewed, although only for patients classified as sensitizers. For repressors, heart rate rose following one presentation and either fell only after three (1978) or continued to rise even after three presentations (1979). Since repression–sensitization scores were again found to correlate with trait anxiety, this result may once more be interpreted as indicating that patients with either a vigilant coping style or high levels of anxiety, profit more from preparation than do avoidant or less anxious patients.

It may be possible to clarify the nature of the relationship between coping style and anxiety by progressing beyond the poorly validated repression–sensitization scale, and adopting a less psychoanalytically influenced measure. For example, it is probably more valid to assess overt preferences for obtaining information about impending stress. Subjects can be divided into monitors, who show a self-reported preference for gathering information or thinking about danger, and blunters, who show a preference for avoiding information and use distraction instead (Miller, 1980). A questionnaire measure of preference for each strategy under a variety of stressful conditions was successfully validated by observing subjects' behaviour given a choice of distracting music or information about possible shock onset. Furthermore, this validated measure related rather poorly, albeit significantly, with the repression–sensitization scale.

Used with gynaecological patients about to undergo colposcopy, Miller (1980) showed that preparatory sensory and procedural information reduced heart rate only when given to monitors; that is, those patients showing a general preference for gathering stress related information. Avoidant patients (blunters) had similarly low heart rates only under the minimal preparation condition. Indeed, for all patients, preparatory information paradoxically increased emotional distress prior to examination, although despite this subjective pain was reduced, particularly in vigilant patients (monitors). Thus, sensory information may successfully reduce perceived pain; but in the case of avoidant patients, who would presumably otherwise control anxiety by distraction, such information may carry an emotional cost.

Somewhat against expectations, given the variety of methods and conditions studied, a reasonable degree of consensus emerges from the literature on coping style. Patients with high fear and/or a vigilant style experience relatively more distress and recover less well from surgery or invasive examinations. However, given preparatory information, such patients benefit relatively more than avoidant patients who may not profit at all from some forms of preparation. Since it has already been concluded that cognitive coping methods may be superior to information alone, the question may be raised as to whether a similar conclusion is justified in the case of these alternative methods. Unfortunately, little data is available. Since cognitive coping frequently emphasizes selective attention being directed towards positive aspects of hospitalization, it would appear to be more compatible with an avoidant coping style. In our own experiment on cognitive coping (Ridgeway and Mathews, 1982), we utilized a measure based on self-estimates of time spent thinking about surgery (vigilance?), but found it ineffective in predicting which patients would respond best to preparation. We suspect that cognitive coping methods are equally acceptable to vigilant monitors as to avoidant blunters, although further research needs to be directed towards this issue.

The most obvious hypothesis to be investigated in such research is that cognitive interventions train vigilant monitors to act more like avoidant blunters, who generally recover more smoothly. At first sight this hypothesis might seem to run counter to the general assumption that information, or the ability to accurately predict events, leads to reduced stress reactions (Averill, 1973). It is also unclear how sensation information can be helpful, while vigilant patients do worse. We assume that the explanation for this last apparent paradox is that vigilant patients are also more generally fearful, and the "information" that they acquire (or imagine) emphasizes possible dangers or disasters that may befall them. Information provided as systematic preparation will, on the contrary, emphasize a more realistic and reassuring view. Thus, informational preparation about sensations is particularly beneficial for vigilant patients, not just because it fits their preferred style, but because it neutralizes and replaces inappropriately fear-arousing ideation.

This explanation also accounts for the earlier apparent contradiction. Whether or not information reduces or increases stress reactions depends on the nature of that information, and more importantly, its significance and implications for the individual. Even highly accurate information may add to stress reactions if it is interpreted to imply a greater threat than previously anticipated, or one that is beyond the coping resources of the individual concerned. Extreme versions of the blunting strategy, such as total avoidance even when active coping is required, must be seen as harmful. On the other hand, processing incoming information and sensations in a relatively benign way, as non-threatening, is assumed to be beneficial, at least as far as recovery from surgery is concerned. It is this aspect of the blunting strategy that we believe leads to a characteristically smoother recovery, and is incorporated in cognitive coping preparation methods.

CONCLUDING DISCUSSION

Our starting point was to question whether the effectiveness of psychological preparation for surgery had been adequately established in controlled experimental studies. At the end of this survey our conclusion is unequivocal: it has. This is not to say that every study has obtained positive results; on the contrary, there are a disconcerting number of failures to show any significant effect of preparation, even in well controlled comparisons.

Clearly, one problem is the nature of the background conditions within which preparation is evaluated. Presumably, the standard and sophistication of psychological care in medical settings is improving, albeit more slowly than might be hoped. If so, then yesterday's experimental intervention becomes today's routine care. In our experience, medical and nursing staff increasingly accept, in principle if not always in practice, that patients should be given information about the surgery they are about to undergo. It thus becomes increasingly difficult to demonstrate the impact of offering additional information in a setting where all patients are routinely provided with at least some basic knowledge.

Even where preparation has been shown to be effective, not all recovery variables show evidence of its impact. It is common to find positive evidence with some variables, such as subjective pain, analgesic usage and length of stay, but less common to find changes in general mood state or medical complications. One implication of this has been discussed earlier, namely that preparation acts indirectly through cognitive and behavioural mediators, rather than directly on autonomic or immunological mechanisms. We also suspect that, depending on the nature of the surgery involved, different recovery variables may be influenced by different types of preparation. For example, the provision of information about sensations seems likely to decrease subjective pain to the extent that it promotes the encoding of such sensations as non-threatening events. Direct evidence supporting this view, and opposed to the accurate expectancy hypothesis, has been reported by Leventhal and his colleagues (Leventhal et al., 1979; Ahles et al., 1983). In laboratory comparisons of distraction, sensation-monitoring or emotion-monitoring, it was found that emotional-encoding heightened discomfort, while sensation-encoding reduced discomfort during a pain tolerance test. Differences were maintained on a second trial with instructions not to employ the same strategy, suggesting the persistence of either the emotional pain schema, or the more neutral sensation schema. Thus, although distraction can be effective in the short-term (see Kanfer and Goldfoot, 1966), in the longer term pain is reduced more by instructions leading to sensations being processed as non-threatening. Sensation information may be less effective, however, in reducing emotional distress during a life-threatening procedure or after major surgery where pain may be severe, but is still only one among many sources of anxiety.

We also believe that different research workers, particularly those from different professional groups, tend to vary considerably in the type of preparation they favour, and incorporate into apparently similar methods. Nursing or medical studies, for example, are very likely to include a great deal of straightforward behavioural instructions within preparation methods described as information. Such instructions can have significant effects in their own right, which may be overlooked in psychological research. If, for example, instructions are given to practice deep breathing, to press gently on the wound area, or to practice walking as soon as possible, preparation effects may reflect mainly the extent to which such advice is followed. Patients complying might be expected to have fewer complications and thus exhibit a more rapid recovery. On the other hand, methods such as cognitive coping are less familiar to medical or nursing staff, and are probably less likely to be adopted by them. Evidence gathered in this review shows, however, that preparation for surgery by training in cognitive coping strategies is probably more effective than are information and/or instructions. It would seem likely that this superiority will prove particularly marked when patients are undergoing a highly threatening procedure likely to provoke a range of disturbing thoughts or worries. Cognitive coping, in which the patient is encouraged to identify their own concerns and to develop an appropriate but more positive reappraisal of their situation, would seem a particularly potent and flexible method appropriate across various types of surgery and patient. As noted earlier, however, procedures involving mainly acute pain during an otherwise non–threatening examination may be sufficiently helped by the provision of sensation information and behavioural instructions.

Since cognitive coping is specifically addressed to fearful thoughts, its effectiveness in reducing worry seems unsurprising. To the extent that pain symptoms and recovery rate may also be affected, however, it becomes necessary to consider what the underlying mechanisms of such effects may be. In the absence of direct evidence we can only speculate, but it has been suggested earlier that many patients may react to surgery with a sense of helplessness, leading to emotional distress, increased pain, and failure to attempt self–help behaviour relevant to recovery. Cognitive coping methods seem an appropriate way of reducing such debilitating consequences, and of promoting a sense of control leading to more satisfaction and self–help behaviour. For example, cognitive methods may also modify the manner in which future events are interpreted, by the same means as the mechanism proposed to account for the effects of sensation information. If post-operative pain is processed as one of a range of events to be interpreted in a benign way (see Ridgeway and Mathews, 1982), then pain complaints and analgesic use may also be reduced. Future research may well substantiate more direct links between emotional distress and failure of physiological or immunological mechanisms involved in healing. The present analysis suggests that, while such links may indeed play a part in explaining how preparation works, more obvious psychological processes may prove sufficient to account for the observed effects.

The possibility that preparation methods can be individually tailored according to the patient's personality has proved an enduring idea. Convincing evidence has accumulated that pre-existing psychological differences do influence recovery, with patients low in anxiety or adopting an avoidant cognitive style recovering better. It also appears probable that such individuals may not profit from additional information, unlike those experiencing high fear or a vigilant coping style. Presumably, non-anxious avoidant patients are naturally using strategies related to cognitive distraction, which facilitate their adaptation to surgery, but which are disrupted by the provision of unsought information. Whether or not this natural style is beneficial or detrimental may depend on whether distraction or related avoidant methods hold up during or after the actual stressful event. We would suggest that with low level or slowly rising pain, or when other anxiety-elevating stimuli are not too intrusive, this strategy is indeed an effective one. Generally speaking, a vigilant or monitoring style would be clearly preferable only where aversive stimuli or external threats cannot be ignored, either because they are too intense, or because the threat demands some action requiring rehearsal or planning. In general, routine surgery does not seem to fit this description, so that vigilance is more disruptive than helpful.

Although we have concluded that the evidence clearly favours the efficacy of sensation information, behavioural instructions (including relaxation) and cognitive coping methods in promoting recovery, our discussion of mechanism has been necessarily less conclusive. Different explanations remain largely untested, and in our view it is to this issue that future research should be directed.

REFERENCES

Ahles, T. A., Blanchard, E. B. and Leventhal, H. (1983). Cognitive control of pain: attention to the sensory aspects of the cold pressor stimulus. *Cogn. Ther. Res.* **7,** 159–178.

Aiken, L. H. and Henrichs, T. F. (1971). Systematic relaxation as a nursing intervention technique with open heart surgery patients. *Nursing Research* **20,** 212–217.

Anderson, K. A. and Masur, F. T. (1983). Psychological preparation for invasive medical and dental procedures. *J. Behav. Med.* **6,** 1–40.

Andrew, J. M. (1970). Recovery from surgery, with and without preparatory instruction, for three coping styles. *J. Personality Soc. Psychol.* **15,** 223–226.

Averill, J. R. (1973). Personal control over aversive stimuli and its relationship to stress. *Psychol. Bull.* **10,** 286–303.

Boore, J. (1978). "Prescription for Recovery." Royal College of Nursing, London.

Borkovec, T. D. and Sides, J. K. (1979). Critical procedural variables related to the physiological effects of progressive relaxation: a review. *Behav. Res. Ther.* **17,** 119–540.

Chapman, J. S. (1970). Effect of different nursing approaches on psychological and physiological responses. *Nursing Rep.* **5,** 1–7.

Cohen, F. and Lazarus, R. S. (1973). Active coping processes, coping dispositions and recovery from surgery. *Psychosom. Med.* **35,** 375–389.

Delong, R. D. (1970). Individual differences in patterns of anxiety arousal, stress-relevant information and recovery from surgery. Doctoral dissertation, University of California, Los Angeles.

Dumas, R. G. and Johnson, B. A. (1972). Research in nursing practice: a review of five clinical experiments. *Int. J. Nursing Stud.,* **9,** 137–149.

Dumas, R. G. and Leonard, R. C. (1963). The effect of nursing on the incidence of post-operative vomiting. *Nursing Res.* **12,** 12–15.

Egbert, L. D., Battit, G. E., Welch, C. E. and Barlett, M. K. (1964). Reduction of post-operative pain by encouragement and instruction of patients: a study of doctor-patient rapport. *New Engl. J. Med.* **270,** 823–827.

Felton, G., Huss, K., Payne, E. A. and Srsic, K. (1976). Pre-operative nursing intervention with the patient for surgery: outcome of three alternative approaches. *Int. J. Nursing Stud.* **13,** 83–96.

Field, P. B. (1974). Effects of tape-recorded hypnotic preparation for surgery. *Inst. J. Clin. Exp. Hypnosis* **22,** 54–61.

Finesilver, C. (1978). Preparation of adult patients for cardiac catheterization and coronary cineangiography. *Int. J. Nursing Stud.* **15,** 211–221.

Flaherty, G. G. and Fitzpatrick, J. (1978). Relaxation technique to increase comfort level of post-operative patients. *Nursing Res.* **27**(6), 352–355.

Fortin, F. and Kirouac, S. (1976). A randomised controlled trial of pre-operative patient education. *Int. J. Nursing Stud.* **13,** 11–24.

Fuller, S. S., Endress, M. P. and Johnson, J. E. (1978). The effects of cognitive and behavioural coping with an aversive health examination. *J. Hum. Stress* **4,** 18–25.

Hayward, J. (1975). "Information—A Prescription against Pain." The study of nursing care project reports, series 2, 5. The Royal College of Nursing, London.

Janis, I. L. (1958). "Psychological Stress: Psychoanalytical and Behavioural Studies of Surgical Patients." Wiley, New York.

Johnson J. E. and Leventhal, H. (1974). Effects of accurate expectations and behavioral instructions on reactions during a noxious medical examination. *J. Personality Soc. Psychol.* **29,** 710–718.

Johnson, J. E., Morrisey, J. F. and Leventhal, H. (1973). Psychological preparation for an endoscopic examination. *Gastrointest. Endosc.* **19,** 180–182.

Johnson, J. E., Rice, V. H., Fuller, S. S. and Endress, M. P. (1978a). Sensory information, instruction in coping strategy, and recovery from surgery. *Res. Nursing Health* **1,** 4–17.

Johnson, J. E., Fuller, S. S., Endress, M. P. and Rice, V. H. (1978b). Altering patients' responses to surgery: an extension and replication. *Res. Nursing Health* **1,** 111–121.

Kanfer, F. H. and Goldfoot, D. A. (1966). Self-control and the tolerance of noxious stimulation. *Psychol. Rep.* **18,** 79–85.

Kaplan, R. M., Atkins, C. J. and Lenhard, L. (1982). Coping with a stressful sigmoidoscopy: evaluation of cognitive and relaxation preparations. *J. Behav. Med.* **5,** 67–82.

Kendall, P. C., Williams, L., Pechacke, T. F., Graham, L. E., Shisslak, C. and Henzoff, N. (1979). Cognitive-behavioral and patient education interventions in cardiac catheterization procedures. The Palo Alto Medical Psychology Project. *J. Consult. Clin. Psychol.* **47**, 49–58.

Langer, E. J., Janis, I. L. and Wolfer, J. A. (1975). Reduction of psychological stress in surgical patients. *J. Exp. Soc. Psychol.* **11**, 155–165.

Leigh, I. M., Walker, J. and Janagathan, P. (1977). Effect of pre-operative anaesthetic visit on anxiety. *Br. Med. J.* **2**, 987–989.

Leventhal, H., Brown, D., Shacham, S. and Engquist, G. (1979). Effects of preparatory information about sensations, threat of pain, and pattern on cold pressor distress. *J. Personality Soc. Psychol.* **37**, 688–714.

Lindeman, C. A. and Stetzer, S. L. (1973). Effect of pre-operative visits by operating room nurses. *Nursing Res.* **22**, 4–16.

Lindeman, C. A. and Van Aernam, B. (1971). Nursing intervention with the pre-surgical patient. The effects of structured and unstructured pre-operative teaching. *Nursing Res.* **20**, 319–332.

Mathews, A. and Ridgeway, V. (1981). Personality and surgical recovery: a review. *Br. J. Clin. Psychol.* **20**, 243–260.

Melamed, B. G. (1977). Psychological preparation for hospitalisation. *In* "Contributions to Medical Psychology" (S. Rachman, ed.), Vol. 1, pp. 43–74. Pergamon Press, Oxford.

Miller, S. M. (1980). When is a little information a dangerous thing? Coping with stressful events by monitoring vs. blunting. *In* "Coping and Health" (S. Levine and H. Ursin, eds). Plenum Press, New York.

Mumford, E., Schlesinger, H. J. and Glass, G. V. (1982). The effects of psychological intervention on recovery from surgery and heart attacks. An analysis of the literature. *Am. J. Health* **72**, 141–151.

Pennebaker, J. W., Burman, M. A., Schaeffer, M. A. and Harper, D. C. (1977). Lack of control as a determinant of perceived physical symptoms. *J. Personality Soc. Psychol.* **35**, 167–174.

Pickett, C. and Clum, G. A. (1982). Comparative treatment strategies and their interaction with locus of control in the reduction of post-surgical pain and anxiety. *J. Consult. Clin. Psychol.* **50**, 439–441.

Reading, A. E. (1982). The effects of psychological preparation on pain and recovery after minor gynaecological surgery: a preliminary report. *J. Clin. Psychol.* **38**, 504–512.

Ridgeway, V. and Mathews, A. (1982). Psychological preparation for surgery: A comparison of methods. *Br. J. Clin. Psychol.* **21**, 243–260.

Schmitt, F. and Woodridge, P. (1973). Psychological preparation of surgical patients. *Nursing Res.* **22**, 108–116.

Shipley, R. H., Butt, J. H. Horwitz, B. and Farbry, J. E. (1978). Preparation for a stressful medical procedure: effect of amount of stimulus pre exposure and coping style. *J. Consult. Clin. Psychol.* **46**, 499–507.

Shipley, R. H., Butt, J. H. and Horwitz, E. A. (1979). Preparation to re-experience a stressful medical examination: effect of repetitious videotape exposure and coping style. *J. Consult. Clin. Psychol.* **47**, 485–492.

Surman, O. S. (1974). Usefulness of psychiatric intervention in patients undergoing cardiac surgery. *Archs Gen. Psychiat.* **30**, 830–835.

Tan, S. Y. and Poser, E. G. (1982). Acute pain in a clinical setting: effects of cognitive behavioural skills training. *Behav. Res. Ther.* **20**, 535–545.

Vernon, D. T. and Bigelow, D. A. (1974). Effect of information about a potentially stressful situation on responses to stress impact. *J. Personality Soc. Psychol.* **29**, 50–59.

Williams, R. G. A., Johnson, M., Willis, L. A. and Bennett, A. E. (1976). Disability: A model and a measurement technique. *Br. J. Prevent. Soc. Med.* **30**, 71–78.

Wilson, J. F. (1981). Behavioral preparation for surgery: benefit or harm? *J. Behav. Med.* **4**, 79–102.

Part Three

Psychological Techniques in the Management of Organic Disorders

Introduction

Medical disorders have attracted the whole gamut of psychotherapeutic procedures, from traditional psychodynamic methods through behaviour therapy to psychophysiological techniques, such as biofeedback and relaxation. These methods have been employed both as alternatives to pharmacological therapy and as supplementary procedures, alleviating the psychological consequences of serious illness. The literature is large, so some selection has proved essential for the purposes of this book. Three important areas of treatment research have therefore been identified, and these are explored in detail by the contributors of the last three chapters.

Johnston (Chapter 9) has provided a review of relaxation, biofeedback and related psychophysiological procedures for the treatment of four common chronic disorders. His conclusions are mixed. While impressive results have been gained for tension and migraine headache and in essential hypertension, clinically useful effects have not been found in bronchial asthma. Unfortunately, few comparisons with conventional medical treatments have been carried out, so the relative efficacy of behavioural procedures is difficult to gauge. Among the behavioural techniques, biofeedback seems to fare poorly in comparison with relaxation or more sophisticated stress management programmes. The psychophysiological rationale underlying many of these treatments is also in doubt. Physiological modifications and therapeutic gains often do not coincide in biofeedback treatment, while the autonomic and neuroendocrine changes during relaxation are inconsistent. The question of how treatments are mediated also emerges in the other contributions to Part III.

Chapters 10 and 11 concern the use of psychological procedures with patients who have suffered an acute life-threatening illness. Behavioural aspects of coronary rehabilitation are discussed by Langosch (Chapter 10). He points out that psychological rehabilitation has several aims, including the secondary modification of risk behaviours such as cigarette smoking and Type A behaviour, the restructuring of social and vocational life, the adjustment to chronic limitations and successful coping with the traumatic event. Since different investigators emphasize various aspects of the rehabilitation phase, the range of techniques explored has been wide. As yet, there is little coherence in this field, but it is interesting that the more successful programmes have concentrated on specific behaviour changes rather than attempting global improvements in well being. Additionally, the stress-management procedures introduced to help patients cope with difficulties in their lives are similar to those described by Johnston in the treatment of psychophysiological disorders.

The last chapter by Grossarth-Maticek and his colleagues summarizes interesting new research into the use of psychotherapy for people with cancer. This area is fraught with methodological hazards, and has already attracted its fair share of unwarranted and sometimes unscrupulous claims of success. The treatment programme developed by the authors arose from prospective psychosocial studies and talking in depth with patients. Although their findings require replication and extension, the two controlled studies decribed in Chapter 11 suggest that psychotherapeutic procedures may significantly delay the course of well established malignancy, sometimes to a remarkable extent. As in the earlier chapters, however, the mechanism responsible for this effect is uncertain.

Neuroendocrine and autonomic processes may be involved in mediating some of the effects produced by the psychological interventions described in these three chapters. The sensitivity of such physiological processes to behavioural stimuli has been outlined in Chapters 3 and 4. Some suggestive evidence emerges from the intervention research as well. For example, Grossarth-Maticek *et al.* find an association between psychotherapy and leucocyte concentration, while Langosch emphasizes the importance of regulating cardiovascular reactions to behavioural challenges. On the other hand, much of the data are not consistent with physiological mechanisms of this nature. Johnston has discussed this problem in detail, noting that many treatment effects appear to be "non specific": that is, procedures with different underlying rationales produce similar responses, and do not operate through anticipated physiological pathways. Similarly, the firmest predictors of benefit identified by Grossarth-Maticek *et al.* in their second study were psychological measures taken after the therapy had been described, but before the start of treatment. The initial positive orientation imparted by the therapist seems to have been as important as psychological changes take place during treatment.

An alternative possibility is that behaviour changes rather than direct physiological modifications are responsible for treatment effects. For example, when patients benefit from biofeedback or relaxation training for migraine, they may not acquire voluntary control over the appropriate vasomotor processes at all; rather, they may become more aware of autonomic reactions and the circumstances in which they are elicited. This may in turn lead people to avoid or restructure potentially disturbing situations, thereby reducing hazards to vasomotor stability. If this type of mechanism is important, it may be more profitable to jettison physiological explanations and concentrate on techniques that are designed to modify these elements of behaviour directly. Langosch has described a number of treatment programmes that aim to help coronary patients precisely through this kind of process.

Important questions about the mechanisms of change remain to be resolved in all the areas discussed in Part III. However, this should not lead us to neglect the real therapeutic benefits accruing from this research. An efficacious result alone does not of course lead to the widespread adoption of any treatment programme. Other factors, such as convenience, the availability of alternative interventions, and sympathies within the prevailing intellectual climate, are all important. Nevertheless, it is to be hoped that the methods described here do not remain academic exercises, but are exploited fully for the benefit of patients and their families.

9

Biofeedback, Relaxation and Related Procedures in the Treatment of Psychophysiological Disorders

D. W. JOHNSTON

Largely because of the interest and excitement generated by the early research on biofeedback and the instrumental control of autonomic responses, the last fifteen years has seen an increasing number of reports of the apparently successful behavioural treatment of a gamut of physical disorders. Much of this research consists of uncontrolled case reports or isolated studies of specific disorders, but there is now sufficient evidence on the behavioural treatment of a few disorders for a preliminary assessment of the success of the behavioural approach.

In this chapter I shall present a selective review of the behavioural treatment of four disorders: tension headache, migraine, essential hypertension and bronchial asthma. Many other conditions have been treated behaviourally, for example, faecal incontinence (Engel et al., 1974), epilepsy (Sterman, 1977) and the symptoms of coronary heart disease (Johnston, 1982a), but these conditions have not received the breadth and depth of research needed for a review that hopes to conclude with something a little less pious than simply that more research is needed. The treatment methods examined are restricted for the same reasons and consist of biofeedback, relaxation training and stress management and, on the rare but welcome occasions when the evidence is available, more complex behavioural and cognitive/behavioural methods. While the chapter is organized primarily by condition, the most popular treatments raise general issues that are best discussed independently of any specific application.

HEALTH CARE AND HUMAN BEHAVIOUR
ISBN 0–12–666460–9

BIOFEEDBACK

Psychophysiological disorders are complex and it is widely believed that many social, psychological and biological factors play an interactive role in the aetiology and maintenance of problems such as essential hypertension and asthma (Weiner, 1977). A treatment approach that acknowledges these complexities may be itself very complex, possibly dauntingly so; biofeedback promises to bypass this complexity, by enabling direct control of the disturbed physiological system. The biofeedback message is clear: if a system is disturbed, let us say a patient's blood pressure is too high, then biofeedback can be used to teach the patient the skill of lowering blood pressure, just as a poor golfer can be taught to improve his swing. Anyone who has attempted to gain proficiency in a sport may be alerted to the problems of this robust approach, and these problems are in no way reduced when this sporting analogy is applied to the control of clinically disturbed systems. When learning to swing a golf club there is reason to believe that the action of swinging such a club is under voluntary control, that coaching will improve that control and that a better and more controlled swing will lead to a better golf shot. The situation is not necessarily the same in the control of disturbed physiological systems or of symptoms assumed to relate to such disturbance. Autonomically innervated systems may not be under voluntary control (although it transpires that most are), biofeedback may not aid such control (as has been found to be the case depressingly often), and even if the system is brought under self-control, such control may not relate to the desired outcome (as appears to be the case in the treatment of tension headache). These three assumptions, viz. that control is possible, that biofeedback is necessary and that the control achieved is relevant, seem necessary but not sufficient for the specific use of biofeedback and will, therefore, form the basis of this review. Clearly biofeedback can still be effective even when none of these assumptions are met, but in such cases it is unlikely that the effects are due to direct physiological control, and other mechanisms for the success must be sought.

RELAXATION TRAINING AND STRESS MANAGEMENT

Conceptually, if not technologically, relaxation training and stress management are more complex forms of treatment than biofeedback. The earliest proponents of relaxation training adopted essentially peripheralist theories of the effects of relaxation (Jacobson, 1938; Gelhorn, 1964). Most modern workers, and certainly most clinicians, assume that at least part of the action of relaxation is central and operates to induce calm and promote improved coping with stress (see Davidson and Schwartz, 1976, for a review of these positions). Because of this and because the most successful clinical research has combined relaxation training with forms of simple stress management (i.e. instructions to apply relaxation skills in stressful situations), the two procedures will be considered jointly in this review. Since it is assumed that relaxation training is a stress reduction method, it is also obviously necessary to assume that the most rational use of relaxation training is in stress related disorders.

Since relaxation training has been applied very widely in laboratory studies and in the treatment of emotional and behavioural disturbance, it might be expected that general conclusions on the power and applicability of the various techniques and the mechanisms involved in their use would be available to guide clinical application. In fact, trawling the relaxation literature produces a disappointing catch and only the most general, and rather dogmatic, conclusions are possible. Three questions of obvious interest arise in the present context.

(i)   Does the type of relaxation used matter?
(ii) Does relaxation training reduce physiological arousal and in particular sympathetic arousal, since this is thought to be central to some of the conditions under review?
(iii) Does relaxation training reduce subjective distress?

While there is an extensive range of relaxation procedures (Hillenberg and Collins, 1982, list over 20), in clinical practice many techniques are used interchangeably or in combination, and it is commonly held that all relaxation techniques operate in approximately the same way and to approximately the same extent. This view has been put most forcibly by Benson (e.g. Benson et al., 1974), but has been countered on both theoretical (Davidson and Schwartz, 1976) and empirical (Borkovec et al., 1975, 1978) grounds. Davidson and Schwartz have provided the most complex typology of relaxation therapies and suggest that anxiety can be dichotomized into cognitive and somatic forms, which are localized hemispherically, and that different forms of relaxation are most appropriate for the various types of anxiety. Most influentially, they have suggested that progressive muscular relaxation should be the most effective treatment for anxiety with a large somatic component. However, research generated by this approach has provided equivocal support at best (Zuroff and Schwartz, 1978; Woolfolk et al., 1982). Borkovec and Sides (1979), in an extensive and influential review of muscular relaxation, make two claims: that live relaxation is better than taped instructions and that more relaxation is better than less. Lehrer (1982), in another extensive review, agrees with the first of these conclusions, but not with the second. A reasonable working view, that appears consistent with the literature on the treatment of physical disorders, is to agree with Benson that all forms of relaxation are approximately equally effective and with Borkovec and Sides that relaxation by a therapist is better than taped instructions.

Three recent reviews have attempted to assess the physiological effect of relaxation training (Borkovec and Sides, 1979; Lehrer, 1982; King, 1980). However, no consensus has emerged and it seems safest to conclude that while relaxation can have physiological effects it does not invariably do so. Consequently, in any specific application the direct effect of relaxation training on physiological activity must still be demonstrated rather than assumed. The effects of relaxation on measures of sympathetic nervous activity have not been convincingly demonstrated either, but the importance and potential generality of such studies demand that they be mentioned briefly. Michaels et al. (1976) could find no difference in plasma noradrenaline between mediators and subjects relaxing without specific instructions. Davidson et al. (1979) did find a decrease in noradrenaline when subjects trained to relax carried out this procedure, but the lack of a control group makes this study difficult to evaluate. Lang et al. (1979) compared very experienced meditators with less experienced practitioners. While the results were somewhat variable, the more experienced meditators were found to have higher urinary adrenaline and noradrenaline, and the authors interpret these results as indicating that meditation leads to increases in sympathetic activity. The non-random allocation of subjects to the treatment comparison in this study seriously weakens this interpretation. Another methodologically troublesome study has been reported by Mathew et al. (1980), who examined catecholamines in 15 anxious patients treated with EMG biofeedback-aided relaxation training and 15 healthy controls. Both adrenaline and noradrenaline reduced significantly in the anxious patients over the four week training period, and there was no comparable reduction in the control subjects. Obviously, the confounding of treatment and patient characteristics in this study makes it unsafe to conclude that relaxation training caused the reduction in catecholamines. A more compelling and sophisticated study has been reported by Hoffmann et al. (1982), who compared subjects receiving Benson's generalized form of relaxation training with self-relaxation in a random allocation study. After thirty days' practice, subjects trained in relaxation produced greater increases in plasma noradrenaline to an exercise challenge, but showed a similar increase in blood pressure compared to self-relaxation subjects. Hoffman et al. interpret this as suggesting that relaxation training decreases adrenergic end-organ responsivity. While this hypothesis is fascinating and requires further study, the very conflicting findings of these experiments suggest that no conclusions about the effects of relaxation on sympathetic activity are at present possible. Nevertheless, it is clear that the simple assumption that relaxation reduces sympathetic activity is unlikely to be fully supported. Such sympathetic effects are, of course, only part of the picture. The work of Obrist in particular (Obrist, 1981) has shown that many physiological changes, particularly those produced in rather undemanding laboratory situations, are associated with increased parasympathetic activity rather than reductions of sympathetic tone. This may also be true of relaxation. However, in some, but not all, of the conditions under review it is clear that relaxation is applied because of its assumed sympathetic effects.

Most reviews have concentrated on the physiological effects of relaxation training, possibly because of the peripheralist origins of some of the techniques. However, the effects of relaxation on subjective arousal and distress have been central to many forms of behaviour therapy since the development of systematic desensitization (Wolpe, 1958). King (1980) makes it clear that relaxation does reduce subjective distress, even in studies in which there is little evidence of physiological change (Borkovec et al., 1978; Lehrer et al., 1980). As mentioned above, there is little support for the belief that some forms of relaxation are more effective in reducing subjective distress and others in altering physiological arousal (e.g. Woolfolk et al., 1982). Nor is it yet clear that relaxation training is superior to convincing placebo conditions in reducing subjective distress (Smith, 1976; Hutchings et al., 1980). This point should be borne in mind when considering the application of relaxation training to psychophysiological disorders.

This general introduction sets the stage for the following discussion of specific conditions. In each condition, while passing mention will be made of the role of psychological factors in the production and maintenance of the condition, the main concern of the review will be to assess if any of the behavioural treatments produce clinically useful changes, and if any of these treatments are more effective than others, either singly or in combination. More detailed discussion of aetiological aspects of these disorders may be found in Chapter 2 (by Kasl) and Chapter 3 (by Steptoe).

TENSION HEADACHE

It is recognized that the classification of headache is currently under increasing challenge (Bakal and Kaganov, 1979), but since tension and migraine headaches have been treated separately in most research it is convenient to continue to do so. The role of stress in tension headache is unclear. Most clinicians believe that psychological stress is central to tension

headache and operates via increased tension in the head and neck musculature, and many patients maintain that tension triggers their headaches
(Friedman, 1979; Feuerstein *et al.*, 1982). There is, however, surprisingly
little empirical evidence to support the view that patients with tension
headache either suffer from more tension or psychological distress than
non-headache sufferers, or that such tension precedes the headache. In
addition, the assumption that tension headache is caused by heightened
muscular tension (EMG) is also certainly unfounded or at least a serious
over-simplification. Martin and Mathews (1978), Anderson and Franks
(1981), Vaughn *et al.* (1976), Feuerstein *et al.* (1982), Van Boxtel and Van
der Ven (1978) among others, could find only trivial and inconsistent
differences between tension headache patients and various control groups in
frontalis and neck EMG at rest and during mild stress. The picture does not
improve if patients are studied during the occurrence of a headache (Martin
and Mathews, 1978; Bakal and Kaganov, 1977), as the levels of muscle
tension seen in patients are still quite unremarkable. Nor does sustained
voluntary contraction of the head musculature produce a headache in
tension headache sufferers (Pearce and Morley, 1981).

Biofeedback

The lack of a clear relationship between muscular tension and tension
headache does little for the rationale underlying frontalis EMG biofeedback
as a treatment for the condition. However, much productive biofeedback
research preceded, and indeed provoked, the research on the mechanisms of
tension headache and is well worth description. Voluntary control of the
striated musculature is obviously possible, but it is much less clear that
EMG biofeedback aids such control. While early studies suggested that
feedback was more effective than various control conditions (Coursey,
1975; Reinking and Kohl, 1975), more recent research has failed to confirm
this difference (Alexander *et al.*, 1977; Siddle and Wood, 1979; Davis, 1980).
Burish *et al.* (1981), in an extensive comparison of EMG biofeedback and
various forms of relaxation, found that feedback was no more effective than
relaxation in lowering EMG or various indices of autonomic arousal at rest;
when stressed, feedback subjects were less able to reduce these autonomic
indices than subjects given relaxation training.

Since it appears that EMG feedback does not have a specific effect on
muscular tension and that such tension may well not relate to tension
headache, it is improbable that EMG feedback has a specific effect on
tension headache. The improbable has not happened. Frontalis EMG
feedback leads to useful, non-specific reductions in tension headache.
Feedback has been shown to be superior to a medication placebo (Cox *et al.*,

1975), self relaxation (Haynes *et al.*, 1975) or an elaborate attention placebo (Holroyd *et al.*, 1980), and to be as effective as relaxation training (Cox *et al.*, 1975; Haynes *et al.*, 1975; Martin and Mathews, 1978). The study by Haynes *et al.* (1975) provides a good example of the procedures used and results obtained with EMG feedback. In this study, 21 student volunteers with tension headache received six twice-weekly sessions of either frontalis EMG feedback or relaxation training, or were simply instructed to relax without further training. Auditory EMG feedback was provided over earphones from the frontalis muscle for approximately twenty minutes on each training session. Relaxation training of similar duration was provided by tape, and while the authors do not provide details of the form of relaxation used it appears that it involved passive muscular relaxation. Subjects were told that they should use the skill they had acquired to prevent and reduce headaches, but the authors do not appear to have instructed subjects to practise regularly between sessions. This is somewhat unusual since clinicians would regard such practice as mandatory. Despite this and also the use of taped relaxation instructions, subjects receiving either biofeedback or relaxation training reduced their headache frequency by similar amounts, from approximately five per week to less than two. There was little reduction of headache frequency in the subjects attempting relaxation unaided and there was no suggestion that feedback was more effective than relaxation training. The size of effects obtained in this study seems broadly in line with those reported by various other authors, and suggest that both biofeedback and relaxation training can produce, both statistically and clinically, significant reductions in headache.

The persistence of the effects of EMG training is open to doubt. Budzynski *et al.* (1973), Hart and Cichanski (1981) and Haynes *et al.* (1975) all report good maintenance of treatment gains up to twelve months after treatment, but Reinking and Hutchings (1981) and Cram (1980) report serious problems with relapse over similar periods. Reinking and Hutchings relate these to patients ceasing to practise the techniques.

Relaxation and Stress Management

The close similarity of the effects of EMG feedback and relaxation training described above suggest that the two procedures operate in a similar way, presumably by reducing the psychological, rather than muscular, tension of headache sufferers. Relaxation may be preferred, if only on the grounds of simplicity, particularly as it is widely held that EMG biofeedback does not generalize well from the muscle groups being fed back to other muscles (Thompson *et al.*, 1981). The effectiveness of relaxation has already been described (Cox *et al.*, 1975; Haynes *et al.*, 1975; Martin and Mathews, 1978), since most of the important studies have used relaxation training as a comparison or control condition in studies of biofeedback. While demonstrating the comparative effectiveness of relaxation training, this unfortunate emphasis has led to a lack of controlled studies that evaluate the non-specific effects of relaxation. The main controlled study used a medication placebo (Cox *et al.*, 1975), possibly a rather inadequate control for some of the attentional and other aspects of relaxation training. The finding by Holroyd *et al.* (1980) that EMG feedback is superior to a psychological placebo might also be expected to apply to relaxation.

Cognitive Behavioural Methods

The final approach to be considered is the very welcome introduction of cognitive behavioural methods in the treatment of tension headache described by Holroyd and his colleagues. The procedures they have developed seek to enable the subject to identify the cognitions occurring before and during stress and periods of headache, and to counter these with methods based on cognitive reappraisal, self-instruction and pleasant imagery. It is worth describing their methods in some detail, since they are more complex than those already described and are likely to be increasingly important, particularly in patients who fail to respond to simple relaxation training. Patients are told that emotional and behavioural problems result from maladaptive cognitions, and that stress-related conditions, such as headache, are no exception to this. In particular, it is made clear that situations are stressful because of the way the patient perceives them and because of his or her expectations about how they should deal with them. A list of stressful situations specific to the patient is constructed, and for each situation the patient and therapist identify: (i) the anxiety cues, (ii) the patient's response to anxiety, (iii) the patient's thoughts before, during and after periods of anxiety, and (iv) the way these thoughts seem to relate to the production and maintenance of the headache. When patients have successfully identified these cognitions and related anxieties, they are taught to interrupt these thoughts with various stratagems, described by Holroyd *et al.* (1977) as "cognitive reappraisal, attention deployment and fantasy". For example, patients might attempt to view the distressing situation differently and ask themselves questions, such as "What am I thinking to induce this distress?", "What are the facts?". They might then attempt to use coping self-statements, such as "Calm down; do not catastrophize", or they might imagine a pleasant scene. In addition, patients are encouraged to identify unrealistic underlying belief systems (such as "I must be liked by everyone") and the thoughts they generate and learn to suppress these thoughts.

In a study using counter-demand instructions, whereby the subject is led to believe that the effects of therapy will be delayed for some time, Holroyd et al. (1977) showed that eight biweekly 45 minute sessions of cognitive behaviour therapy was more effective than frontalis EMG feedback. On measures of headache frequency, intensity and duration the cognitive behavioural treatment was superior, the results being seen most clearly on a composite score derived by multiplying duration of headache by intensity (the latter measured on a 0–10 scale). On this measure, the cognitive behavioural treatment led to reductions from a score of 92 to 25 while the comparable reduction in the biofeedback group was from 102 to 76. There were no reductions in subjects in a wait list control condition. Subjects receiving biofeedback did show greater reductions in frontalis EMG level, but this apparently conferred no therapeutic advantage. The effects of biofeedback on headache appeared somewhat poorer than those reported by others, which may indicate that biofeedback operates primarily via non-specific effects that are eradicated by counter-demand instructions. If true, this has obvious implications both for biofeedback and for relaxation training, which I have argued is so similar in its effects. The results of a further study, using a group version of the cognitive behavioural technique, were somewhat less satisfactory, since although the cognitive approach led to substantial reductions in headache so did a non-specific discussion group (Holroyd and Andrasik, 1980). The authors argue that the discussion group evolved their own rather idiosyncratic version of cognitive therapy and that this mediated therapeutic gains. While this view has attractions, the alternative possibility, that the effects of treatment were entirely due to non-specific effects, must also be considered and a final answer obviously awaits further investigations. Holroyd and Andrasik (1982) report that the treatment gains obtained with cognitive therapy are maintained over a two-year follow-up.

Tension headache can be treated by behavioural methods. A variety of procedures produce substantial and useful reductions in headache frequency, intensity and duration. The patients in most of these studies had previously been treated pharmacologically, presumably either with analgesics or anxiolytics, without much benefit, and it is likely that many patients seeking a behavioural treatment of headache will have already attempted these other remedies. Direct comparisons of behavioural and pharmacological treatments are rare, but Paiva et al. (1982) have reported an interesting, albeit somewhat limited, comparison of EMG feedback and diazepam in tension headache patients. During the period of active treatment both reduced headache by comparable amounts. However, during the follow-up period, when medication was discontinued, EMG feedback was superior. As might be expected, headaches recurred in the medically treated patients when they ceased taking medication. I would, therefore, argue that a form of behavioural treatment should be seriously considered for all sufferers of chronic tension headache. Which form of behavioural therapy is less clear; none have demonstrated a strong advantage in the studies I have described, and indeed the possibility that the effects are largely non-specific has not yet been ruled out. That being said, relaxation training has obvious practical attractions. The success of Holroyd and his colleagues' cognitive approach, particularly if it is independently replicated, suggests that it might be worth supplementing relaxation with these more complex methods in patients who fail to respond to the simpler approach.

MIGRAINE

It is the belief of many clinicians and their patients that migraine is precipitated by tension and stress. Parnell and Cooperstock (1979) found anxiety and worry among the most common reported precipitants of migraine, and Henryk-Gutt and Rees (1973) found stress to precede approximately 50% of migraines over a two-month period. While such data is difficult to interpret in the absence of control information, it provides some evidence that migraines are precipitated by stress. The presumed mechanism for such an effect is some form of vascular instability in migraineurs which is triggered by sympathetic over-activity; but while such instability has been investigated a number of times its exact nature remains obscure. For example, Bakal and Kaganov (1977) and Price and Tursky (1976) have shown a vasoconstriction in the temporal arteries in response to stress in migraineurs, in contrast to a vasodilation in headache-free controls. On the other hand, Cohen et al. (1978) could find no difference between migraineurs and controls on an indirect measure of extracranial blood flow, and Feuerstein et al. (1982) also failed to find any differences on a variety of vascular and other psychophysiological measures in migraineurs and controls while they underwent a battery of sttrsors. Therefore, while stress may well play a role in migraine and may even do so by inducing vascular changes, the mechanisms are as yet unclear and undemonstrated.

Biofeedback

Biofeedback for migraine has taken one of two forms: either feedback of hand temperature to enable subjects to warm their hands or feedback of aspects of blood flow in the temporal arteries. The rationale for hand-warming is uncompelling and based on the serendipidous observation that a subject attempting such a task with the aid of temperature feedback reported a reduction in migraine (Sargent *et al.*, 1973). Procedures aimed at controlling the size of the temporal artery have the more obvious aim of counteracting the vasodilatation associated with the painful aspects of migraine. A number of studies in healthy volunteers have shown that skin temperature from various sites on the body can be controlled in quite precise ways (Roberts *et al*, 1973; Steptoe *et al.*, 1974). However, temperature biofeedback is not invariably more effective than purely verbal instructions (Surwit and Fenton, 1980). Most worrying from the point of view of therapeutic application is that increases in hand temperature, as distinct from decreases, may be difficult to achieve (Surwit *et al.*, 1976; Ohno *et al.*, 1977).

The comparative ease with which decreases in temperature can be learnt suggest that feedback to decrease blood flow in the temporal artery may be more readily carried out. Unfortunately, most research on blood flow in healthy volunteers has concentrated on blood flow in the hand and these findings may not generalize to the temporal artery. Johnston (1977a) and Naliboff and Johnson (1978) found control of skin blood flow to be possible and largely confined to decreases in flow. Johnston, in addition, found that while feedback tended to be better than instructions this effect was not reliable. Simpson and Nelson (1976) found skin blood flow feedback to be superior to relaxation instructions in increasing skin blood flow. Overall, such studies suggest that the control of the vascular system with biofeedback is possible, but it is unlikely that skin temperature feedback is more effective than relaxation training in enabling increases in temperature. The data on blood flow feedback is scanty and not entirely consistent, but it is possible that such feedback is more effective than verbal instructions in enabling self-control of blood flow.

Controlled research in general suggests that, while temperature biofeedback does lead to reduction in headache, there is little reason to believe that it is an essential component of such treatment. Blanchard *et al.* (1978) have described a paradigmatic study. Thirty-seven patients experiencing at least two migraine headaches per month were randomly assigned to skin temperature training, relaxation training or a wait list condition. Patients were seen twice weekly for six weeks with approximately thirty minutes of each session spent in active treatment. Visual feedback of finger tip temperature was provided in combination with brief autogenic training, and subjects were instructed to practice what they had been taught in the laboratory for five to ten minutes two or three times per day. Feedback was not provided during these home practice sessions. Relaxation training was a modified version of Jacobson progressive muscular relaxation and again subjects were instructed to practise at home. Relaxation training was slightly more effective than skin temperature training on some measures of migraine headache at the end of treatment, but these differences quickly disappeared during the follow-up. Both treatments were better than self-monitoring. The results were seen most clearly on a headache index calculated by averaging on a weekly basis the intensity of headache assessed four times per day on a 0–8 scale. On this measure, both biofeedback and relaxation reduced the index from approximately 0.8 to 0.25, while there was no reduction in the wait condition. Rather untypically of studies in this area, headache frequency did not decrease more in the treated groups.

Cohen et al. (1980) compared a variant of hand temperature feedback involving the simultaneous cooling of the forehead with a variety of other feedback procedures. All were found to be modestly and equally effective in reducing migraine headache, including procedures such as EEG alpha feedback that had no detectable effect on the physiological parameters being considered. LaCroix et al. (1983) report contrary findings in a study of in-patient migraineurs in which they compared intensive training in hand warming, EMG frontalis feedback and relaxation. While all procedures led to a reduction in headache this occurred more rapidly in the group receiving thermal feedback. Over a six-month follow-up period relaxation and thermal feedback subjects continued to improve. Kewman and Roberts (1980) reported a double blind comparison of hand temperature increase and decrease. While the results were not fully reported, it appears that there was little difference in temperature control or headache activity between increase and decrease subjects. Gauthier et al. (1981) compared finger temperature increase and decrease in an un-blind study, in which temporal artery warming and cooling were also examined. All four conditions were equally effective in reducing migraine frequency, although only hand temperature control in fact proved possible. This study supports Kewman and Roberts' conclusion that the effects of temperature training are non-specific placebo effects.

The use of feedback of temporal artery size has been more specific in its effects. Friar and Beatty (1976) compared decreases in temporal artery flow with decreases in finger blood flow, and as might be predicted, headache duration was reduced by temporal artery feedback. Bild and Adams (1980) found that both temporal artery feedback and frontalis EMG feedback reduced headache frequency, but that the vascular feedback was slightly more effective. Elmore and Tursky (1981) claim that temporal artery flow feedback is more effective than skin temperature feedback in altering some aspects of headache pain. They argue that the reduction in the size of the temporal artery is the result of increased sympathetic activity, while the hand temperature increase is associated with reduced sympathetic activity. Knapp (1982) disagrees vigorously with this, and argues that both procedures lead to reduced sympathetic arousal. Elmore and Tursky do report that hand temperature training was associated with a decrease in flow in the temporal artery, an embarrassment for their position. In a rather impressive study, Allen and Mills (1982) examined the ability of migraineurs to control temporal artery flow with feedback during the occurrence of a migraine. Subjects were able to increase and decrease flow during such a period and the expected variations in pain occurred: an important demonstration that the mechanisms thought to be involved in clinical outcome studies can, in fact, operate.

In the studies that have produced reliable reductions in headache, follow-ups of twelve months have been reported, and the results in general sugggest that the gains made during treatment are maintained (Blanchard *et al.*, 1978; Bild and Adams, 1980; Cohen *et al.*, 1980) or even that further improvements occur (LaCroix *et al.*, 1983).

Both skin temperature training and vasomotor feedback from the temporal artery are associated with reductions in migraine headache and these effects persist for at least one year after treatment. While the effects are not entirely consistent across studies, there is little reason to believe that temperature feedback is more effective than relaxation training, at least in long-term outcome. There are insufficient studies on the comparative effectiveness of temporal artery feedback for any general conclusions to be drawn. However, the initial findings and rationale for this approach are positive and appealing and suggest that it should be explored further, possibly in combination with other procedures such as relaxation training. As Elmore and Tursky (1981) and others have argued, reductions in temporal artery size are not likely to be part of the general relaxation response (see above), and more may be achieved by combining treatments with different modes of action rather than by attempting to summate essentially similar de-arousing treatments. This suggests that the combination of relaxation training to reduce the frequency of migraine and vasomotor feedback from the temporal artery to deal with the migraines once they have occurred is a possibility that is worth further exploration.

Relaxation and Stress Management

There is suggestive evidence in the studies reviewed earlier and indirect evidence from at least two studies that relaxation training reduces the frequency of migraine (Blanchard *et al.*, 1979; LaCroix *et al.*, 1983). Mitchell and White (1977) have shown that a combination of treatments in which relaxation dominates also reduces migraine. Both Blanchard *et al.* and Mitchell and White have shown this decrease was greater than that produced by self-monitoring alone, which had little effect. However, studies involving more powerful control conditions are lacking, and the strong suggestion that the effects of biofeedback are non-specific raises similar doubts about relaxation, if only by association.

Behaviour Therapy

More complex behavioural methods have been applied with very encouraging results in the treatment of migraine by Mitchell and his colleagues. Mitchell and Mitchell (1971) compared a combination of systematic desensitization and assertive training with relaxation in a small group of intractable migraneurs. The combination of behaviour therapies was found to be more effective in reducing the frequency and duration of headache than relaxation training. In a second study, systematic desensitization and assertive training were compared with desentization alone and untreated controls. Again, the combination of behaviour therapies was the most effective. Mitchell and White (1977) report a careful study of a complex form of behaviour therapy. In this study 12 migraineurs received a treatment package that became increasingly complex at each of four stages. These stages were: (i) self-monitoring of migraine headache; (ii) self-monitoring of headache and associated emotional events (two hours training on such self-monitoring was provided for each subject); (iii) various forms of taped relaxation training and imaginal systematic desensitization were added to the self-monitoring; (iv) further tape-recorded versions of various behavioural techniques were provided. These procedures were designed to deal with what the authors describe as surplus (e.g. tension, emotional outbursts) or deficit behaviours (e.g. timidity and fatigue). They included material on positive self-talk, thought-stopping, assertive training, imaginal modelling, *in vivo* desensitization and rational thinking. Subjects were instructed to use these techniques on a cafeteria basis as seemed appropriate and patient understanding of the techniques and their use was monitored at regular meetings. The four stages in this treatment programme were implemented sequentially in three-month blocks, with three patients stopping at each stage of treatment (i.e. all twelve patients received stage one but only three received all four stages). All subjects monitored headaches for the 48 weeks of the study. The results are impressive. Patients started with a headache frequency of approximately 13 headaches per month and this remained constant through the first two stages of self-monitoring, but dropped to approximately seven when the first stage of the behavioural treatment was introduced. It dropped to approximately two headaches per week when the complete behavioural package was implemented. Subjects who only monitored headaches (stages one and two) throughout the twelve months showed no reductions. Although small, this is an important study that cries out for replication and extension. If confirmed, it corroborates Holroyd's work on tension headache, and suggests that there may be considerable gains to be made in the treatment of headache by the use of complex but entirely conventional behavioural techniques, and that the concentration on biofeedback and relaxation training that has to date dominated this literature may be unnecessarily limiting.

I have argued in this section that the behavioural treatment of migraine can be effective and clinically useful. An obvious question arises as to whether there are specific individuals for whom particular behavioural approaches are most appropriate, or for whom pharmacological approaches should be offered, at least initially. Unfortunately there appear to be no comparative studies of the power of the various pharmacological treatments for migraine and the behavioural methods I have described. Clearly, elaborate behavioural treatment is not an attractive possibility for patients who experience very infrequent migraines. For the moderate to severe migraineurs typically seen in these studies, behavioural methods are a reasonable possibility, particularly as most of the patients will already have received medication and found it wanting. Furthermore, the most common medications for migraine, based on ergotamine derivatives, do not reduce the frequency of migraine but only affect its duration and intensity. I have argued that relaxation should, and to some extent does, affect the frequency of migraine. I, therefore, do not think it is unduly optimistic to suggest that relaxation training and more complex behavioural methods have a role to play in the treatment of migraine. While many questions remain un-answered, clinicians should not be hesitant about applying the techniques I have described.

ESSENTIAL HYPERTENSION

Unlike most of the other conditions under consideration, the role of stress in essential hypertension has been the subject of considerable empirical interest, and there is now impressive, although of course incomplete, evidence that stress plays a part in the hypertension of at least some individuals. Laboratory studies with lower animals have shown that blood pressure (BP) is elevated in animals exposed to harsh experimental conting-encies (Forsyth, 1971), especially in genetically susceptible animals (Lawler et al., 1980) and in mice placed in stressful situations of social conflict (Henry et al., 1975). Laboratory studies with humans have also shown large elevations in BP caused by a variety of stressors, particularly those involving active coping (Obrist et al., 1978), and such effects are enhanced in subjects with a family history of hypertension (Hastrup et al., 1982).

Non-experimental studies have shown that intuitively stressful events, such as battle experience (Graham, 1945) are associated with elevated BP, while studies of working populations have shown that both redundancy (Kasl and Cobb, 1970) or working in stressful jobs (Cobb and Rose, 1973) are associated with elevated BP. Sokolow et al. (1970) used ambulant monitoring techniques to show that BP in some hypertensives was elevated during periods of stress or time pressure. The mechanisms underlying these effects, and the basis of essential hypertension in general, are still hotly disputed (see Steptoe, 1981), but most most would agree that sympathetic nervous stimulation is likely to be involved at some stage.

Biofeedback

Both systolic and diastolic BP can be controlled voluntarily by normotensives (Shapiro et al., 1969, 1972), but it is very doubtful if decreases in pressure or of correlates of pressure, such as pulse transit time (PTT; Steptoe et al., 1976; Marie et al., in press), are aided by feedback compared to simpler verbal methods. Steptoe (1976, 1978), Steptoe and Ross (1982), Shapiro (1973), Surwit et al. (1977) and Lutz and Holmes (1981) all failed to find any clear superiority of feedback over a variety of procedures not involving feedback in lowering BP, although Fey and Lindholm (1978) found the combination of relaxation and feedback to be more effective than either procedure alone. Steptoe (1977) and Marie and Johnston (in preparation) both found PTT feedback to be more effective than simple instructions when due allowance was made for the arousing effects of feedback procedure itself. Lo and Johnston (in press) found that feedback of the product of heart rate (HR) and PTT conferred a slight advantage in increasing PTT (lowering systolic blood pressure) over relaxation training. While the latter studies suggest avenues for future research, overall the results indicate that at best only marginal advantages accrue from the use of cardiovascular feedback.

These studies have examined subjects in peaceful, relaxing conditions. In contrast, Steptoe (1978) and Steptoe and Ross (1982) have compared PTT feedback and relaxation training during arousing cognitive tasks and find both to be equally effective in reducing cardiovascular arousal. Johnston et al. (1982) have examined cardiovascular feedback during dynamic exercise and have found that HR-PTT product feedback, described above, was more effective than a variety of control conditions in reducing the pressor response to exercise. Marie and Johnston (in preparation) could find no difference between PTT feedback and instructions in reducing the pressor response to isometric exercise. Therefore, only in the case of dynamic exercise is there convincing evidence that PTT feedback aids control compared to alternative methods.

On the basis of the findings from healthy volunteers, one cannot be optimistic about the effects of blood pressure feedback in aiding BP control in hypertensive patients, and the results have indeed been unimpressive. Surwit *et al.* (1977), Frankel *et al.* (1978) and Blanchard *et al.* (1978) all found that various types of blood pressure feedback and other procedures were almost totally ineffective in lowering BP. Two studies have reported a slight superiority of feedback over alternative methods. Glasgow *et al.* (1982) have reported that a very simple form of blood pressure feedback used at home led, when combined with relaxation training, to reductions in pressure that were not found with relaxation or biofeedback alone. However, the amount of training offered in this study was very brief, consisting of one session of either relaxation instruction or instruction in how to use a standard sphygmomanometer to provide a form of systolic blood pressure feedback. In addition, the reductions seen were only obtained on a few of a large number of measures of BP. Despite these weaknesses, the use of home blood pressure feedback is a welcome innovation and further exploration of this technique, particularly in comparison with a more realistic version of relaxation training, would be worthwhile. Goldstein *et al.* (1982) contrasted blood pressure feedback with relaxation training, self-monitoring or anti-hypertensive medication. In general, medication was most effective, but on some of the measures feedback was more effective than relaxation or self-monitoring, both of which were ineffective.

This study nicely highlights a problem that runs through many biofeedback studies with hypertensives. In the majority of them, while feedback has been found to be of little effect this is also true of the alternative behavioural treatments used for control or comparison purposes. However, these results are anomalous, since many researchers investigating relaxation and stress management have shown such procedures do indeed lower BP. I have suggested elsewhere that the poor performance of behavioural treatments in biofeedback studies (Johnston, 1982b) may be due to over-elaborate and stressful psychophysiological measurement, the low BP of the patients, and the limited emphasis placed on practical application of relaxation in these studies. Be that as it may, at the moment there is no firm basis for advocating biofeedback as a treatment for hypertension. If the evidence from studies of volunteers is drawn on then, there is little reason to believe that feedback should be either more or less effective than alternative procedures, though the results of the training of subjects under various forms of stress suggests that this approach may be worth extending to clinical studies of hypertensive patients.

Relaxation and Stress Management

Methods that are based predominantly on relaxation and stress management, although sometimes including a form of biofeedback, have been applied with great vigour to the treatment of hypertension. Patel and her colleagues have shown that a combination of relaxation, meditation, yogic breathing exercises, skin conductance feedback, stress management and health education can lead to clinically valuable reductions in BP in both medicated (Patel and North, 1975) and unmedicated (Patel et al., 1981) hypertensives; reductions that might enable patients to avoid the necessity of taking anti-hypertensive medication. Untreated patients show much smaller reductions in BP. Similar findings have been reported by Taylor et al. (1977), Brauer et al. (1979), and Bali (1979), who have compared relaxation training with various forms of supportive psychotherapy. Brauer et al. have also confirmed the expectation from the general literature on relaxation that live relaxation is more effective than taped. Southam et al. (1982) have shown, using a semi-automatic ambulatory measurement technique, that after relaxation training BP is lower throughout the working day.

In a very recent study we (Irvine et al., in preparation) compared the Patel relaxation package with an elaborately constructed control condition involving mild exercise training and training in cognitive alertness, which attempted to control for many of the non-specific aspects of Patel's procedure. Our version of Patel's treatment is representative of the effective forms of relaxation training. Patients were seen individually for ten weekly sessions of approximately 45 minutes. The first two sessions were spent in patient education, which involved discussion of hypertension, its effects, and the role of stress in its production. A brief commercial film on the role of stress was shown. The remaining eight sessions were spent on passive relaxation exercises, simple instructions in regular breathing and skin conductance feedback. On the second training session, but only on that session, Jacobsonian muscle tension was incorporated in an attempt to improve the patient's awareness of muscle tension. However, the patient was instructed not to use muscle tension as part of his or her regular relaxation procedures. Meditation, firstly to a pleasant scene and then to a simple verbal cue, was introduced on session 4 and on subsequent sessions training was given in relaxing in response to stress and to a number of common environmental cues. For example, patients would be instructed to place small coloured adhesive dots on everyday objects, such as a watch or telephone, and instructed that they should relax briefly every time they noticed the coloured dot. In addition, patients were encouraged to practise relaxation for approximately 20 minutes twice daily.

Thirty-two hypertensives, 16 medicated and 16 unmedicated, were randomly allocated to either relaxation or to the control procedure. The control condition received as much attention and structure as the relaxation training, and was equally acceptable to patients. Nevertheless, relaxation led to a larger reduction in BP, as assessed both by nurses blind to the treatment condition and the patients' therapist. Irvine *et al.* failed to find any reliable difference between the control condition and relaxation on BP measures taken by the patients daily in their own homes. This was almost certainly related to the lower BP that patients displayed under these circumstances. In this study, patients were followed up for three months, at which time gains were maintained. This is a general finding, since studies by Patel (Patel and North, 1975; Patel *et al.*, 1981) have shown sustained changes over a six-month period, while Bali (1979) reported continued BP control over twelve months.

Anxiety Management Training

As was noted earlier, most forms of relaxation incorporate some form of stress management and for that reason the two procedures have been grouped together. Stress management usually consists of instruction in the application of relaxation skills in the face of environmental stressors. Anxiety management training (AMT) takes this one stage further and incorporates anxiety induction procedures into the training. Jorgensen *et al.* (1981) describe an initial study of the use of such procedures in hypertensives. Eighteen medicated hypertensive patients were assigned either to AMT or a wait list control condition. After six weeks of treatment, both systolic and diastolic BP decreased more in the AMT than control group; the latter did not change. Paradoxically, the pressor response to a cognitive stressor was increased after AMT. This is unexplained and appears to contradict the findings from other studies that relaxation-related procedures either reduce the pressor response (Patel *et al.*, 1975) or leave it unchanged (Irvine *et al.*, in preparation; Goldstein *et al.*, 1982). Jorgensen *et al.*'s study is preliminary and lacks adequate control conditions, but may offer an interesting way forward in this field if it receives appropriate replication and extension.

There is now convincing evidence that relaxation and related procedures can lower BP in hypertensives. Some have argued that much stronger effects can be obtained with anti-hypertensive medication (Andrews *et al.*, 1982) than with either the behavioural treatments described here or other non-pharmacological treatments involving dietary change and weight loss. We (Johnston and Steptoe, 1982) dispute this interpretation of the clinical trial data and also, rather more importantly, have pointed out that even if anti-hypertensive drugs are shown to be capable of producing larger decreases in pressure, this does not necessarily indicate that they are the treatments of choice. The aim of treatment with hypertensives is to produce in the patient a BP level that is associated with an acceptable risk of cardiovascular disease. If a diastolic BP of 90 or below is taken as a criterion, then treatment packages such as Patel's may be quite appropriate for many patients. In her studies she has consistently shown, and we have replicated, pressure reductions from 160/100 to 140/90. This means that the average patients at the end of treatment is at or near the normotensive range. Few would propose that moderate or severely hypertensive individuals should be denied anti-hypertensive medication, but many would side with Oliver (1982) in his concern about the long term effects of anti-hypertensive medication on patients with only mild elevations in BP, and hence only mild elevations in cardiovascular risk. For such patients, behavioural treatment of the type that I have described offers an attractive alternative or adjunct to pharmacological therapies.

BRONCHIAL ASTHMA

Bronchial asthma was once considered a psychophysiological disorder *par excellence*. Heightened arousal, produced either by suggesting that neutral substances are, in fact, allergic (e.g. Luparello *et al.*, 1968) or by more conventional laboratory stressors such as distressing films (Mathé and Knapp, 1971; Weiss *et al.*, 1976), can produce increased respiratory resistance in asthmatics compared with non-asthmatic subjects. The effect on asthmatic attacks of the presumed reduction in family stress caused by separating asthmatic children from their parents has been documented by Purcell *et al.* (1969). However, in an excellent review of many aspects of asthma, Alexander (1981) points out that as research becomes increasingly sophisticated the evidence for psychological factors playing a primary role in asthma diminishes steadily. Writing in a rather similar vein Kinsman *et al.* (1980) have pointed out that only a minority of asthmatics respond to stress, at least as induced by suggestion, with bronchial spasm, and hence the role of stress reduction methods in asthma may be limited. The physiological mechanisms involved in the production of asthmatic attacks are complex and beyond the scope of this chapter, but it may be worth noting that asthmatic symptoms are worsened by increased parasympathetic activity and reduced by sympathetic activity. This fact has guided some behavioural approaches to therapy.

Biofeedback

Direct feedback of total respiratory resistance using the forced oscillation technique has been examined by Steptoe et al. (1981), who found a small effect favouring feedback in normals, but very little evidence that feedback aided control in asthmatic subjects. Vachon and Rich (1976) in a series of four experiments on asthmatic patients demonstrated that contingent feedback of total respiratory resistance did enable subjects to decrease their resistance, whereas non-contingent feedback did not. These two studies are both too limited and inconsistent for any conclusion to be drawn. It is tempting to suggest that future research is needed on these techniques, but experience suggests that if only two papers have appeared in six years on the use of an appealing gadget in a common condition, then there is a real possibility that it has been tried and found wanting by others.

Kotses et al. (1976, 1978) have examined the use of EMG feedback from the frontalis muscle and found that a reduction in facial muscle tension is associated with an increase in peak expiratory flow (PEF). Kotses and Glaus (1981) suggest that there may be a specific link between reduced tension in the facial muscles and decreased vagal tone to the bronchi, and hence reduced bronchial constriction; however, this mechanism is highly speculative. It is also worth mentioning that the measure of pulmonary function used, PEF, is effort-related and may well be susceptible to placebo and expectancy effects. It cannot, therefore, be regarded as entirely satisfactory in the absence of less reactive measures of pulmonary functioning, such as are available from the whole body plethysmograph. This criticism applies to virtually all studies in this section.

Harding and Maher (1982) also attempted to reduce vagal effects on the bronchi, in their case by training subjects in heart rate acceleration. They argue, with some plausibility, that this response is associated with decreased vagal input to the heart. Harding and Maher trained eight asthmatic subjects to increase their HR markedly over several sessions of training. Control subjects received one session of training in the maintenance of HR at a constant level. Both PEF and, more importantly, diary measures of asthmatic attacks and medication, suggest that the experimental subjects had benefitted from the feedback procedure, while the control subjects had not. This study is not entirely satisfactory methodologically since the experimental subjects received more training than the controls, and more subjects appear to have been dropped from the experimental group for various reasons. However, the simplicity and novelty of the approach suggests that it is worth further work.

Relaxation and Stress Management

At first sight, the use of relaxation training with asthmatics does not have a compelling rationale, since it is commonly assumed that relaxation operates by decreasing the sympathetic and increasing the parasympathetic outflow in the autonomic nervous system. However, the mechanisms underlying relaxation are mysterious, and it is possible that the central calming action or improved coping with stress associated with relaxation might well have beneficial effects in asthma, as it does in other conditions. In fact, the effects of relaxation training on asthma have been disappointing. Alexander and his colleagues in a series of studies have shown that relaxation can produce relatively trivial increases in forced expiratory volume over one second (FEV$_1$), another effort-related measure of pulmonary function (Alexander, 1972; Alexander *et al.*, 1972). This finding was replicated by Hock *et al.* (1978). Unfortunately, more satisfactory measures of pulmonary functioning do not show these beneficial effects (Alexander *et al.*, 1979).

Behaviour Therapy

More complex behavioural techniques have been used in the treatment of asthma for some time. Alexander (1981) has provided a good review of approaches based on the operant tradition; more germane to the concern of this paper are attempts to apply systematic desensitization and assertive training in this condition. Results with systematic desensitization are somewhat puzzling and disappointing. Moore (1965) compared systematic desensitization and relaxation training given in two ways, and found greater increases in PEF in the subjects receiving desensitization. Alexander (1981) commenting on this study, pointed out that PEF was measured very infrequently, a hazardous procedure when trying to assess as variable a condition as asthma. Yorkston and his colleagues have reported two studies (Yorkston *et al.*, 1974, 1979) in which systematic desensitization and relaxation were contrasted. In the first of these, 14 patients were allocated to the two treatments and FEV$_1$ was found to be significantly improved following systematic desensitization, while there was no change after relaxation. Furthermore, on a two-year follow-up by psychiatric interview, the patients who had received desensitization were judged as having received more clinical benefit, and to have reduced their medication to a greater extent. In their second study, Yorkston *et al.* added a third group who received systematic desensitization plus a form of *in vivo* desensitization, whereby they were taught to breathe against a progressively increasing resistance. This modification to the desensitization technique had no detectable effects, but again they report that systematic desensitization improved pulmonary function and also that subjects receiving desensitization reduced medication to a greater extent and reported less respiratory symptomatology. In this study, the positive effects of desensitization were confined to patients receiving steroids.

Against these generally rather hopeful findings have to be put the disappointing results of the study by Miklich *et al.* (1977). They argue that previous studies have not provided a firm basis for evaluating the clinical usefulness of systematic desensitization, and they sought to do this in an in-patient study of severely asthmatic children. Eighteen patients received systematic desensitization, while seven received the standard treatment regime of the institution. In both groups, FEV_1 measured twice daily decreased slightly (possibly the result of the institution's policy of withdrawing steroid medication from in-patients). This reduction in FEV_1 was greater in the control condition, suggesting that systematic desensitization had offset the effects of steroid withdrawal. However, daily measures of asthmatic symptomatology showed the opposite pattern, i.e. a greater reduction symptomatology in the control group. These contradictory findings are difficult to reconcile; indeed, the authors take the unusual step of admitting that "We ourselves are not in agreement on whether the results of the experimental subjects . . . are clinically useful. We are in agreement, however, that, even at best, systematic desensitization by reciprocal inhibition appears to have no more than an ancillary role in the management of asthma. All our subjects left the study as they entered it: chronically ill, moderately severe asthmatics." (Miklich *et al.*, 1977). It is unclear if the difference between this study and the other positive studies is due to some important difference between the methods of treatment, the patient populations, or to the methodological inadequacies of the positive studies.

Hock *et al.* (1978) compared assertive training with relaxation training, standard medical treatment or a placebo control in asthmatic boys. They found that such training did little to improve pulmonary functioning (as measured by FEV_1), and was associated with an increased frequency of asthmatic attacks. As mentioned above, relaxation training led to an improvement in pulmonary functioning and a temporary reduction in asthmatic attacks, while a combination of assertive training and relaxation training produced an intermediate result. There is, therefore, no reason on the basis of this study to suggest that assertive training would be appropriate for asthmatic boys in general.

The use of behavioural methods in the treatment of asthma has been disappointing. Feedback methods have been tried tentatively with little success, while clinical studies of relaxation training, systematic desensitization and assertive training have either failed to demonstrate convincing clinical improvements or have produced inconsistent results. These inconsistencies may relate to the methodological inadequacies of the studies. Kinsman *et al.* (1980) have argued that the heterogeneity of the asthmatic response to stress has to be acknowledged in the design of treatment trials, and suggest that behavioural treatment should be restricted to patients with highly reactive bronchi who also respond to stress with emotional arousal. This and other behavioural analyses of the factors associated with asthmatic attacks in individual patients might well improve patient selection, and provide a more malleable problem for the behavioural approach.

OVERVIEW

In the preceding sections, I have considered four different conditions. Behavioural methods have produced useful symptom control of tension and migraine headache and have lowered blood pressure. Only in the treatment of asthma has little been achieved. These gains are substantial and would have appeared quite remarkable only fifteen years ago. They must, therefore, be credited as very considerable successes for the behavioural approach. These successes have come about in a slightly unexpected manner; in particular, the failure of biofeedback to measure up to its early promise, or at least to the claims of some of its more enthusiastic supporters, is quite striking.

I noted earlier that this whole field was based on the enthusiasm aroused by biofeedback and related procedures, yet there is hardly any evidence that feedback has a *specific* effect, although it may have a beneficial non-specific effect. The failure to find convincing evidence that biofeedback in clinical practice adds to the methods of control that are available without feedback casts doubt on the skills model that was implicit in much biofeedback research, a doubt that is not confined to the clinical situation (Johnston, 1977b). Recent research has shown that under some circumstances, in which the accurate control of autonomic responses is required, a version of the skills model of biofeedback is applicable (Johnston and Lethem, 1981). However, such situations are far from the type of clinical problems we have been considering in this chapter.

Complete pessimism about the likely effects of biofeedback are not totally justified, as under some circumstances feedback does appear to have a specific effect. When the arousing effects on a feedback display and task are allowed for, then feedback is more effective than some purely verbal methods (Steptoe, 1977; Marie and Johnston, in preparation). There is related evidence that feedback is more effective than relaxation training during some forms of stress (Johnston *et al.*, 1982). The use of biofeedback to reduce the physiological effects of stressful or arousing situations is clearly an area requiring further exploration, particularly as many psychophysiological disorders are regarded as stress-related. Self-control during periods of stress would be of much greater clinical utility than the ability to control physiological functions under non-stressful or restful conditions. In addition, the use of biofeedback to foster changes that are unlikely to be produced by relaxation, such as responses mediated by increases in sympathetic nervous tone, is an area that requires more vigorous investigation. It is somewhat unfortunate that most investigators have chosen to emphasize those features of biofeedback that seem to be shared by other procedures, such as relaxation, rather than exploit its uniqueness.

A corollary of the non-specific effects of biofeedback is the good showing of relaxation training and stress management in three of the four conditions under consideration. The literature on the general effects of relaxation training does not encourage optimism about the likely success of such methods with psychophysiological disorders; but in fact such procedures appear to have powerful effects that are associated with impressive and useful clinical changes. The mechanisms underlying these therapeutic successes and the effective components of the total treatment and stress management package are still unclear and have to be evaluated. While in practically all the conditions some form of controlled trial of relaxation has been reported, these are in many instances rather weak, isolated studies. Only in the treatment of essential hypertension can a convincing case be made for the proposition that relaxation training and stress management have important specific effects. A priori there is no reason why this should not be true of the other conditions, but in the case of migraine in particular there is a strong suggestion that non-specific effects play a very large part in the therapeutic gains achieved both by relaxation training and skin temperature feedback. Given that headaches are common and that relaxation training appears to be an attractive treatment, sophisticated efforts to explore the non-specific effects of relaxation in this condition are urgently required.

If, as seems likely, psychophysiological disorders have a complex relationship with stress and other behavioural factors, then it is at least arguable that apparently simple treatments such as relaxation and stress management may not be optimally effective. Other more complex procedures that attempt more radical alterations in the patient's response to stress may be more effective. Behaviour therapy and cognitive behaviour therapy now offer many possible therapeutic approaches, some of which are gaining acceptance in the treatment of a variety of behavioural problems. The research generated by the cognitive behavioural approach of Holroyd and Mitchell is not extensive, but there is empirical support to bolster the already considerable intellectual attractions of a cognitive behavioural approach to stress-related disorders. It is to be hoped that the future will see further work on these and related approaches in all the conditions we have been considering. An attractive feature of these more complex approaches is that they incorporate detailed analysis of the situations that actually influence the patient's psychophysiological disturbance. Treatment can, therefore, be tailored to the requirements of the individual patient. If such matching of patients and treatment is important, and most behaviour therapists believe it to be so, then this has implications for the interpretation of the type of outcome trial that is the basis of this review. Such trials normally only enable one to comment on the comparative effectiveness of a particular treatment on the average patient. While it would be a bold (or ignorant) clinician who persistently used a treatment that had been shown to be ineffective in clinical trials, it should be recalled that even with the most effective behavioural treatments some patients respond poorly. On the other hand, the treatments that do not appear to have widespread advantages are occasionally effective with individual patients. For example, while I have argued that in the treatment of tension headache EMG biofeedback has no specific advantage over relaxation training, it might still be perfectly appropriate to use biofeedback in patients with very high levels of muscular tension, particularly if they have failed to respond to relaxation training.

A major problem in the use of complex behavioural approaches in this field is the lack of adequate evidence on how stress produces or affects these physiological disorders. It is hoped that future behavioural work on aetiology, maintenance and treatment of these conditions will not be carried out in isolation, and that the impressive empirical gains made in the last fifteen years may be put on a more secure intellectual basis: a basis that may be necessary for their continued rational application in the face of the fadism and mysticism to which practitioners in this field are endemically prone.

ACKNOWLEDGEMENTS

During the preparation of this chapter the writer was in receipt of a grant from the Medical Research Council.

REFERENCES

Alexander, A. B. (1972). Systematic relaxation and flow rates in asthmatic children: relationship to emotional precipitants and anxiety. *J. Psychosom. Res.* **16,** 405–410.
Alexander, A. B. (1981). Behavioural approaches to the treatment of bronchial

asthma. *In* "Medical Psychology: Contributions to Behavioural Medicine" (C. P. Prokop and L. A. Bradley, eds), pp. 373–394. Academic Press, Orlando, New York and London.

Alexander, A. B., Miklich, D. R. and Hernskoff, H. (1972). The immediate effects of systematic relaxation training on peak expiratory flow in asthmatic children. *Psychosm. Med.* **34**, 388–394.

Alexander, A. B., White, P. D. and Wallace, H. M. (1977). Training and transfer effects of training effects in EMG biofeedback. *Psychophysiology* **14**, 551–559.

Alexander, A. B., Cropp, G. J. A. and Cahi, H. (1979). Effects of relaxation training on pulmonary mechanics in children with asthma. *J. Appl. Behav. Anal.* **12**, 27–35.

Allen, R. A. and Mills, G. K. (1982). The effects of unilateral plethysmographic feedback of temporal artery activity during migraine headache pain. *J. Psychosom. Res.* **26**, 133–140.

Anderson, C. D. and Franks, R. D. (1981). Migraine and tension headache: is there a physiological difference? *Headache* **21**, 63–71.

Andrews, G., McMahon, S., Austin, C. and Byrne, D. (1982). Hypertension; comparison of drug and non-drug treatments. *Br. Med. J.* **284**, 1523–1526.

Bakal, D. A. and Kaganov, J. A. (1977). Muscle contraction and migraine headache: a psychophysiological comparison. *Headache* **17**, 208–215.

Bakal, D. A. and Kaganov, J. A. (1979). Symptom characteristics of chronic and non-chronic headache sufferers. *Headache* **19**, 285–289.

Bali, L. R. (1979). Long term effect of relaxation on blood pressure and anxiety levels in essential hypertensive males: A controlled study. *Psychosom. Med.* **41**, 637–646.

Benson, H., Beary, J. F. and Carol, M. P. (1974). The relaxation response. *Psychiatry* **37**, 37–46.

Bild, R. and Adams, H. E. (1980). Modification of migraine headaches by cephalic blood volume pulse and EMG biofeedback. *J. Consult. Clin. Psychol.* **48**, 51–57.

Blanchard, E. B., Theobald, D. E., Williamson, D. A., Silver, B. V. and Brown, D. A. (1978). Temperature biofeedback in the treatment of migraine headaches. *Arch. Gen. Psychiat.* **35**, 581–588.

Blanchard, E. R., Miller, S. T., Abel, C. C., Haynes, M. R. and Wicker, R. (1979). Evaluation of biofeedback in the treatment of essential hypertension. *J. Appl. Behav. Anal.* **12**, 99–110.

Borkovec, T. D. and Sides, J. K. (1979). Critical procedural variables related to the physiological effects of progressive relaxation: a review. *Behav. Res. Ther.* **17**, 119–125.

Borkovec, T. D., Kaloupek, D. G. and Slama, K. (1975). The facilitive effect of muscle tension-release in the relaxation therapy of sleep disturbance. *Behav. Ther.* **6**, 301–309.

Borkovec, T. D., Grayson, J. B. and Cooper, K. M. (1978). Treatment of general tension: subjective and physiological effects of progressive relaxation. *J. Consult. Clin. Psychol.* **46**, 518–528.

Brauer, A., Horlick, L. F., Nelson, B., Farquhar, J. U. and Agras, W. S. (1979). Relaxation therapy for essential hypertension: a Veterans Administration out patients study. *J. Behav. Med.* **2**, 21–29.

Budzynski, T. H., Stoyva, J. M., Adler, C. S. and Mullaney, D. J. (1973). EMG biofeedback and tension headache: a controlled outcome study. *Psychosom. Med.* **35**, 484–496.

Burish, T. G., Hendrix, E. M. and Frost, R. O. (1981). Comparison of frontal EMG biofeedback and several types of relaxation instructions in reducing multiple indices of arousal. *Psychophysiology* **18**, 594–602.

Cohen, M. J., Ricles, W. H. and McArthur, D. L. (1978). Evidence of physiological response stereotypy in migraine headache. *Psychosom. Med.* **40**, 344–354.

Cohen, M. J., McArthur, D. L. and Rickles, W. H. (1980). Comparison of four biofeedback treatments for migraine headaches: physiological and headache variables. *Psychosom. Med.* **42**, 463–480.

Coursey, R. D. (1975). Electromyograph feedback as a relaxation technique. *J. Consult. Clin. Psychol.* **43**, 825–834.

Cox, D. J., Freundlich, A. and Meyer, R. G. (1975). Differential effectiveness of electromyograph feedback, verbal relaxation instructions, and medication placebo with tension headaches. *J. Consult. Clin. Psychol.* **433**, 892–898.

Cram, J. R. (1980). EMG biofeedback training and the treatment of tension headaches: a systematic analysis of treatment components. *Behav. Ther.* **11**, 699–710.

Davidson, D. M., Winchester, M. A., Taylor, C. B., Alderman, E. A. and Engels, N. B. (1979). Effects of relaxation therapy on cardiac performance and sympathetic activity in patients with organic heart disease. *Psychosom. Med.* **41**, 303–309.

Davidson, P. O. and Schwartz, G. E. (1976). The psychobiology of relaxation and related states, a multi-process theory. *In* "Behaviour Control and Modification of Physiological activity" (D. I. Mostofsky, ed.), pp. 399–442. Prentice-Hall, New York.

Davis, P. J. (1980). Electromyographic biofeedback: generalisation and relative effects of feedback, instructions and adaptation. *Psychophysiology* **17**, 604–612.

Elmore, A. M. and Tursky, B. (1981). A comparison of two psychophysiological approaches to the treatment of migraine. *Headache* **21**, 93–101.

Engel, B. T., Nikoomanesh, P. and Schuster, M. M. (1974). Operant conditioning of rectosphincteric responses in the treatment of fecal incontinence. *New Engl. J. Med.* **290**, 646–649.

Feuerstein, M., Bush, C. and Corbisiero, R. (1982). Stress and chronic headache: a psychophysiological analysis of mechanisms. *J. Psychosom. Res.* **26**, 167–182.

Fey, S. G. and Lindholm, E. (1978). Biofeedback and progressive relaxation: effects on systolic and diastolic blood pressure and heart rate. *Psychophysiology* **15**, 239–247.

Forsyth, R. P. (1971). Regional blood flow changes during 72-hour avoidance schedules in the monkey. *Science* **173**, 546–548.

Frankel, B. L., Patel, D. J., Horwitz, D., Friedwald, M. T. and Gaardner, K. P. (1978). Treatment of hypertension with biofeedback and relaxation techniques. *Psychosom. Med.* **40**, 276–293.

Friar, L. R. and Beatty, J. T. (1976). Migraine: management by operant conditioning of vasoconstriction. *J. Consult. Clin. Psychol.* **44**, 46–53.

Friedman, A. P. (1979). Characteristics of tension headache: a profile of 1420 cases. *Psychosomatics* **20**, 451–461.

Gauthier, J., Bois, R., Allaire, D. and Drolet, M. (1981). Evaluation of skin temperature biofeedback training at two different sites on migraine. *J. Behav. Med.* **4**, 407–420.

Gellhorn, E. (1964). Motion and emotion: The role of proprioception in the physiology and pathology of the emotions. *Psychol.* **71**, 457–472.

Glasgow, M. S., Gaardner, K. R. and Engel, B. T. (1982). Behavioural treatment of high blood pressure: II Acute and sustained effects of relaxation and systolic blood pressure biofeedback. *Psychosom. Med.* **44**, 155–171.

Goldstein, I. B., Shapiro, D., Thananopavarn, C. and Sambhi, M. P. (1982). Comparison of drug and behavioural treatments of essential hypertension. *Health Psychol.* **1**, 7–26.

Graham, J. D. P. (1945). High blood pressure after battle. *Lancet* **i**, 239–240.

Harding, A. V. and Maher, K. R. (1982). Biofeedback training of cardiac acceleration; effects on airway resistance in bronchial asthma. *J. Psychosom. Res.* **26**, 447–454.

Hart, J. D. and Chichanski, K. A. (1981). A comparison of frontal EMG biofeedback and neck EMG biofeedback in the treatment of muscle-contraction headache. *Biofeedback and Self-Regulation* **6**, 63–74.

Hastrup, J. L., Light, K. C. and Obrist, P. A. (1982). Parental hypertension and cardiovascular responses to stress in healthy young adults. *Psychophysiology* **19**, 615–622.

Haynes, S. N., Griffin, P., Mooney, D. and Parise, M. (1975). Electro-myographic biofeedback and relaxation instructions in the treatment of muscle contraction headaches. *Behav. Ther.* **6**, 672–678.

Henry, J. P., Stephens, P. M. and Santisteban, G. A. (1975). A model of psychosocial hypertension showing reversibility and progression of cardiovascular complications. *Circulation Res.* **36**, 156–164.

Henryk-Gutt, R. and Rees, W. L. (1973). Psychological aspects of migraine. *J. Psychosom. Res.* **17**, 141–153.

Hillenberg, J. B. and Collins, F. L. (1982). A procedural analysis and review of relaxation training research. *Behav. Res. Ther.* **20**, 251–260.

Hock, R. A., Rodgers, C. H., Reddi, C. and Kennard, D. V. (1978). Medico-psychological interventions in male asthmatic children: An evaluation of physiological change. *Psychosom. Med.* **40**, 210–215.

Hoffman, J. W., Benson, H., Arns, P. A., Stainbrook, G. L., Landsberg, L., Young, J. B. and Gill, A. (1982). Reduced sympathetic nervous system responsivity associated with the relaxation response. *Science* **215**, 190–192.

Holroyd, K. A. and Andrasik, F. (1980). Coping and the self-control of chronic tension headache. *J. Consult. Clin. Psychol.* **46**, 1036–1045.

Holroyd, K. A. and Andrasik, F. (1982). Do the effects of cognitive therapy endure? A two year follow-up of tension headache sufferers treated with cognitive therapy. *Cognit. Ther. Res.* **6**, 325–334.

Holdroyd, K. A., Andrasik, F. and Westbrook, T. (1977). Cognitive control of tension headache. *Cognit. Ther. Res.* **1**, 121–133.

Holroyd, K. A., Andrasik, F. and Noble, J. (1980). A comparison of EMG biofeedback and a credible pseudotherapy in treating tension headache. *J. Behav. Med.* **3**, 29–39.

Hutchings, D. F., Denney, D. R., Basgall, J. and Houston, B. K. (1980). Anxiety management training and applied relaxation training in reducing general anxiety. *Behav. Res. Ther.* **18**, 181–190.

Irvine, J., Johnston, D. W., Jenner, D. and Marie, G. V. A controlled trial of relaxation and stress management in essential hypertension. Manuscript in preparation.

Jacobson, E. (1938). "Progressive Relaxation." University of Chicago Press, Chicago.

Johnston, D. W. (1977a). Feedback and instructional effects in the voluntary control of digital pulse amplitude. *Biol. Psychol.* **5**, 159–171.

Johnston, D. W. (1977b). Biofeedback, verbal instructions and the motor skills analogy. In "Biofeedback and Behaviour" (J. Beatty and H. Legewie, eds), pp. 331–341. Plenum Press, New York.

Johnston, D. W. (1982a). The behavioural treatment of the symptoms of ischaemic heart disease. In "Behavioral Treatment of Disease" (R. Surwit, R. Williams, A. Steptoe and R. Biersner, eds), pp. 115–127. Plenum Press, New York.

Johnston, D. W. (1982b). Behavioural treatment in the reduction of coronary risk factors: Type A behaviour and blood pressure. *Br. J. Clin. Psychol.* **21**, 281–294.

Johnston, D. W. and Lethem, J. (1981). The production of specific decreases in interbeat interval and the motor skills analogy. *Psychophysiology* **18**, 288–300.

Johnston, D. W. and Steptoe, A. (1982). Non-drug treatments of hypertension. *Br. Med. J.* **285**, 1046.

Johnston, D. W., Lo, C. R., Marie, G. V. and Van Jones, J. (1982). Self-control of interbeat interval and pulse transit time at rest and during exercise. A preliminary report. *Acta Med. Scand.* **660**(suppl.), 238–243.

Jorgensen, R. S., Houston, B. K. and Zoravski, R. M. (1981). Anxiety management training in the treatment of essential hypertension. *Behav. Res. Ther.* **19**, 467–474.

Kasl, S. V. and Cobb, S. (1970). Blood pressure changes in men undergoing job loss: A preliminary report. *Psychosom. Med.* **32**, 19–32.

Kewman, D. and Roberts, A. H. (1980). Skin temperature biofeedback and migraine headaches: A double-blind study. *Biofeedback and Self-Regulation* **5**, 327–346.

King, N. J. (1980). The therapeutic utility of abbreviated progressive relaxation: A critical review with implications for clinical practice. In "Progress in Behaviour Modification (M. Hersen, R. M. Eisler and P. M. Miller, eds), Vol. 10, pp. 147–182. Academic Press, Orlando, New York and London.

Kinsman, R. A., Dirks, J. F., Jones, N. F. and Dahlem, N. W. (1980). Anxiety reduction in asthma: four catches to general application. *Psychosom. Med.* **42**, 397–405.

Knapp, T. W. (1982). Evidence for sympathetic deactivation by temporal vasoconstriction and digital vasodilation-biofeedback in migraine patients: A reply to Elmore and Tursky and a new hypothesis. *Headache* **22**, 233–236.

Kotses, H. and Glaus, K. D. (1981). Application of biofeedback to the treatment of asthma: a critical review. *Biofeedback and Self-Regulation* **6**, 573–593.

Kotses, H., Glaus, K. D., Crawford, P. L., Edwards, J. E. and Scherr, M. S. (1976). Operant reduction of frontalis EMG activity in the treatment of asthma in children. *J. Psychosom. Res.* **20**, 453–459.

Kotses, H., Glaus, K. D., Bricel, S. K., Edwards, J. E. and Crawford, P. L. (1978). Operant muscular relaxation and peak expiratory flow rate in asthmatic children. *J. Psychosom. Res.* **22**, 17–23.

LaCroix, J. M., Bock, J. C. and Lavis, S. (1983). Biofeedback and relaxation in the treatment of migraines: Comparative effectiveness and physiological correlates. *J. Neurol. Neurosurg. Psychiat.* **46**, 525–532.

Lang, R., Dehof, K. A., Meurer, W. and Kaufmann, J. (1979). Sympathetic activity and transcendental meditation. *J. Neural Transmiss.* **44**, 117–135.

Lawler, J. M., Barker, G. F., Hubbard, J. W. and Allen, M. T. (1980). The effects of conflict on tonic levels of blood pressure in the genetically borderline hypertension rat. *Psychophyiology* **17**, 363–370.

Lehrer, P. M. (1982). How to relax and how not to relax: a re-evaluation of the work of Edmund Jacobson-I. *Behav. Res. Ther.* **20,** 417–428.

Lehrer, P. M., Schoicket, S., Carington, P. and Woolfolk, J. M. (1980). Psychophysiological and cognitive responses to stressful stimuli in subjects practising progressive relaxation and clinically standardised meditation. *Behav. Res. Ther.* **18,** 293–303.

Lo, C. R. and Johnston, D. W. (in press). The self control of the cardiovascular response to exercise using feedback of the product of interbeat interval and pulse transmit time. *Psychosom. Med.*

Luparello, T. J., Lyons, H. A., Bleecker, E. R. and McFadden, E. R. (1968). Influences of suggestion on airway reactivity in asthmatic subjects. *Psychosom. Med.* **30,** 819–825.

Lutz, D. J. and Holmes, D. S. (1981). Instructions to change blood pressure and diastolic blood pressure feedback: their effects on diastolic blood pressure, systolic blood pressure and anxiety. *J. Psychosom. Res.* **25,** 479–485.

Marie, G. V. and Johnston, D. W. The self-control of pulse transit time at rest and during isometric exercise. Manuscript in preparation.

Marie, G. V., Lo, C. R., Van Jones, J. and Johnston, D. W. (in press). The relationship between pulse transit time and arterial blood pressure during dynamic and static exercise. *Psychophysiology.*

Martin, P. R. and Mathews, A. M. (1978). Tension headache: psychophysiological investigation and treatment. *J. Psychosom. Res.* **22,** 389–399.

Mathe, A. A. and Knapp, P. A. (1971). Emotional and adrenal reactions to stress in bronchial asthma. *Psychosom. Med.* **33,** 323–340.

Mathew, R. S., Ho, B. T., Kralik, D., Taylor, D., Semchuk, K., Weinman, M. and Claghorn, J. L. (1980). Catechol-O-Methyltransferase and catecholamines in anxiety and relaxation. *Psychiat. Res.* **3,** 85–91.

Michaels, R. R., Huber, M. J. and McCann, D. S. (1976). Evaluation of transcendental meditation as a method of reducing stress. *Science* **192,** 1242–1244.

Miklich, D. R., Renne, C. M., Creer, T. L., Alexander, A. B., Chai, H., Davis, M. H., Hoffman, A. and Danker-Brown, P. (1977). The clinical utility of behaviour therapy as an adjunctive treatment for asthma. *J. Allergy Clin. Immunol.* **60,** 285–294.

Mitchell, K. R. and Mitchell, D. M. (1971). Migraine: an exploratory treatment application of programmed behaviour therapy techniques. *J. Psychosom. Res.* **15,** 137–157.

Mitchell, K. R. and White, R. C. (1977). Behavioural self-management: an application to the problem of migraine headaches. *Behav. Ther.* **8,** 213–221.

Moore, N. (1965). Behaviour therapy in bronchial asthma: a controlled study. *J. Psychosom. Res.* **9,** 257–276.

Naliboff, B. D. and Johnson, H. J. (1978). Finger pulse amplitude and frontalis EMG: effects of single and two system biofeedback training. *Biofeedback and Self-Regulation* **3,** 133–143.

Obrist, P. A. (1981). "Cardiovascular Psychophysiology." Plenum Press, New York.

Obrist, P. A., Light, K. C., McCubbin, J. A., Hutcheson, J. S. and Hoffer, J. L. (1978). The relationship among heart rate, carotid dP/dt and blood pressure in humans as a function of the type of stress. *Psychophysiology* **15,** 102–115.

Ohno, Y., Yoshihaura, T., Takeya, T. and Ikemi, Y. (1977). Modification of skin temperature by biofeedback procedures. *J. Behav. Ther. Exp. Psychiat.* **8,** 31–34.

Oliver, M. F. (1982). Risks of correcting the risks of coronary disease and stroke with drugs. *New Engl. J. Med.* **306**, 297–298.

Paiva, T., Nunes, J. S., Moreira, A., Santos, J., Teixeira, J. and Barbosa, A. (1982). Effects of frontalis EMG biofeedback and diazepam in the treatment of tension headache. *Headache* **22**, 216–220.

Parnel, P. and Cooperstock, R. (1979). Tranquillisers and mood elevators in the treatment of migraine: An analysis of the Migraine Foundation Questionnaire. *Headache* **19**, 78–84.

Patel, C. (1975). Yoga and biofeedback in the management of "stress" in hypertensive patients. *Clin. Sci. Molec. Med.* **48**(suppl.), 171–174.

Patel, C. and North, W. R. S. (1975). Randomised controlled trial of yoga and biofeedback in the management of hypertension. *Lancet* **ii**, 93–95.

Patel, C., Marmot, M. G. and Terry, D. J. (1981). Controlled trial of biofeedback-aided behavioural methods in reducing mild hypertension. *Br. Med. J.* **282**, 2005–2008.

Pearce, S. and Morley, S. (1981). An experimental investigation of pain production in headache patients. *Br. J. Clin. Psychol.* **20**, 275–281.

Price, K. P. and Tursky, B. (1976). Vascular reactivity of migraineurs and non-migraineurs: a comparison of responses to self-control procedures. *Headache* **16**, 210–217.

Purcell, K., Brady, K., Chai, H., Muser, J., Molk, L., Gordon, N. and Means, J. (1969). The effect of asthma in children of experimental separation from family. *Psychosom. Med.* **31**, 144–164.

Reinking, R. H. and Kohl, M. L. (1975). Effects of various forms of relaxation training on physiological and self report measures of relaxation. *J. Consult. Clin. Psychol.* **43**, 595–600.

Roberts, A. H., Kewman, D. G. and MacDonald, H. (1973). Voluntary control of skin temperature: unilateral changes using hypnosis and feedback. *J. Abnorm. Psychol.* **82**, 163–168.

Sargent, J., Greene, E. and Walters, E. (1973). Preliminary report on the use of autogenic feedback training in the treatment of migraine and tension headache. *Psychosom. Med.* **35**, 129–135.

Shapiro, D. (1973). Role of feedback and instructions in the voluntary control of human blood pressure. *Jap. J. Biofeedback Res.* **1**, 2–9.

Shapiro, D., Tursky, B., Gershon, E. and Stern, M. (1969). Effects of feedback and reinforcement on control of human systolic blood pressure. *Science* **163**, 588–590.

Shapiro, D., Schwartz, G. E. and Tursky, B. (1972). Control of diastolic blood pressure in man by feedback and reinforcement. *Psychophysiology* **9**, 296–304.

Siddle, D. A. T. and Wood, L. (1979). Effects of frontalis EMG feedback and reinforcement on frontalis EMG level. *Biol. Psychol.* **9**, 227–236.

Simpson, D. D. and Nelson, A. E. (1976). Specificity of finger pulse volume feedback during relaxation. *Biofeedback and Self-Regulation* **1**, 433–443.

Smith, J. C. (1976). Psychotherapy effects of transcendental meditation with controls for expectation of relief and daily sitting. *J. Consult. Clin. Psychol.* **44**, 630–637.

Sokolow, M., Werdegar, D., Perloff, D. B., Cowan, R. M. and Brenenstuhl, H. (1970). Preliminary studies relating portably recorded blood pressures to daily life in patients with essential hypertension. "Psychosomatics in Essential Hypertension" (M. Koster, H. Musaph and P. Visser, eds), pp. 164–189. Karger, Basel.

Southam, M. A., Agras, W. S., Taylor, C. B. and Kraemer, H. C. (1982).

Relaxation training: blood pressure during the working day. *Arch. Gen. Psychiat.* **39,** 715–717.

Steptoe, A. (1976). Blood pressure control: a comparison of feedback and instructions using pulse transit time feedback. *Psychophysiology* **13,** 528–536.

Steptoe, A. (1977). Voluntary blood pressure reductions measured with pulse transit time: training conditions and reaction to mental work. *Psychophysiology* **14,** 492–498.

Steptoe, A. (1978). The regulation of blood pressure reactions to taxing conditions using pulse transit time feedback and relaxation. *Psychophysiology* **15,** 429–438.

Steptoe, A. (1981). "Psychological Factors in Cardiovascular Disorders." Academic Press, London, Orlando and New York.

Steptoe, A. and Ross, A. (1982). Voluntary control of cardiovascular reactions to demanding tasks. *Biofeedback and Self-Regulation* **7,** 149–166.

Steptoe, A., Mathews, A. and Johnston, D. W. (1974). The learned control of differential temperature in the human earlobe: Preliminary study. *Biol. Psychol.* **1,** 237–242.

Steptoe, A., Smulyan, H. and Gribbin, B. (1976). Pulse wave velocity and blood pressure: calibration and applications. *Psychophysiology* **13,** 488–493.

Steptoe, A., Phillips, J. and Harling, J. (1981). Biofeedback and instructions in the modification of total respiratory resistance: an experimental study of asthmatic and non-asthmatic volunteers. *J. Psychosom. Res.* **25,** 541–551.

Sterman, M. B. (1977). Clinical implications of EEG biofeedback training: A critical appraisal. *In* (G. E. Schwartz and J. Beatty, eds.), pp. 389–411. "Biofeedback: Theory and Research" Academic Press, Orlando, New York and London.

Surwit, R. S. and Fenton, C. H. (1980). Feedback and instructions in the control of digital skin temperature. *Psychophysiology* **17,** 129–132.

Surwit, R. S., Shapiro, D. and Feld, J. L. (1976). Digital temperature autoregulation and associated cardiovascular changes. *Psychophysiology* **13,** 236–241.

Surwit, R. S., Hager, J. L. and Feldman, T. (1977). The role of feedback in voluntary control of blood pressure in instructed subjects. *J. Appl. Behav. Anal.* **10,** 625–631.

Taylor, C. B., Farquhar, J. W., Nelson, E. and Agras, W. S. (1977). Relaxation therapy and high blood pressure. *Arch. Gen. Psychiat.* **34,** 339–342.

Thompson, J. K., Haber, J. D. and Tearnan, B. H. (1981). Generalisation of frontalis electromyographic feedback to adjacent muscle groups: A critical review. *Psychosom. Med.* **43,** 19–24.

Vachon, L. and Rich, E. S. (1976). Visceral learning in asthma. *Psychosom. Med.* **38,** 122–130.

Van Boxtel, A. and Van der Ven, J. R. (178). Differential EMG activity in subjects with muscle contraction headaches related to mental effort. *Headache* **17,** 233–237.

Vaughn, R., Pall, M. L. and Haynes, S. N. (1976). Frontalis EMG response to stress in subjects with frequent muscle contraction headaches. *Headache* **16,** 313–317.

Weiner, H. (1977). "Psychobiology and Human Disease." Elsevier, New York.

Weiss, J. H., Lyness, J., Molk, L. and Riley, J. (1976). Induced respiratory change in asthmatic children. *J. Psychosom. Res.* **20,** 115–123.

Wolpe, J. (1958). "Psychotherapy by Reciprocal Inhibition." Stanford University Press, Stanford.

Woolfolk, R. L., Lehrer, P. M., McCann, B. S. and Rooney, A. J. (1982). Effects of progressive relaxation and meditation on cognitive and somatic manifestations of daily stress. *Behav. Res. Ther.* **20,** 461–467.

Yorkston, N. J., McHugh, R. B., Brady, R., Serber, M. and Sergeant, H. G. S. (1974). Verbal desensitisation in bronchial asthma. *J. Psychosom. Res.* **18,** 371–376.

Yorkston, N. J., Eckert, E., McHugh, R. B., Philander, D. A. and Blumenthal, M. N. (1979). Bronchial asthma: improved lung function after behaviour modification. *Psychosomatics* **20,** 231–237.

Zuroff, D. C. and Schwartz, J. C. (1978). Effects of transcendental meditation and muscle relaxation on trait anxiety, maladjustment, locus of control and drug use. *J. Consult. Clin. Psychol.* **46,** 264–271.

10

Behavioural Interventions in Cardiac Rehabilitation

WOLFGANG LANGOSCH

CARDIOLOGICAL COMPLICATIONS FOLLOWING ACUTE MYOCARDIAL INFARCTION

Myocardial infarction is usually a manifestation of coronary insufficiency, which is defined as an imbalance between the demand and supply of oxygen (Büchner, 1939). Coronary sclerosis leading to stenosis or occlusion generally makes up the morphological basis for coronary insufficiency. If acute coronary insufficiency is maintained over a long period of time considerable necrosis of the myocardium may result, whereas a passing acute coronary insufficiency only leads to the occurrence of angina pectoris (Roskamm, 1982). Myocardial infarction may, therefore, be regarded as a complication of a chronic coronary disease (Kalusche, 1982).

Many patients, however, do not experience any typical angina pectoris pains directly prior to infarction. Schweizer *et al.* (1977) report that only 20% of their infarction patients suffered pectanginal symptoms before onset of infarction. During an acute myocardial infarction, however, 80% of the patients questioned reported experiencing considerable pain. Such pain is often accompanied by anxiety and depression that may continue for several hours or even days (Kalusche, 1982).

Approximately 80% of deaths resulting from infarction occur before the victims reach the hospital. In this early phase of acute myocardial infarction, two complications determine the outcome: onset of rhythmic disturbances and hyperactivity of the sympathetic and parasympathetic nervous systems. Accordingly, within the first four hours after infarction onset, ventricular extrasystoles are exhibited in 93% of cases, bradyrhythmia in 40%, and ventricular fibrillation in 15.5% (Kalusche, 1982). Since the introduction of

HEALTH CARE AND HUMAN BEHAVIOUR
ISBN 0–12–666460–9

coronary care units, the mortality rate subsequent to hospitalization has dropped considerably, although is still stands at 15% (Meltzer, 1969).

The long-term prognosis of the post-infarct patient is dependent on the severity of angina pectoris, the size of the myocardium, occurrence of rhythmic disturbances, number of diseased coronary vessels, as well as the condition of the ventricles. Accordingly, the survival rate after a 10 year period is 97% for patients with one-vessel disease, 79% for two-vessel disease, and 66% for three-vessel disease with normal ventricular functioning. With pathological ventricular functioning the survival rates are 85%, 58% and 40% for the same groups respectively (see Parker, 1978). Moret *et al.* (1981) report that over a period of ten years, 38% of their patients are free of angina pectoris and reinfarction. In contrast, 34% complained of angina pectoris pain, 9% experienced reinfarction, and in 6% both angina pectoris and reinfarction occurred. Although the mortality rate is lower in younger patients, Stürzenhofecker *et al.* (1981) found that amongst males suffering an infarction before the age of 40, the mortality rate of 2.7% per year over a period of four years was higher than that expected by chance.

PSYCHOLOGICAL RESPONSE TO INFARCTION

In light of the various cardiac complications that occur not only in the acute, but also in the chronic phases of myocardial infarction, it is not surprising that many patients have considerable difficulty in coping with all stages of the illness. Following the acute phase of illness, the post infarction patient is confronted with the consequences of physical impairment, intense pain, and the experience of just surviving a severely life-threatening event (Kazemier, 1981).

The severity of the infarction is not, however, the primary determinant of the psychological reaction (Nagle *et al.*, 1976). The presence of angina pectoris pain may be significant. Langosch and Brodner (1979) carried out a one-year follow-up study with 87 post-infarction patients. They reported that patients with angina pectoris rate themselves as significantly less assertive, as receiving less recognition and respect, over-meticulous, tense, reserved if not socially inhibited, and socially less successful. Physical fitness may play an important role in the psychological differences between patients with and without angina pectoris, since these differences tend to increase in parallel with physical fitness ratings (Langosch *et al.*, 1980).

Upon returning home, post-infarction patients often report a change in mood, leading to depression (Hackett and Cassem, 1982). Wishnie *et al.* (1971) report that of 24 patients who reported that they were looking forward to returning home, 21 rated themselves as anxious or depressed during the first month following their return.

With increasing chronicity of illness, psychological adjustment to changed living conditions becomes more important (see Zaitsev, 1976). Various follow-up studies have shown the importance of this adjustment for post-infarction patients. Mayou *et al.* (1978a) report that two months after infarction 72% of patients complain of impairment in their subjective state and 53% of moderate distress; anxiety and depression were the most frequently reported symptoms among these patients. Upon follow-up after one year, 66% of these patients report impaired subjective state, whereas 64% still experienced moderate distress (Mayou *et al.*, 1978b). In a follow-up study with 289 post-infarction patients conducted one year after the event, Croog and Levine (1977) observed that 50.5% of their patients rated themselves as discouraged or depressed, 30% report that their lives were not yet back to normal and 55.6% continued to complain of bodily disturbances.

Medert-Dorscheidt and Myrtek (1977) describe extensive disturbances in the subjective states of post-infarction patients two years after hospitalization. Three years after discharge, the patients' psychological state was markedly worse compared to their ratings conducted during hospitalization (Langosch, 1980). Apparently, most post-infarction patients are only partially successful in coping with chronic illness. On returning home, post-infarction patients experience further disturbances in well-being as well as having to deal with physical deterioration. The patient is subjected to quite specific constraints on physical activity. These "functional limitations" often lead to a contradiction between patients and their families about his or her expected and actual capabilities. Such discrepancies may elicit psychosocial effects that induce patients to perceive themselves as "handicapped" (Kallinke, 1982). This syndrome is common amongst the chronically ill, and not specific to cardiac patients (Stocksmeier, 1976; Viney and Westbrook, 1981).

TASKS AND GOALS OF CARDIAC REHABILITATION

The acute myocardial infarction may be viewed as a life crisis that unexpectedly and dramatically interrupts the patient's daily routine, simultaneously evoking anxiety and depression. Following infarction, not only is it important that patients avoid further cardiac complications like reinfarction and angina pectoris, but they must reintegrate themselves into daily living despite illness. The patient must find a lifestyle that is compatible with functional limitations, as well as with the effects of chronic illness on family and vocation.

The task of rehabilitative therapy in cardiology is to provide assistance to these patients. According to the World Health Organisation definition, cardiac rehabilitation is the sum of all measures needed to provide the best possible bodily, psychological and social conditions for the patient to regain as normal a position in society, and as active and productive a life as possible. In accordance with this idea, the following three phases have been differentiated (see König, 1982): *Phase I* consists of the hospitalization period directly following infarction, and lasting until discharge (see Chapter 7); *Phase II* consists of immediate rehabilitation following discharge and ends when the patient goes back to work (i.e. is capable of rejoining daily life in so far as this is possible in view of coronary insufficiency and physical limitation, and *Phase III* is concerned with life following vocational and social reintegration.

What psychological and behavioural aspects are important in successful cardiological rehabilitation? First, it is essential to reduce the standard risk factors that are dependent on behaviour, i.e. smoking, high cholesterol diet, lack of physical activity, etc. By reducing such risk factors the likelihood of reinfarction or a progression in coronary sclerosis is reduced (Epstein and Wilhelmsen, 1982; Stürzenhofecker *et al.*, 1981). Improved compliance with medications may further serve this goal. Another recently recognized risk factor is the Type A behaviour pattern (see Review Panel, 1981). This not only doubles the risk of initial myocardial infarction (Brand, 1978), but also increases the risk of reinfarction (Jenkins, 1976; Jenkins *et al.*, 1971). The Type A behaviour pattern is characterized according to Rosenman and Friedman (1977) by a profound sense of time urgency, as well as by enhanced aggressiveness and drive that often merges into hostility. Therefore, the second step is the reduction in Type-A response patterns, in an effort to improve the prognosis of the post-infarction patient. Siegrist *et al.* (1982) have shown that patients experiencing reinfarction exhibit significantly higher frequencies of psychosocial risk factor constellations, demonstrate extensive Type A behaviour, are subjected to more intensive vocational stress elicited by the organizational structure and activity, and experience more changes in life events, than patients without reinfarction. Furthermore, Langosch *et al.* (1983) reported that post-infarction patients who exhibit a progression in coronary sclerosis have been subjected to more intense vocational stress than those who regress. In light of this, not only is a reduction in the psychosocial risk factor constellations important, but an improvement in patients' capacities to master their environments successfully.

Thirdly, post-infarction patients should be trained to cope with psychosocial stress without exhibiting heightened cardiovascular responses. The relevance of these to pathological processes has been discussed by Steptoe in Chapter 3. This goal may be achieved in two ways. First, patients should be trained the better to discriminate situations in which a change in behaviour can bring about a reduction in challenge from those in which behavioural change leads to no reduction. Secondly, patients should acquire methods that allow them to avoid cardiovascular hyperreactivity during stressful confrontations, and to regain psychophysiological stability as quickly as possible after arousing episodes.

Finally, post-infarction patients should be assisted in constructing their environments so that they receive more social and emotional support during stressful events. The importance of the individual's ability to cope successfully with stressful events is supported by findings reported by Cay et al. (1975; 1976). These indicate that 75% of post-infarction patients who successfully managed earlier life crises went back to work after an average of 68 days, whereas 55% of patients rated as psychologically unstable rejoined the work force after an average of 92 days.

Coronary rehabilitation should not only attempt to reduce risk factors and Type-A behaviour patterns, to enhance compliance and to develop behavioural strategies to cope with stressful events, but it should also attempt to assist patients in dealing with their traumatic illness and in adjusting to their chronic functional limitations. Furthermore, proper rehabilitation should reduce the severe anxiety patients experience concerning the possible occurrence of cardiological complications. Pancheri et al. (1978) have shown that patients diagnosed as showing "no improvement" 7–10 days after admission to a coronary care unit were characterized as individuals who were subjected to more intensive psychosocial stress, were more emotionally labile, and reacted to their infarction with more anxiety. Cay et al. (1973) and Cay (1982) have found that 52% of patients exhibiting little or no emotional arousal during hospitalization were back to work within four months, whereas only 32% of those showing anxiety and depression during their hospital visit went back to their jobs during the same period. Successful recovery also appears to be dependent on the severity of the emotional impairment: 88% of patients who described themselves as adequately coping with their acute illness went back to work, in comparison with only 31% of those depicted as responding with considerable emotional arousal. The importance of coping with illness has also been emphasized by others (see Degree-Coustry, 1976; Degree-Coustry and Grevisse, 1982; Langosch et al., 1983).

A fourth step in cardiac rehabilitation is, therefore, to assist the post-infarction patient in coping with the traumatic event of illness, reducing the likelihood of chronic anxiety and depression. It is evident that psychotherapeutic measures should be taken as early as possible. Furthermore, it should be noted that the change from clinic to home represents an extraordinarily stressful event. This has been documented by the observation of psychological disturbances occurring in patients returning home (see

Wishnie *et al.*, 1971). Langosch and Brodner (1984) have reported that, even after a one-year period, considerable worsening of the patient's psychological state may be observed. Thus a fifth step in coronary after-care is the preparation of patients for their discharge from hospital. In addition, psychotherapeutic assistance may be continued following the patient's return home. In this way, the post-infarction patient can cope more adequately with changed living conditions.

Since the marriage partner is usually the most significant person for the chronically ill patient, the marriage partner should be incorporated into the psychotherapeutic consultation. The family must also be assisted through the crises that come about during chronic illness. Cay (1982) has shown that anxious over-protective behaviour on the part of a male coronary patient's wife may hinder successful rehabilitation.

REDUCTION OF RISK BEHAVIOURS

Wenger (1982) has emphasized the goal of education and counselling is the provision of information concerning coronary disease and its management, thereby allowing the patient to become responsible for his or her future state of health. In the coronary care unit, the patient should already have been informed in simple terms of diagnosis, and we assume that this enhances the patient's ability to adjust to the threatening situation. Subsequently, an in-hospital education programme should be conducted. We view this as the essential foundation of rehabilitation during the in-patient care period. Cromwell and Levenkron provide more details of this aspect in Chapter 7. According to Wenger's recommendations, the patient is first informed about cardiac functioning and the atherosclerotic process. The patient is advised to take steps that will enhance future prognosis. These may include a change in dietary habits, cessation of smoking, increases in physical activity, and a return to work as soon as possible. Sexual problems are dealt with in joint meetings with the spouse. Family members are also consulted on the patient's diet, i.e. proper preparation of low-cholesterol meals, and the need to suspend tobacco consumption. Furthermore, the patient is informed about the various medications that should be taken at home. Whenever severe angina pectoris occurs, the patient is advised to visit the nearest hospital. Finally, the patient is warned about the multitude of problems to be expected following discharge, such as over protectiveness on part of the family members and occupational difficulties arising from physical limitations. Family members are advised to assist patients in adjusting to their changed life style, and not to pamper them. No data are yet available about the effectiveness of this programme, so no definite conclusion can be drawn here.

Young *et al.* (1982) describe a rehabilitation intervention programme that consists of the following elements:

(i) Educating patients, and when possible their spouses, about the standard risk factors and their possible control; informing patients about the nature of coronary disease, myocardial infarction, the expected recovery, as well as the use of medications, their effects and side effects. This information can be provided by trained nurses or a health team, and written material or audiovisual aids may also be employed.

(ii) Educating and instructing the patient and spouse as to proper nutrition. This can be performed by a dietitian.

(iii) Gradually increasing physical activities. Exercises may be conducted daily by a physical therapist, and can begin in the coronary care unit.

(iv) Instructing the patient about progressive self-monitoring of movements; heart rate and other symptoms are emphasized.

(v) Consultation about work prospects; a vocational counsellor can be engaged here.

Young *et al.* (1982) compared 100 patients who participated in this rehabilitation programme with 100 controls. The results indicate that the intervention group demonstrated significantly more knowledge about their condition, coronary disease, risk factors, symptoms and medications than did controls. Three months after infarction, the rehabilitation group followed their prescribed diets more frequently, engaged in more gymnastic exercises and took more walks, lost more weight, exhibited lower serum cholesterol levels, reported less intensive angina pectoris pain, had less severe symptoms of congestive heart failure, and more frequently quit smoking when compared to controls. One year after infarction, however, the intervention group showed a general decline in compliance, leaving significant differences only for dietary habits, frequency of gymnastic participation, and serum cholesterol. A state-trait anxiety questionnaire administered 18 months following discharge suggested a trend towards lower anxiety scores in the experimental group. No differences were, however, evident between patient groups for frequency of reinfarction, mortality rate, and the rate of going back to work. Overall, the study showed that patients tend to take up old living habits following discharge from the clinic. To bring about long-term effects, a rehabilitation programme should be more comprehensive and should incorporate social reinforcement of desired behavioural adjustments.

Egger (1980) maintains that the essential goals of in-patient rehabilitation are changes in behaviours that foster secondary prevention. These goals were pursued in behaviour-therapeutic group sessions. Participation in the group directly after admission and just prior to discharge was mandatory for all patients, whereas all other sessions were voluntary. The goal of the initial interview with patients was to establish active co-operation between patient and hospital personnel, as well as to engender an interest in managing their disease. The aim of the final interview prior to release was to motivate patients to comply with rehabilitative measures, and to anticipate difficulties related to illness, family and job.

Further group sessions concerned the following: life with coronary disease (the goal here is to relieve the patient of anxiety and insecurity by actively coping with illness and evaluating prospects for the future); behavioural risk factors involved in ischaemic heart disease (e.g. Type A behaviour patterns, excessive eating, lack of physical activity, as well as chronic stress arising from life events); problems arising from chronic functional impairments limitations, as well as those stemming from vocational reintegration or early retirement; smoking, the goal being either reduction of consumption or quitting altogether; sexual behaviour following myocardial infarction, the aim here being the reduction of anxiety concerning sexual activity. All group sessions were conducted in a relaxed manner, focusing on a specific theme. In addition, autogenic training was carried out in small groups. Over a period of three weeks, two hour-long sessions were held each week. The effectiveness of this programme is evident in some data reported by Egger: upon release in 1977, 90% of patients receiving the regime had stopped smoking and 75–90% of all patients were interested in the group session concerning sexuality. Further findings that indicate the long-term success of this regime have, however, not been presented.

MODIFICATION OF TYPE A BEHAVIOUR PATTERNS

Friedman (1979) argues that Type A behaviour can only be successfully modified in patients following infarction. The results of the studies conducted by Roskies et al. (1978, 1979), Jenni and Wollersheim (1979) and Suinn and Bloom (1978) that attempted to modify certain aspects of Type A behaviour in subjects without coronary disease, confirm this argument. Only after patients suffer infarction are they able to recognize that the emotional stress elicited by "driving too hard and too relentlessly" is a coronary risk. They no longer attempt to deny that Type A behaviour may increase their susceptibility to ischaemic heart disease, and increase the likelihood of anxiety-inducing symptoms (e.g. angina pectoris, dyspnoea, easily tired). The reduction of Type A behaviours is further complicated by increased hostility. Enhanced hostility is exhibited in 20–30% of all post-infarction patients. Since hostility evidently decreases with age, successful modifications of Type A behaviour in young coronary patients may prove even more difficult (see Friedman, 1979). Moreover, it is uncertain which aspects of Type A behaviour should receive the highest priority in behavioural modification, since all elements of Type A behaviour cannot be equated with coronary disease (see Roskies, 1980). After conducting a principle-component factor analysis, Matthews *et al.* (1977) concluded that the factors "competitive drive" and "impatience" were of primary importance for the occurrence of myocardial infarction. It is not known, however, whether or not these factors are vital to the prevention of reinfarction.

One possible means of avoiding the need to specify therapeutic goals would be to reshape the fundamental beliefs, values and attitudes that underlie Type A behaviour (Rosenman and Friedman, 1977). Another alternative would be to modify the psychophysiological responses thought to link Type A behaviour and coronary heart disease (see Chapter 3).

Blumenthal *et al.* (1980) showed that regular participation in an exercise programme led to an attenuation of Type A behaviour in patients. These results place into doubt the notion that a philosophical reorientation is an essential prerequisite for the successful modification of Type A behaviour. Suinn (1974) reported data on the effects of his "cardiac-stress management" programme. This programme consists of training the patient to identify the early signs of bodily tension and to relieve this tension using relaxation techniques. In addition, patients are asked to imagine situations in which they respond with alternative forms of behaviour instead of their normal Type A patterns. This therapy programme, consisting of only five hours, brought about not only positive psychological effects in patients two to four weeks following infarction (e.g. 83% reported increased control over tension, 50% thought that the therapy enhanced their ability to change old living habits), but also led to physiological change (i.e. significant reduction in serum cholesterol levels compared with controls). A follow-up study endorsed these findings, in that both intervention groups ($n_I = 10$, $n_{II} = 17$) produced considerable decreases in cholesterol and triglyceride levels following therapy in comparison with controls ($n = 10$). Suinn failed to report, however, on the extent to which Type A behaviour was modified by the regime.

Friedman *et al.* (1982) presented a preliminary report of a study encompassing a five-year observation period of post-infarction patients. The patient sample consists of 1035 male and female patients under the age of 64 years who suffered their first or most recent infarction within a six-month period prior to the initiation of the investigation. All patients were either non-smokers or ex-smokers and showed no signs of diabetes. Nine hundred and sixty eight live in the San Francisco Bay area, and 92% agreed to be randomly designated to one of two intervention groups, while the remaining 84 patients agreed to act as controls. In order to ensure that not all controls were familar with the Type A concept (well-known in the Bay area), and therefore, attempting to alter behaviour on their own, 67 additional controls were recruited from within a one hundred mile radius of San Francisco.

Two hundred and seventy were assigned to "Cardiological Counselling" and 614 to the "Type A Behaviour Counselling". Since a higher number of drop-outs were expected in the latter group, more patients were assigned to it initially. The Cardiologic Counselling groups each consisted of 12 patients. During the first three months, a session was held once a fortnight; in the following three months the groups met just once a month, and subsequently they met once every two months. Every third month, either a psychiatrist or a clinical psychologist was present during the session and offered counselling concerning the management of anxiety, depression or phobic reactions. The sessions were conducted by a cardiologist who attempted to enhance the patients' compliance with diet, physical exercise, and medication. The Type A Behavioural Counselling groups consisted of ten patients each, and met each week for the first two months, then once a fortnight for the next two months, and finally once a month. Every third month, a cardiologist participated in the group session, and answered questions concerning cardiovascular functioning. The group leaders were either psychiatrists, clinical psychologists or cardiologists, all of whom had prior counselling experience. Patients who either missed three sessions in a row or refused to follow the advice of their group leaders were classified as drop-outs. After a period of one year, 213 of 270 patients were still in the Cardiologic Counselling group, 514 remained in the Type A Behavioural Counselling group, and 124 were still available in the control condition. Of the patients that dropped out, 124 were willing to participate in the annual check-ups, and therefore, may be considered as additional controls.

In the intervention groups, 4.4% of the patients suffered reinfarction after the first year, 20 of these 43 reinfarctions leading to death. The reinfarction and mortality rates were significantly lower in the intervention groups than in controls. Compared with the 8.9% reinfarction rate in the control group, only 2.9% suffered infarction in the Type A Behavioural Counselling group. The reinfarction rate in the Type A Behavioural Counselling group was also 55% lower than amongst drop-outs. The patients suffering reinfarction were higher on risk factors, such as angina pectoris pain, coronary insufficiency, hypertension, arrhythmia, two or more previous infarctions, and a higher score on the Peel-index. The lower reinfarction rate in the Type A Behavioural Counselling group cannot be accounted for by their level on these risk factors, since the three groups do not differ significantly at the beginning of the study.

Some further findings are reported by Thorensen *et al.* (1982). The second year recurrence rate was lower in the Type A Behavioural Counselling group than in the Cardiological Counselling groups or in the control group (2.9% vs. 4.6% vs. 5.4%). The annual rate during the third year was 1.2% for the Type A Behavioural Counselling group compared to 5.7% in the Cardiological Counselling group. Subjects who had a recurrence during the first year were significantly higher on the hostility component of the videotaped structured interview ($P < 0.05$), but not higher on their total interview score.

Participants in the Type A Behavioural Counselling group reported a change in Type A behaviour pattern (as assessed by questionnaire) of about 14% ($P < 0.001$); by contrast, members of the Cardiological Counselling group and control subjects reported slight but not significant improvements over the first year (4.5% and 3.5% respectively). Subjects in Type A Behavioural Counselling groups also showed substantial changes in Type A interview scores (31%) compared to initial levels. This difference was significantly greater than that seen in the Cardiological Counselling and control groups ($P < 0.001$).

These results suggest that the lower rate of fatal and non-fatal recurrences is associated with successful changes in the Type A behaviour pattern, and also in hostility, one major Type A component. It should be noted, however, that patients participating in the investigation were not assigned to intervention or control groups at random. Those receiving therapy may differ from controls in terms of motivation to change old living habits. Furthermore, patients resistant to change were dropped from the intervention groups, while no equivalent action was taken in the control condition. This may contribute to outcomes favouring the intervention groups.

ENHANCEMENT OF STRESS-MANAGEMENT SKILLS

A study was conducted by Fielding (1979), in which 70 post-infarction patients under the age of 60 years participated in a psychotherapeutic intervention programme. Thirteen per cent refused to participate, while 24% consented and then changed their minds. The remaining 45 were randomly assigned to one of four groups: the first group met for six counselling sessions lasting one-and-a-half hours, the second group met for group sessions followed by relaxation training, the third group underwent six control check-ups without any additional therapy, and the fourth group received neither check-ups nor therapy. Group counselling consisted of discussing techniques of stress and anxiety management, supplemented by additional medical advice. In the check-up, only control group patients were administered standard interviews in which the interviewer was advised to remain neutral. Data were collected for all groups prior to and following the intervention or observation period, as well as at 6 and 12 months after myocardial infarction.

The results of this study suggested that significant differences were present over the various test periods on symptom scores from the Beck Depression Inventory. Whereas 25% of the patient group receiving only check-ups and 15% of the control group without check-ups suffered reinfarction, none of the patients in the intervention groups developed new infarctions. These differences in reinfarction rate may have been due firstly to the psychotherapeutic intervention, and secondly to differences in family history of heart disease. No relationship was found between the severity of disease and the psychological questionnaire data. This led the author to conclude that the psychological response to myocardial infarction is largely independent of the severity of disease.

Juli and Brenner (1977) presented a behaviour therapy group training programme for coronary in-patients. In the initial phase, the patients were introduced to a psychosomatic model of ischaemic heart disease, in which the significance of Type A behaviour, psychological stress and life style was explained. Subsequently, individual behaviour analyses were conducted in the group. The goal of these analyses was to reduce the stresses confronting each patient. With the aid of role paying, risk behaviour patterns were replaced by a new repertoire intended to increase patients' self-control over their behaviour in critical situations. The programme continued for about ten hours.

A follow-up study at two years revealed that 90% of the 58 patients questioned showed a moderate to considerable change in attitudes and behaviour; 80% of spouses confirmed these reports. In another group of 49 patients, behaviour and attitude ratings made prior to infarction were compared with those collected two years after infarction. The patients were found to be more capable of delegating work, were less dependent on recognition from others, were less perfectionistic, and worked less overtime and less on weekends following therapy.

Brenner (1980, 1981) has conducted further group therapy programmes with coronary patients. The therapeutic goals consist of differentiating self-perception and self-exploration, reducing an idealistic self-image, reducing inner tension and responses to stress, enhancement of behavioural and attitudinal flexibility, reassessing socially and emotionally challenging stimuli, and enhancing personal responsibility for health and self-control. Brenner's group therapy is based on behaviour therapy but also incorporates concepts and methods derived from client-centered therapy, rational-emotive therapy, and thematic-centered therapy as described by Cohn.

A follow-up study was conducted three years following discharge, in which two patient groups were compared. The first group consisted of patients who participated in at least seven group therapy sessions; they were considered to be high on self-control and self-responsibility scores prior to therapy. Patients with less self-control and self-responsibility who chose not to take part in behaviour therapy formed the control group. The primary results of the follow-up survey show that patients with more "psychological insight" and more "health-oriented self-responsibility" exhibited seven times less infarction and a four-fold decrease in mortality over patients showing impaired "psychological insight" or less "health-oriented self-responsibility". The group differences on mortality rate were significant and on reinfarction highly significant. Furthermore, patients receiving therapy manifest fewer stress-related disturbances, more frequently quit smoking, and more frequently preferred to return to work by working just part-time at first. Approximately one third of all patients in both groups reported that they were still under considerable stress. The patients participating regularly in therapy reported, however, that their behaviour and attitude towards stressful events had changed, whereas the controls reported only changes in behaviour. Unfortunately, the dependent variables selected to indicate illness behaviour were not always differentiated from cardiac complications. Furthermore, since the data concerning reinfarction and mortality were strictly based on the reports of patients or family, it is possible that in some cases apparent infarctions may have been spuriously identified as genuine. In addition, patients were not assigned to groups at random, so both psychological and medical differences may have been present prior to therapy. The results of this study must, therefore, be treated with caution.

Langosch et al. (1982a,b) compared three patient groups. The first consisted of 32 patients who participated in stress management training, the second group consisted of 28 patients taking part in relaxation training, and the third was a control group of 30 patients. The stress management training programme consisted of eight sessions conducted over a period of two weeks. The programme, based on psychosomatic concepts, consisted of:

(i)   discriminating somatic and psychological tension,
(ii) reducing impairments in subjective state by means of relaxation techniques,
(iii) recognizing symptoms of psychophysical overload and negative self-talk in response to challenging events,

(iv)   increasing competence in taking responsibility for stress management,
 (v)   discerning insecure behaviour, and
(vi)   developing and practising behavioural alternatives in the imagination.

The relaxation group was trained during the same period of time and learned relaxation techniques, such as muscular relaxation, meditative breathing patterns and autogenic training. After completion of therapy, positive psychological changes were evident in both intervention groups compared with controls. Patients receiving therapy were less anxious about social exchanges, were less hurried and more patient, and were more convinced that they were now capable of managing stress. Furthermore, the patients who participated in the relaxation training reported that they were able to reduce their devotion to work and rated themselves as significantly more self-assured than did controls. It should be emphasized that participants did not differ on initial psychological data or on cardiological findings.

A follow-up study conducted six months after discharge indicated that 74% of the patients who took part in stress management training and 65% of patients from the relaxation group were back to work, while 10% in the stress-management group and 31% in the relaxation group had suffered further cardiac complications. Questionnaire data suggested that patients showed less social anxiety, exhibited less competitive behaviour at work, showed less devotion to work, and were less irritable than before therapy. Although patients in the stress management group still reported being able to manage stressful events, patients in the relaxation group reported a decline in their ability to cope with stress. Patients further reported spending more time on various leisure activities, such as walking, reading and hobbies than they did prior to illness. The majority of patients also indicated that they utilized the behaviour therapeutic techniques that they had acquired during treatment.

It may, therefore, be concluded that an improvement in psychological factors such as self-confidence, social anxiety, as well as in various components of Type A behaviour are relevant to coronary disease. Furthermore, some of these positive psychological modifications are stable at six months. The primary difference between the two forms of intervention appears to lie in the enhanced ability of patients trained in stress management to discriminate specific situational cues that signal the use of self-control techniques. Stress management training thus appears to increase patients' ability to engage in self-control procedures. Both interventions also appear to reduce the previously mentioned deterioration of subjective state commonly observed following discharge.

Herzog *et al.* (1982) have recently described a rather complex group therapy consisting of 15 sessions, each lasting about 90 minutes with three sessions per week. The general goal of this intervention is the formation of health-oriented attitudes and behaviour. More specifically, the following aims were defined: reduction of the insecurity and anxiety induced by the clinical setting, modification of the various attitudes held by patients concerning cardiac rehabilitation, treatment of the emotional effects of infarction, reduction of anxiety and insecurity about the future, and recognition of self-destruction response patterns. In addition, patients were encouraged in alternative strategies concerning risk behaviour and stress management, and acquired a battery of self-control skills including practical anti-stress measures, perception of inner conflict and its role in pathogenesis, reduction of anxiety concerning sexual activity following infarction, reorientation of vocational ambitions, anticipation of problems that might occur upon renewing social contacts, and recognition of meaningful leisure time activities. This comprehensive programme, of which stress management is just one, albeit a central component, is further supplemented by lectures on risk factors, stress, the effects and side-effects of medication, the basics of physical therapy, and coronary diseases. Unfortunately, little information is as yet available about the effectiveness of the programme. Of patients participating thus far, 90% rate the programme itself as "interesting and meaningful" and 86% believe that the techniques and information acquired have had "a considerable effect on their behaviour". Assessment of the effectiveness of the intervention cannot, however, be based on such data.

ASSISTANCE IN COPING WITH TRAUMATIC ILLNESS

The management of traumatic illness has already been described as one of the many goals of intervention programmes. The following section focuses on some salient aspects of this issue.

Gruen (1975) investigated the extent to which psychotherapeutic measures initiated during the hospitalization period have an effect on the recovery process. A group of 70 post-infarction patients were randomly assigned either to an intervention or a control group. The intervention, consisting of medical and psychotherapeutic counselling, was initiated the day after admission and was conducted six times per week during intensive care and subsequently five times per week. Findings indicate that the intervention group required a shorter intensive care period and also an overall shorter hospitalization period compared with controls. During the second week of hospitalization, fewer supraventricular arrhythmia, fewer symptoms of fatigue and less depression were observed in the patients

receiving therapy. Ratings administered on the eleventh day of hospitalization confirmed the positive effects of intervention: in-patients receiving
therapy reported themselves as less inhibited, less depressed and anxious, as
well as more interested in social contact. An interview conducted four
months following infarction by the family physician showed that more
patients in the intervention group had returned to normal daily activities,
and that they also demonstrated less anxiety. The results of this investigation suggest that well-defined psychotherapeutic measures do contribute to
an improvement in the patient's ability to manage the trauma of severe
illness.

PROMOTING ADJUSTMENT TO CHRONIC ILLNESS

Naismith *et al.* (1979) carried out a study in which patients were counselled
on the third day following infarction by a rehabilitation team consisting of a
physician and nurse. Psychological counselling continued for the next six
months when deemed necessary, first in the hospital and then at home.
Both patient and spouse were encouraged during these sessions to speak
freely about their anxieties and difficulties. The 68 "comprehensively
rehabilitated" patients were then compared to controls who received
normal care following infarction. At six months, the "comprehensively
rehabilitated" patients were deemed more socially independent, and they
returned to working life earlier. The rehabilitation was evidently most
successful in a subsample of "introverted neurotics". The authors, therefore, suggest that comprehensive rehabilitation should be directed primarily
towards introverted neurotic patients, and may be less effective in stable
extraverts.

Ibrahim *et al.* (1974) offered patients the opportunity to participate in
psychotherapeutic intervention shortly after discharge from hospital. A
total of 58 patients who received psychotherapy once a week over a
one-year period was compared with 60 controls. Nine patients of the
intervention group discontinued attendance at the sessions, a drop-out rate
of 15.5%. Controls (16.6%) who did not attend the semi-annual check-ups
were also considered drop-outs.

The patients receiving psychotherapy were similar to controls in the
severity of disease, assessed by the Peel-index, and in various socio-
economic factors. The therapists attempted to encourage exchange of
emotions and attitudes among group members, but patients were either not
able or willing to explore their emotional state.

Results of questionnaires directly after treatment and six months after
completion of intervention revealed that the degree of "social alienation"

was significantly reduced in the psychotherapy group. Interestingly, this effect was not observed in the wives of these patients. Leisure activities, family and vocational concerns were changed similarly in both groups. A reduction in competitive behaviour was observed in patients immediately following intervention, but not sustained at six months. Physiological variables showed no significant differences between intervention and control groups. However, a division of the severely ill (Peel-index score of ⩾12) from remaining patients indicated that the survival rate was considerably higher in the severe subgroup who participated in psychotherapy compared with controls. Of the severely ill patients receiving therapy, 93% were still alive at one year follow-up, compared with 74% of controls. Although approximately the same number of patients had to be readmitted to hospital in the two groups, patients in the intervention group needed on average 26 days of care, compared with 36 days for controls.

Rahe et al., (1973) presented results of an out-patient after-care programme for post-infarction patients. Patients were advised about risk behaviours and were also offered an opportunity to participate in group therapy. The programme consisted of four to six 90 minute sessions conducted once a fortnight during the first three months following infarction. Counselling dealt with physiological and psychological aspects of myocardial infarction, as well as relevant rehabilitative goals. Of the total 60 patients examined, 38 were randomly assigned to the intervention and 22 to the control group. All patients were less than 60 years old and had suffered only one infarction; on medical grounds, they were considered capable of going back to work after rehabilitation.

During the group sessions, patients supposedly gained insight into the stresses that preceded their infarction, especially unrealistic occupational goals (e.g. considerable overtime, excessive feelings of responsibility, ambition, time pressure induced by deadlines, competitive tendency). Patients were also confronted with their own defence mechanisms, such as denial. Other problems, such as returning home and going back to work, were dealt with in the group sessions. The authors emphasized how the mutual, and often humorous, support given in the group enhanced a more realistic estimate of future difficulties, as well as increasing the self-confidence of patients.

Only 3% of patients receiving therapy experienced cardiac complications (insufficiency, coronary bypass, reinfarction, death) during the first six months, compared with 24% of controls. After 18 months, 19% of patients receiving therapy and 58% of the controls had experienced at least one cardiac complication. None of the patients in the intervention group suffered reinfarction, whereas ten controls had another infarction, two of these leading to death (Rahe et al., 1975). Four years after infarction, the positive effects of the intervention were still evident. However, no significant differences were found between the frequency of coronary insufficiency or the number of bypass operations in the two groups. Patients receiving therapy were more likely to have returned to work. Members of the intervention group in work had reduced the number of hours they worked, whereas controls showed no significant reductions. They also reported feeling that they were under less time pressure than before (Rahe et al., 1979).

Little research has been carried out into the involvement of spouses in coronary rehabilitation. Adsett and Bruhn (1968) reported a small study, but the drop-out rate was considerable and the controls were poorly matched. The role of the spouse in rehabilitation has yet to be determined systematically.

DISCUSSION

Blanchard and Miller concluded in 1977 that coronary rehabilitative programmes that include psychotherapeutic measures have certain advantages over programmes without any psychological components. The present review lends further support to this conclusion. Unfortunately, few studies in the literature have tested the long-term effects of interventions. There appears to be a considerable discrepancy between theory and practical applications in cardiac rehabilitation (see Frank et al., 1979).

One difficulty lies in establishing the criteria for success or failure. Physiological variables, standard risk factors, or data concerning cardiac complications, are frequently employed. But if there is no evidence of changes in behaviour or attitude following therapy, links between physiological or cardiac changes and psychotherapeutic interventions must remain conjectural.

Generally, no studies have shown negative effects of psychotherapeutic interventions. Thus it may be concluded that such procedures may be administered to the post-infarction patient without any danger of damaging health. This conclusion is limited, however, to the therapies discussed above: counselling, supportive psychotherapy, relaxation training and various behaviour therapies. Generalization to other forms of therapy, especially those that elicit psychophysiological activation, such as flooding or implosion, should not and cannot be made here.

Furthermore, it is apparent that intensive group dynamic techniques or explorative psychotherapeutic methods are not called for in coronary patients. The formation of an adequate working relationship between patient and therapist is seldom possible, due to the modest ability of these patients in such skills as introspection or toleration of frustration (see Goldschmidt, 1980).

Positive psychological effects have been observed in most studies not only immediately following therapy, but also six months after infarction. The results of the study conducted by Langosch et al. (1982a,b) suggest, however, that these "positive" effects may well just be attenuations of the normally severe psychological impairments following infarction. Patients appear to be more concerned with reducing their working hours and with increasing the range of their leisure activities than they were prior to infarction. Vocational reintegration is apparently influenced in various ways. In some studies, patients successfully completing therapy went back to work earlier (Langosch et al., 1982a,b; Naismith et al., 1979), whereas in other studies a positive effect was seen in patients who did not rush back to work (Brenner 1980, 1981).

The most impressive findings are those showing positive cardiological effects of psychological intervention, especially in severe cases. In several studies (Brenner, 1980, 1981; Fielding, 1979; Friedman et al., 1982; Gruen, 1975; Ibrahim et al., 1974; Rahe et al., 1975, 1979), patients receiving treatment manifest significantly fewer cardiac complications, especially reinfarction or death, and required less hospitalization during rehabilitation than controls. However, these findings cannot always be unequivocally interpreted, since illness behaviour may not be delineated from the illness itself (Cohen, 1979). Nevertheless the positive effects of psychological interventions are even more robust when one considers that reductions in nicotine abuse or excessive bodyweight were not necessarily achieved (Ibrahim et al., 1974; Rahe et al., 1979). In view of the evidence (Langosch et al., 1983) for an association between the progression of coronary stenosis and various psychosocial variables, further research into the potential effectiveness of behavioural treatments on coronary functioning is required. Such research demands a thorough examination of patients before and after intervention, to confirm whether cardiac complications such as infarction or reinfarction are exhibited or whether progression or regression in coronary atherosclerosis has occurred following therapy.

It should, however, be borne in mind that at best 80% of patients participating in intervention programmes are truly motivated. Before the treatment is completed, approximately 15% will have dropped out. Care must, therefore, be taken to enhance the motivation of patients, and to keep them from dropping out before completion.

Further rigorous empirical investigations are required in order to identify the crucial elements of the various forms of therapy. The current trend of continuously introducing new forms of therapy or new combinations of pre-existing therapies does not appear to reflect genuine progress. These new therapy packages have seldom incorporated the existing body of empirical findings adequately. The superiority of these new programmes has yet to be demonstrated critically in experimental studies.

REFERENCES

Adsett, C. A. and Bruhn, J. G. (1968). Short-term group psychotherapy for post-myocardial infarction patients and their wives. *Can. Med. Ass J.* **99**, 577–584.

Blanchard, E. B. and Miller, S. T. (1977). Psychological treatment of cardiovascular disease. *Arch. Gen. Psychiat.* **34**, 1402–1413.

Blumenthal, J. A., Williams, R. S., Williams, R. B. and Wallace, A. G. (1980). Effects of exercise on the type A (coronary prone) behavior pattern. *Psychosom. Med.* **42**, 289–296.

Brand, R. J. (1978). Coronary-prone behavior as an independent risk factor for coronary heart disease. *In* "Coronary-prone Behavior" (T. M. Dembroski, S. M. Weiss, J. L. Shields, S. G. Haynes and M. Feinleib, eds), pp. 11–24. Springer-Verlag, Berlin.

Brenner, H. (1980. Themzentierte Gespräche und Verhaltensübungen zur Einstellungsund Verhaltensänderung von Herzinfarktpatienten. *In* "Psychosoziale Probleme und psychotherapeutische Interventionsmöglichkeiten bei Herzinfarktpatienten" (W. Langosch, ed.), pp. 201–226. Minerva Publikation, München.

Brenner, H. (1981). Herzinfarkt und Selbstverantwortung. *Prävention* **4**, 13–18.

Büchner, F. (1939). "Die Coronarinsuffizienz". Steinkopff, Dresden.

Cay, E. L. (1982). Psychological problems in patients after a myocardial infarction. *Adv. Cardiol.* **22**, 108–112.

Cay, E. L., Dugard, P. and Philip, A. E. (1973). Return to work after a heart attack. *J. Psychosom. Res.* **17**, 1–13.

Cay, E. L., Gardner, A. V., Vetter, N. J. and Philip, A. E. (1975). Rehabilitation after a heart attack: the team approach. Proc. 3rd Congr. Int. College Psychosom. Med., Rome.

Cay, E. L., Philip, A. E. and Aitken, C. (1976). Psychological aspects of cardiac rehabilitation. *In* "Modern Trends in Psychosomatic Medicine" (O. W. Hill, ed.), pp. 330–346. Butterworth, London.

Cohen, F. (1979). Personality, stress and the development of physical illness. *In* "Health Psychology—a Handbook" (G. C. Stone, F. Cohen and N. E. Adler, eds), pp. 77–112. Josey-Bass, San Francisco.

Croog, S. H. and Levine, S. (1977). "The Heart Patient Recovers'. Human Sciences Press, New York.

Degree-Coustry, C. (1976). Psychological problems in rehabilitation programmes. *In* "Psychological Approach to the Rehabilitation of Coronary Patients" (U. Stocksmeier, ed.), pp. 32–34. Springer-Verlag, Berlin.

Degree-Coustry, C. and Grevisse, M. (1982). Psychological problems in rehabilitation after myocardial infarction: non-institutional approach. *Adv. Cardiol.* **29**, 126–131.

Egger, J. (1980). Psychologische Gruppenarbeit mit Herzinfarktpatienten. *Öst. Ärztetg.* **35**, 419–426.

Epstein, F. H. and Wilhelmsen, L. (1982). Do the standard risk factors alter their role after the first myocardial infarction? In "Controversies in Cardiac Rehabilitation" (P. Mathes and M. J. Halhuber, eds), pp. 18–20. Springer-Verlag, Berlin.

Fielding, R. (1979). Behavioural treatment in the rehabilitation of myocardial infarction patients. In "Research in Psychology and Medicine" (D. J. Oborne, M. M. Gruneberg and J. R. Eiser, eds), pp. 176–182. Academic Press, London, Orlando and New York.

Frank, K. A., Heller, S. S. and Kornfeld, D. S. (1979). Psychological intervention in coronary heart disease. Gen. Hosp. Psychiat. 1, 18–23.

Friedman, M. (1979). The modification of Type A behavior in post-infarction patients. Am. Heart J. 97, 551–560.

Friedman, M., Thoresen, C. E., Gill, J. J., Ulmer, D., Thompson, L., Powell, L., Price, V., Elek, S. R., Rabin, D. D., Breall, W. S., Piaget, G., Dixon, T., Bourg, E., Levy, R. A. and Tasto, D. L. (1982). Feasibility of altering Type A behavior pattern after myocardial infarction. Recurrent coronary prevention project study: methods, baseline results and preliminary findings. Circulation 66, 83–92.

Goldschmidt, O. (1980). Überlegungen zur Frage der Behandelbarkeit der Herzinfarktpatienten. Psych 6, 563–573.

Gruen, W. (1975). Effects of brief psychotherapy during the hospitalization period on the recovery process in heart attacks. J. Consult. Clin. Psychol. 43, 223–232.

Hackett, T. P. and Cassem, N. H. (1982). Adjusting to coronary artery disease: coping with the problems of convalescence following myocardial infarction. In "Controversies in Cardiac Rehabilitation" (P. Mathes and M. J. Halhuber, eds), pp. 85–91. Springer-Verlag, Berlin.

Herzog, M., König, K., Maas, A. and Neufert, R. (1982). Gesundheitserziehung und Gruppenarbeit in der Rehabilitation von Patienten mit Herzinfarkt im Rahmen der Anschlußheilbehandlung. Rehabilitation 21, 8–12.

Ibrahim, M. A., Feldman, J. G., Sultz, H. A., Staiman, M. G., Young, L. G. and Dean, D. (1974). Management after myocardial infarction: a controlled trial of the effect of group psychotherapy. Int. J. Psychiat. Med. 5, 253–269.

Jenkins, C. D. (1976). Recent evidence supporting psychologic and social risk factors for coronary disease. New Engl. J. Med. 294, 987–994 and 1033–1038.

Jenkins, C. D., Zyzanski, S. J., Rosenman, R. H. and Cleveland, G. L. (1971). Association of coronary-prone behavior scores with recurrence of coronary heart disease. J. Chron. Dis. 24, 601–611.

Jenni, M. A. and Wollersheim, J. P. (1979). Cognitive therapy, stress management training and the Type A behavior pattern. Cog. Ther. Res. 3, 61–73.

Juli, D. and Brenner, H. (1977). Ein verhaltenstherapeutisch orientiertes Modell für die Gruppenarbeit mit Herzinfarktpatienten. Herz/Kreisl. 9, 661–669.

Kallinke, D. (1982). Psychotherapie bei chronisch körperlichen Krankheiten. In "Grundbegriffe der Psychotherapie" (R. Bastine, ed.), pp. 200–203. Edition Psychologie, Weinheim.

Kalusche, D. (1982). Klinik des Herzinfarkts. In "Herzkrankheiten. Pathophysiologie, Diagnostik, Therapie" (H. Roskamm and H. Reindell, eds), pp. 962–995. Springer-Verlag, Berlin.

Kazemier, M. (1981). Cardiac disease and the trauma it inflicts on the patient's "body esteem". In "Psychosomatic Cardiovascular Disorders-when and how to treat?" (P. Kielholz, W. Siegenthaler, P. Taggart and A. Zanchetti, eds), pp. 147–153. Hans Huber, Bern.

König, K. (1982). Kardiologische Rehabilitation. In "Herzkrankheiten. Pathophysiologie, Diagnostik, Therapie" (H.Roskamm and H. Reindell, ed.), pp. 1512–1516. Springer-Verlag, Berlin.

Langosch, W. (1980). Ergebnisse psychologischer Verlaufsstudien bei Herzinfarkt-Patienten (Ein- und Drei-Jahres-Katamnese). *In* "Psychosoziale Probleme und psychotherapeutische Interventionsmöglichkeiten bei Herzinfarktpatienten" (W. Langosch, ed.), pp. 99–114. Minerva Publikation, München.

Langosch, W. and Brodner, G. (1979). Ergebnisse einer psychologischen Verlaufsstudie an Herzinfarkt-Patienten. *Ztschrft. Klin. Psychol.* **8**, 256–269.

Langosch, W. and Brodner, G. (1984). Persönlichkeits- und Befindlichkeitsveränderungen von Herzinfarktpatienten in Abhängigkeit von Erkrankungsdauer und Untersuchungssetting im Vergleich zu einer Kontrollgruppe chronisch Kranker. *Ztschrft. Klin. Psychol.* **13**, in press.

Langosch, W., Prokoph, J. H. and Brodner, G. (1980). Der psychologische Screeningbogen für Patienten mit Myocardinfarkt (PSM) bei verschiedenen kardiologischen Diagnosegruppen. *In* "Der Herzinfarkt als psychosomatisches Geschehen in der Rehabilitation" (C. F. Fassbender and E. Mahler, eds), pp. 89–124. Boehringer, Mannheim.

Langosch, W., Brodner, G. and Michallik-Herbein, U. (1981). Psychological and vocational aspects in postinfarction patients below the age of 40. *In* "Myocardial Infarction at Young Age" (H. Roskamm, ed.), pp. 187–195. Springer-Verlag, Heidelberg.

Langosch, W., Seer, P., Brodner, G. and Kallinke, D. (1982a). Stationäre Verhaltenstherapie mit Koronarkranken: Ergebnisse einer vergleichenden Untersuchung. *In* "Therapieforschung für die Praxis 3" (J. C. Brengelmann and G. Bühringer, eds), pp. 141–166. Gerhard Röttger Verlag, München.

Langosch, W., Seer, P., Brodner, G., Kallinke, D., Kulick, B. and Heim, P. (1982b). Behavior therapy with coronary heart disease patients: results of a comparative study. *J. Psychosom. Res.* **26**, 475–484.

Langosch, W., Brodner, G. and Borcherding, H. (1983). Psychological and vocational long-term outcomes of cardiac rehabilitation with postinfarction patients under the age of forty. *Psychother. Psychosom.*, **40**, 115–128.

Matthews, K. A., Glass, D. C., Rosenman, R. H. and Bortner, R. W. (1977). Competitive drive, pattern A, and coronary heart disease: A further analysis of some data from the Western Collaborative Group Study. *J. Chron. Dis.* **30**, 489–498.

Mayou, R., Williamson, B. and Foster, A. (1978a). Outcome two months after myocardial infarction. *J. Psychosom. Res.* **22**, 439–445.

Mayou, R., Foster, A. and Williamson, B. (1978b). Psychosocial adjustment in patients one year after myocardial infarction. *J. Psychosom. Res.* **22**, 447–453.

Medert-Dornscheidt, G. and Myrtek, M. (1977). Ergebnisse einer Zwei-Jahres-Katamnese an Herz-Kreislaufkranken nach einem Heilverfahren. *Rehabilitation* **16**, 207–217.

Meltzer, L. E. (1969). The present status and future direction of intensive coronary care. *In* "Coronary Heart Disease" (A. N. Brest, ed.), pp. 177. Davies, Philadelphia.

Moret, P., Gutsweiller, F. and Junod, B. (1981). Coronary artery disease in young adults under 35 years old: risk factors (Swiss survey). *In* "Myocardial Infarction at Young Age" (H. Roskamm, ed.), pp. 17–22. Springer-Verlag, Berlin.

Nagle, R., Morgan, D., Bird, J. and Bird, J. (1976). Interaction between physical and psychological abnormalities after myocardial infarction. *In* "Psychological

Approach to the Rehabilitation of Coronary Patients" (U. Stocksmeier, ed.), pp. 84–88. Springer-Verlag, Berlin.

Naismith, L. D., Robinson, J. F., Shaw, G. B. and MacIntyre, M. M. (1979). Psychological rehabilitation after myocardial infarction. Br. Med. J. **67,** 439–442.

Pancheri, P., Bellaterra, M., Matteoli, S., Christofori, M., Polissi, C. and Puletti, M. (1978). Infarct as a stress agent: life history and personality characteristics in improved versus not-improved patients after severe heart attack. J. Hum. Stress **4,** 16–42.

Parker, J. O. (1978). Prognosis in coronary artery disease. Arteriographic, ventriculographic and hemodynamic factors. Cleveland Clin. Q. **45,** 145–146.

Rahe, R. H., Tuffii, C. F., Suchor, R. J. and Arthur, R. J. (1973). Group therapy in the outpatient management of post-myocardial infarction patients. Psychiat. Med. **4,** 77–78.

Rahe, R. H., O'Neill, T. O., Hagan, A. and Arthur, R. J. (1975). Brief group therapy following myocardial infarction: eighteen months follow up of a controlled trial. Psychiat. Med. **6,** 349–358.

Rahe, R. H., Ward, H. and Haynes, V. (1979). Brief group therapy in myocardial infarction rehabilitation: Three-to-four-year follow-up of a controlled trial. Psychosom. Med. **41,** 229–241.

Review Panel On Coronary-Prone Behavior and Coronary Heart Disease (1981). Coronary-prone behavior and coronary heart disease: critical review. Circulation **63,** 1199–1215.

Rosenman, R. H. and Friedman, M. (1977). Modifying type A behaviour pattern. J. Psychosom. Res. **21,** 323–331.

Roskamm, H. (1982). Pathophysiologie der Coronarerkrankungen. In "Herzkrankheiten. Pathophysiologie, Diagnostik, Therapie" (H. Roskamm and H. Reindell, eds), pp. 907–919. Springer-Verlag, Berlin.

Roskies, E. (1980). Considerations in developing a treatment program for the coronary-prone (type A) behavior pattern. In "Behavioral Medicine: Changing Health Life-style" (P. Davidson and S. M. Davidson, eds), pp. 299–333. Brunner/Mazel, New York.

Roskies, E., Spevack, M, Surkis, A., Cohen, C. and Gilman, S. (1978). Changing the coronary-prone (type A) behavior pattern in a non-clinical population. J. Behav. Med. **1,** 201–215.

Roskies, E., Kearney, N., Spevack, M., Surkis, A., Cohen, C. and Gilman, S. (1979). Generalizability and durability of treatment effects in an intervention program for coronary-prone (type A) managers. J. Behav. Med. **2,** 195–207.

Schweizer, W., Renggli, I. and Zutter, W. (1977). Einleitung, Methodik, Patienten. In "Der Myokardinfarkt im Stadtspital" (F. Burkart, B. Heierli, R. Ritz, I. Renggli, O. F. Scheidegger, W. Schweizer and W. Zutter, eds), pp. 5–10. Schweiz. med. Wschr. **107,** (Suppl. 6).

Siegrist, J., Dittmann, K., Rittner, K. and Weber, I. (1982). The social context of active distress in patients with early myocardial infarction. Soc. Sci. Med. **16,** 443–453.

Stocksmeier, U. (1976). Medical and psychological aspects of coronary heart disease. In "Psychological approach to the Rehabilitation of Coronary Patients" (U. Stocksmeier, ed.), pp. 9–19. Springer-Verlag, Berlin.

Stürzenhofecker, P., Samek, L., Droste, C., Gohlke, H., Petersen, G. and Rostamm, H. (1981). Prognosis of coronary heart disease and progression of coronary arteriosclerosis in postinfarction patients under the age of 40. In

"Myocardial Infarction at Young Age" (H. Roskamm, ed.), pp. 82–91. Springer-Verlag, Berlin.

Suinn, R. M. (1974). Behavior Therapy for cardiac patients. *Behav. Ther.* **5**, 569–571.

Suinn, R. M. and Bloom, L. L. (1978). Anxiety management training for pattern A behavior. *J. Behav. Med.* **1**, 25–35.

Thorensen, C. E., Friedman, M., Gill, J. K. and Ulmer, D. K. (1982). The recurrent coronary prevention project. Some preliminary findings. *Acta. Med. Scand.* **660**, (suppl.) 172–192.

Viney, L. L. and Westbrook, M. T. (1981). Psychological reactions to chronic illness-related disability as a function of its severity and type. *J. Psychosom. Res.* **25**, 513–523.

Wenger, N. K. (1982). Patient and family education and counseling: a requisite component of cardiac rehabilitation. *In* "Controversies in Cardiac Rehabilitation" (P. Mathes and M. J. Halhuber, eds), pp. 108–114. Springer-Verlag, Berlin.

Wishnie, H. A., Hackett, T. P. and Cassem, N. H. (1971). Psychological hazards of convalescence following myocardial infarction. *J. Am. Med. Ass.* **215**, 1292–1296.

Young, D. T., Kottke, T. E., McCall, M. M. and Blume, D. (1982). A prospective controlled study of in-hospital myocardial infarction rehabilitation. *J. Cardiac Rehab.* **2**, 32–40.

Zaitsev, V. P. (1976). Classification of psychic changes in m.i. patients in connection with problems of rehabilitation. *In* "Psychological Approach to the Rehabilitation of Coronary Patients" (U. Stocksmeier, ed.), pp. 101–107. Springer-Verlag, Berlin.

11

Psychotherapy Research in Oncology

RONALD GROSSARTH-MATICEK, PETER SCHMIDT, HERMANN VETTER and SIGRID ARNDT

Interest in the psychological aspects of cancer and its management has increased rapidly over recent years (Fox, 1981). The aim of our research programme is to study the interaction between psychosocial and organic risk factors in cancerogenesis. Using multivariate statistical analyses of prospective and retrospective studies, it has been possible to demonstrate that both sets of factors are involved in the development and progress of malignancies. In order to test the proposition that psychosocial risk factors play a causal role in the disease process, two intervention trials have also been carried out. The present chapter outlines some aspects of this research programme. The personality characteristics of cancer patients that were identified in prospective studies are first described. The two intervention studies in which attempts were made to modify psychosocial factors using psychotherapy are then outlined. In the first study, three different types of therapy were applied to women with breast cancer: behaviour therapy, analytic depth psychotherapy and Creative Novation Therapy (a method developed by Grossarth-Maticek). The interaction between chemotherapy and psychotherapy was also examined. The second study was another controlled trial, in which the effect of Creative Novation Therapy administered by therapists with different degrees of experience was assessed.

PERSONALITY CHARACTERISTICS AND CANCER

A prospective study of psychosocial characteristics associated with the development of cancer was performed in a Yugoslavian town with a

HEALTH CARE AND HUMAN BEHAVIOUR
ISBN 0–12–666460–9

population of 14 000 (Grossarth-Maticek, 1980). The sample consisted of 1353 subjects; they were recruited by selecting the oldest person in every second house in the town. Most of the subjects were between 50 and 65 years old. Psychosocial data were recorded between 1965 and 1966, using a questionnaire and an observation catalogue. Height, weight, blood pressure and data on cigarette smoking were also collected. Further medical information was recorded periodically between 1969 and 1976. Ten years after starting the study, a physician assessed the occurrence of different diseases in the sample, and also recorded diagnoses on the death certificates. A total of 117 men and 87 women had developed cancer over this period; cancer of the lung, stomach, rectum and prostate predominated amongst males, while breast, uterine and cervical cancer occurred in 69% of females. This study was later replicated in Heidelberg, using a cross-sectional analysis of a random sample of 1026 subjects.

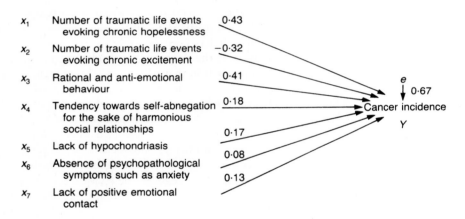

Fig. 1   Determinants of cancer incidence.

Figure 1 summarizes the characteristics associated with cancer incidence. The figures are standardized, partiallized regression coefficients, while the error term represents the square root of the residual variance of cancer incidence. All the predictors included in Fig. 1 are statistically significant ($P < 0.01$). Cancer patients appear to strive to fulfil the expectations of significant others. They tend to idealize the person closest to them, while at the same time showing low self esteem and lack of assertion. Such people seem to be well adjusted on the surface. They report no violent outbreaks of anger, few anxieties and a poor fantasy life, and behave in a rational, unemotional fashion. They have a strong need for harmonious relationships, and this is intensified in times of conflict. They tend to deny any inhibition of emotional expression, and are socially conformist.

These results are consistent with Bastiaans' concept of hysteria and psychosomatic disease (Bastiaans, 1967, 1974). According to this theory, many psychiatric symptoms result from attempts by neurotic individuals to escape hysteria or the free expression of emotion. This avoidance of excess emotion can be traced back to early childhood. Such children experience rejection by their parents, and respond by trying to fulfil the exaggerated demands of the mother for grown-up behaviour. We suggest that cancer patients too, learn that they have to make every effort to fulfil the expectations of others in order to gain their love. They feel that they cannot live without the approval of a beloved, idealized person; in childhood this may be the mother, but the focus may later shift to a spouse, the patient's own child, or even a colleague at work. On the experience of loss, other severe life events or even shocking behaviour by the beloved person, the patient realizes that his or her efforts are useless, and reacts with chronic hopelessness.

These notions are consistent with other studies of coping and survival among cancer patients. Much of the research into the personality traits of cancer patients has been methodologically weak, with retrospective designs and assessments by investigators who were not blind to diagnosis (Morrison and Paffenbarger, 1981). However, Greer and Morris (1975) administered structured interviews and standarized tests to 160 consecutive admissions for breast tumour biopsy, then compared those subsequently found to have cancer with benign breast disease. Breast cancer was associated with an apparently life-long tendency to suppress anger. This suppressed anger was shown to correlate with elevations of serum IgA (Pettingale et al., 1977). Similar factors may affect survival after diagnosis. Greer et al. (1979) found that survival five years after the diagnosis of breast cancer was significantly related to psychological responses assessed at three months. Women considered on the basis of a structured interview to show "denial" or "fighting spirit" had a better prognosis than those displaying "stoic acceptance" or "helplessness/hopelessness". Similarly, Derogatis et al. (1979) found that women with breast cancer who survived more than one year had higher ratings on measures of hostility and anger than those who died within the first year.

The results of these studies suggested to us that psychotherapeutic interventions aimed at modifying these characteristics might not only improve the quality of patients' lives, but might prolong their survival time.

PREVIOUS PSYCHOTHERAPY RESEARCH IN ONCOLOGY

Psychotherapeutic interventions in cancer have taken several forms. Many clinicians have been concerned with the psychiatric sequelae of a diagnosis of cancer, and have developed counselling procedures to aid adjustment to the disease. These range from the group procedures pioneered by Yalom and associates (1977) to the comprehensive rehabilitation programmes developed in Israel by Izsak *et al.* (1973). These and other procedures are reviewed elsewhere (Meyerowitz, 1980; Holland and Rowland, 1981); they share many characteristics with the coronary rehabilitation programmes described in Chapter 10 by Langosch. The present chapter concerns the use of psychotherapy in the treatment of cancer, rather than as an aid to rehabilitation and adjustment. Research in this area was pioneered by LeShan and LeShan (1971) and Bahnson (1976). More complete descriptions have been published by Simonton *et al.* (1980). Their technique has three parts. In the central part, patients are trained in muscular relaxation and regular breathing, and this is coupled with mental imagery. The imagery, which includes visualization of white cells acting on the malignancy, is intended to desensitize the patients about cancer, increase the flexibility of thinking and release anger and resentment. Patients are encouraged to develop a sense of mastery over the disease. The second part consists of counselling, which includes assertiveness training to improve emotional outlets, goal setting, guided fantasy about disease recurrence and death, and the clarification of underlying beliefs and fears. Thirdly, patients are educated about the benefits of physical exercise. Simonton *et al.* (1980) report that patients undergoing this procedure survive rather longer than would have been expected from national statistics; however, controlled studies have not been performed. The effects on survival time may be products of improved patient motivation, greater confidence in treatment and positive expectancies. Indeed, a survey of the international literature suggests that no quasi-experimental research has been performed in this area. Factors such as the nature of the psychotherapy, the personality of the therapists, contra-indications for therapy and the interaction with medical treatments have not been evaluated. Most of the literature describes preliminary results based on case studies. Randomized designs with appropriate allocation of patients to treatment and control groups have not been reported. In our research programme, we have therefore undertaken two clinically-controlled randomized quasi-experimental studies, in order to investigate the effects of psychotherapy and its interaction with medical treatment.

The psychotherapies investigated in these studies are based on concepts derived from the aetiological research described above (Grossarth-Maticek *et al.*, 1982, 1983a,b). Our assumption is that the development of cancer is related to disturbances of inter-personal relationships in patients. Therapies that present behavioural alternatives to patients will enable them to express their emotional needs more effectively. It is argued that a failure to express these needs is central to the problem. Not only the behaviour but the values and assumptions associated with it may require analysis and restructuring. Since anxiety was negatively associated with cancer incidence in the prospective study summarized earlier, it is suggested that awareness and verbalization of anxiety may be valuable to the psychotherapeutic process. The dimension of hopelessness may be countered by an intense will to live, while survival may also be enhanced by increased self esteem. In summary, we conceptualize the goals of the psychotherapy as increasing the will to live, reducing hopelessness, increasing anxiety and self esteem, and releasing the expression of feelings and emotional needs.

THE FIRST PSYCHOTHERAPY EXPERIMENT

The following hypotheses were examined in this study. First, it was postulated that cancer patients who have undergone psychotherapy will survive for longer than those not treated. Secondly, different psychological interventions will vary in their effects on survival time, according to their impact on the psychosocial variables mentioned above. Thirdly, it was hypothesized that psychotherapy and chemotherapy have a synergistic effect on survival time. Finally, it is possible that the effects of psychotherapy may be mediated by alterations in immune function.

Three different types of psychotherapy were compared in this study:

(i) *Behaviour Therapy* This treatment was performed by three experienced behaviour therapists. Therapists and patients together developed a list of desirable and undesirable behaviours. Desirable behaviours (such as the ability to speak freely to strangers) were encouraged in a progressive step-by-step fashion. Undesirable symptoms (such as the wish to run away at the sight of strangers) were modified by imagery and desensitization, in the hope of extinguishing them from the patient's repertoire.

(ii) *Depth Psychotherapy* Three therapists with an orientation towards depth psychology and classical psycho-analysis carried out this procedure. Emphasis was placed on the genesis of psychosocial maladjustments. The psychological problem was considered to result from a sequence of traumatic experiences in early childhood. During sessions, therapists and patients explored the origin and dynamics of their behaviour, and through the revival of early trauma, patients gained insight into the original fixation. It is assumed in this form of psychotherapy that lasting changes in behaviour can only emerge with alteration in these basic problems.

(iii) *Creative Novation Therapy* (Novation means the substitution of a new obligation for an old one.) This therapy has been developed by Grossarth-Maticek for use with cancer patients. It is a form of cognitive behaviour therapy, uniting the principles of learning underlying conventional behavioural techniques with certain psychodynamic concepts. The therapy is designed to "hysterize" the patient, i.e. it enables the patient to express needs that have previously been inhibited, and to engage in more satisfying social interactions. It is assumed that undesirable behaviour patterns are guided by cognitive–emotional programmes (values and assumptions) which can be modified. Through a careful analysis, the conflicting needs of the patient are identified. These are considered to be approach–avoidance conflicts, but are also similar to double-binds (e.g. "I love my husband who died two years ago. I believe that I cannot live without him, therefore, I wish to die to be reunited with him. But I also love to live and to have good relations with my children."). The next therapeutic step is to define with the patient alternative behaviour and patterns of cognitive interpretation. No attempt is made to dismantle the structure of emotional needs (as in depth psychotherapy), but rather to bring resolution by substitution of new cognitive programmes (e.g. "I love my mother but I have always thought I would betray her if I loved another woman. Now I realize that I am able to love both at the same time. Therefore, I do not feel guilty any more."). Relaxation and suggestion are used to emphasize these alternative cognitive interpretations. In addition, a programme of concrete behavioural changes is developed with the patient, and he or she is encouraged to work on these at home.

The design of the study is outlined in Fig. 2. One hundred and seventy-nine women with breast cancer and visceral metastases, to whom a Doxorubicin (adriblastine or adriamycin) combination chemotherapy had been proposed, were asked whether they would like to receive psychotherapy at the same time. Seventeen refused psychotherapy, and another 56 declined chemotherapy. Fifty of the women who acccept chemotherapy were divided into pairs, matched on age, social background, extent of cancer and medical treatment. A similar procedure was applied to 50 of those who refused chemotherapy, while the remainder were excluded from the design. One member of each pair was chosen at random to be treated with psychotherapy, while the other received no psychotherapy. A 2×2 design was

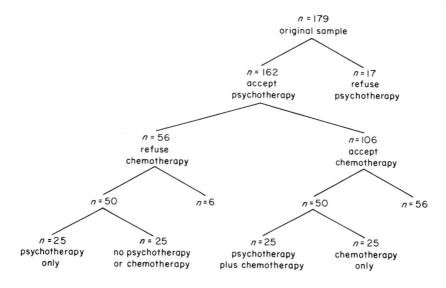

Fig. 2 Selection of the four groups for Experiment 1.

therefore completed (psychotherapy/no psychotherapy; chemotherapy/no chemotherapy) with 25 women in each condition. Patients were allocated to the different psychotherapies at random. Twenty-four patients received Creative Novation Therapy, 12 underwent depth psychotherapy, while the remaining 14 were treated with behaviour therapy. Patients who accepted or refused chemotherapy were distributed proportionately to the different therapies.

The sequence of events is summarized in Table 1. Before treatment, self-ratings of psychosocial parameters were made, predominantly using 9-point scales. These were repeated at appropriate phases of the study. More details of these measures are provided below. Chemotherapy consisted of Doxorubicin (adriamycin) in combination with other agents. Doxorubicin was combined with cyclophosphamide (Endoxana) in seven pairs, with fluorouracil in 13 pairs, and with vincristine in one pair. The remaining four pairs received a combination of Doxorubicin, fluorouracil, vincristine, cyclophosphamide and prednisolone. Chemotherapy was administered in three to four week cycles and repeated between four and nine times. Thirty hours of psychotherapy was provided, as shown in Table 1. Various alterations were made in chemotherapy as appropriate. The outcome variables included the interval between surgery and the detection

TABLE 1 Temporal description of first experiment

t_0	Diagnosis of breast cancer
	↓
t_1	Operation
	↓
t_2	Radiation or adjuvant chemotherapy
	↓
t_3	Diagnosis of visceral metastases
	↓
t_4	Combination chemotherapy proposed
	↓
t_5	Refusal or acceptance of chemotherapy and psychotherapy
	↓
t_6	Ten hours of psychotherapy
	↓
t_7	First cycle of combination chemotherapy
	↓
t_8	Ten hours of psychotherapy
	↓
t_9	Second cycle of combination chemotherapy
	↓
t_{10}	Ten hours of psychotherapy
	↓
t_{11}	Third cycle of combination chemotherapy
t_{12}. . . .	

of metastases or new recidivism and the interval between metastases and death. These two intervals in combination comprise the total survival time. The results presented here concern the relationship between intervention variables (chemotherapy and psychotherapy) and outcome variables (total survival time, changes in leucocyte concentration and lymphocyte percentage, and changes in psychosocial variables). Multiple linear regression and analyses of variance or covariance were employed in the statistical analyses.

The mean survival time of all 100 patients was 15.7 months, with a standard deviation of 7.3 months. Total survival times ranged from 6 to 38 months. The relationship between psychotherapy, chemotherapy and survival time is summarized in Table 2. Chemotherapy alone increased survival time by 2.80 months ($P < 0.001$), while psychotherapy alone increased survival by 3.64 months ($P < 0.001$). If the two effects were additive, one would expect a survival time of $11.28 + 2.80 + 3.64 = 17.72$ months for the group with combined therapies. However, the mean survival time of the chemotherapy plus psychotherapy group was 22.40 months, exceeding the additive value by 4.68 ($P < 0.05$). This indicates that

TABLE 2 Survival time in months of women in the four conditions

| | | Chemotherapy | | |
		no	yes	totals
Psychotherapy	no	mean = 11.28 $n = 25$	mean = 14.08 $n = 25$	mean = 12.68
	yes	mean = 14.92 $n = 25$	mean = 22.40 $n = 25$	mean = 18.66
totals		mean = 13.10	mean = 18.24	grand mean = 15.67 $n = 100$

a positive interaction between chemotherapy and psychotherapy takes place, and that they operate synergistically.

Since chemotherapy was not randomly assigned to subjects, it is possible that differences in the initial values of metastases detection time or psychosocial variables contribute to the pattern of results. These factors were, therefore, controlled by multiple regression. In the case of chemotherapy, the results of this procedure depended on the method of analysis. If chemotherapy was analysed as a dummy variable (yes–no), its effects after controlling for initial values of metastases detection time and psychosocial variables was no longer significant. If, on the other hand, chemotherapy was analysed in terms of the number of treatment periods (which frequently extended beyond the three cycles illustrated in Table 1), it retained its statistical significance. In contrast, the effects of psychotherapy were scarcely reduced by controlling for these initial factors; this is to be expected, since psychotherapy was randomly allocated to subjects. After controlling for initial values and metastases detection time, the interventions taken together account for 37% of the variance in survival time.

The impact of psychotherapy on the intervening variables (both psychosocial and physiological) that may mediate effects are illustrated in the path diagram shown in Fig. 3. Again, the coefficients reported are standardized, partiallized regression coefficients, indicating the strength of the relationships between psychotherapy and different target variables, after controlling for initial values. Psychotherapy had a significant effect on the six psychosocial variables thought to be significant in the process. It led to an increase in the will or drive to live, self esteem and anxiety, a decrease in the wish to die, less inter-personal or social repression, and less blocking of emotional expression. Psychotherapy was also associated with a less negative response to the side-effects of chemotherapy, and an increase in the lymphocyte percentage.

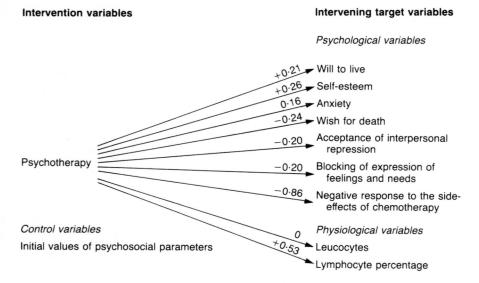

Fig. 3   Psychotherapy, physiological and psychosocial variables.

Figure 4 summarizes the relationship of intervening psychosocial variables with survival time. Changes in the psychosocial variables (controlling for their initial values) were added to the multivariate analysis of survival time. The error term (e) is the square root of the unexplained variance. In this analysis, psychotherapy no longer has a significant effect; this suggests that the effects of psychotherapy were mediated through the psychosocial variables. Chemotherapy has a significant effect when assessed in terms of number of treatment periods. The factors included in Fig. 4 are ordered according to their statistical significance ($P < 0.05$, $F = 3.64$). The most significant variable was "change in pathological social interactions". The unexpected positive association of "blocking of expression of feelings and needs" is presumably due to multi-collinearity. Figure 4 suggests that our model was very successful in terms of a proportion of variance explained; only 17% of variance was not accounted for. The adjusted squared multiple correlation of all the variables with survival time is 0.79. This means that 79% of the variance can be attributed to initial conditions, interventions and their effects.

The three forms of psychotherapy were not equivalent in their effects. The mean survival time in months of patients in the three conditions is shown in Table 3. Creative Novation Therapy led to significantly longer survival than either of the other procedures ($P < 0.001$). This difference

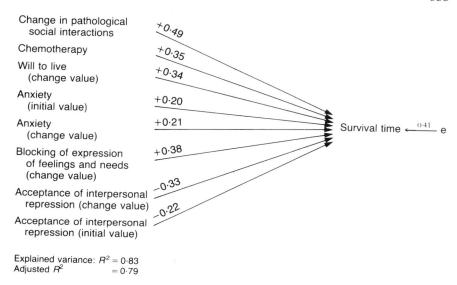

Change in pathological
social interactions   +0.49

Chemotherapy   +0.35

Will to live
(change value)   +0.34

Anxiety
(initial value)   +0.20

Anxiety
(change value)   +0.21   Survival time ←—0.41— e

Blocking of expression
of feelings and needs
(change value)   +0.38

Acceptance of interpersonal   −0.33
repression (change value)
                                      −0.22
Acceptance of interpersonal
repression (initial value)

Explained variance: R^2 = 0.83
Adjusted R^2 = 0.79

Fig. 4 Determinants of survival time.

remains significant even when initial conditions are controlled by analysis of covariance. Similar differences between the therapies were found in respect of changes in psychosocial variables. Deep psychotherapy was also weaker than behaviour therapy in the majority of measures.

It was considered necessary to involve the families of 12 patients who were receiving Creative Novation Therapy. When initial conditions were controlled statistically, family therapy was associated with a marginally significant improvement in survival time. Patients' perceptions of psychotherapy were assessed through a 10-item questionnaire, administered

TABLE 3 Survival time according to type of psychotherapy

Type of psychotherapy	Survival time in months	
Behaviour therapy	mean	15.29
	n	14
Creative Novation Therapy	mean	23.54
	n	24
Depth psychotherapy	mean	12.83[a]
	n	12
Total	mean	18.66
	n	50

[a]Compare with the row mean of 12.68 for non-psychotherapy subjects in Table 2.

at the end of treatment; each was scored with a 9-point rating scale. However, these items showed a strong uni-dimensional pattern, so that a single score was constructed. Principally, this represents acceptance and belief in the therapists, the impression that important issues have been taken up in therapy, and that new feelings, thoughts and behaviour have been acquired. This combined score was strongly associated with survival time ($r^2 = 0.69$) and also with positive changes in the psychosocial variables.

Overall, the results suggest that psychotherapy may have a valuable effect on the prognosis of women with breast cancer. Procedures based on depth psychotherapy had little or no effect on survival. Perhaps these depth techniques improve insight into existing personality deficits, rather than producing immediate alterations in behaviour. Such methods may take many years to produce behaviour changes, since patients are required to reconstruct their personalities before they can expect behaviour changes. In addition, patients frequently become distressed soon after the beginning of therapy, as they begin to acknowledge the magnitude of their difficulties. Depth psychotherapy needs a considerable amount of time, and this is something that metastatic cancer patients cannot afford. Indeed, we would argue that psychotherapies that uncover psychological problems without presenting simultaneous cognitive and behavioural alternatives may even increase the sense of hopelessness experienced by patients.

There was only a modest prolongation in survival time from patients given behaviour therapy. This may be due to the fact that behaviour is modified without taking into account the psychological needs, values and assumptions associated with the behaviour. It may be that for this reason, the alterations in behaviour are neither satisfying nor stable. Our results suggest that psychotherapy may affect prognosis, only if it influences those psychosocial variables that are relevant in aetiology. Modifications in lymphocyte function were also observed, suggesting that effective psychotherapy influences the immune system in a positive way.

THE SECOND PSYCHOTHERAPY EXPERIMENT

The second intervention study was designed to explore a number of hypotheses. The first was that cancer patients who have undergone psychotherapy have a better prognosis than those not treated by psychotherapy; essentially, this was an attempt to replicate the results of the first study. Secondly, we postulated that Creative Novation Therapy has a stronger effect on survival, via the specified psychosocial variables, than other psychotherapies. Thirdly, it was hypothesized that the effects of Creative Novation Therapy on outcome will depend on the degree of training that therapists have undertaken.

Four groups of psychotherapy patients were compared, both with each other and with no psychotherapy controls. Three groups received Creative Novation Therapy from therapists with different degrees of experience. Group 1 ($n = 13$) was treated by Grossarth-Maticek. Group 2 ($n = 13$) was treated by therapists who had undertaken a 100 hour training course on the principles and practice of Creative Novation Therapy. Group 3 ($n = 13$) was treated by therapists who had received an introduction to Creative Nova-tion Therapy over an eight hour course, but applied their conventional therapeutic procedures to these principles. Group 4 ($n = 10$) received either depth psychotherapy or behaviour therapy, and their therapists were not provided with any information about the principles of Creative Novation Therapy.

The participants in the trial were 98 patients with regional lymph metastases, treated radiologically after surgery. All patients had agreed to receive psychotherapy for 20 h during radiotherapy (for further details of the medical treatments and data see Grossarth-Maticek *et al.*, 1983c). Patients were placed in matched pairs, and one member of the pair was assigned at random to psychotherapy; the other acted as a control. The four psychotherapy groups were comparable in terms of age, sex, type of cancer, the extent of regional lymph metastases and surgery. Patients were fol-lowed up for 94 months.

The main results concerning the effectiveness of psychotherapy are shown in Tables 4 and 5. Total survival times for the four therapy groups are given in Table 4. It can be seen that the greatest difference between therapy and control was found in Group 1. In the case of Group 4,

TABLE 4 Total survival time in the four conditions

		n	Mean	Standard deviation	Mean difference (psychotherapy control)	Standard Deviation of difference
Creative Group 1	Therapy	13	55.15	35.56	9.39	12.36
	Control	13	45.77	30.97		
NovationGroup 2	Therapy	13	52.08	33.75	6.77	15.08
	Control	13	45.31	31.60		
Therapy Group 3	Therapy	13	48.85	30.85	4.84	17.15
	Control	13	44.00	28.60		
Other psycho-therapy Group 4	Therapy	10	30.80	17.59	−14.20	19.30
	Control	10	45.00	29.72		

TABLE 5   Mean pair differences (psychotherapy minus control) by treatment condition

Therapy group	no. of pairs	X = Time from diagnosis to occurrence of distant metastases	Y = Time from occurrence of distant metastases to death	Z = Total survival time $X + Y$
Creative	1	13	15.8 $n = 12; P = 0.009$	-8.0 $n = 12$; n.s.	9.4 $n = 13$ (10) $P = 0.018$
Novation	2	13	4.1 $n = 11; P = 0.42$	3.8 $n = 11$; n.s.	6.8 n.s.
Therapy	3	13	-3.4 $n = 11$; n.s.	5.6 $n = 11$; n.s.	4.8 n.s.
Other therapies	4	10	-19.5 $n = 10; P = 0.003$	5.3 $n = 10$; n.s.	-14.2 $P = 0.045$

psychotherapy was evidently associated with a poorer prognosis than no psychotherapy. These results are extended in Table 5, where mean pair differences (therapy minus control) are shown for three outcome criteria: time from diagnosis to occurrence of distant metastases, time from occurrence of distant metastases to death, and total survival time. These results indicate that patients given psychotherapy in Group 1 lived for an average of 9.4 months longer than their paired controls; this difference is significant ($P < 0.018$). On the other hand, the total survival time of psychotherapy patients in Group 4 was significantly less (mean 14.2 months, $P < 0.05$) than that of paired controls. Some differences for intermediate variables were also observed. The pair difference in time from diagnosis to occurrence of distant metastases was significant for Group 1 ($P < 0.009$), and also for Group 4 ($P < 0.003$). In none of the groups were there significant differences in the interval between the occurrence of distant metastases and death. Comparing the groups, analysis of variance indicated that survival time was significantly different in the four conditions. However, there were no reliable differences in total survival time between Groups 1, 2 and 3.

These data suggest that Creative Novation Therapy has a positive effect on survival in patients with advanced cancer. This effect was not reliably associated with degree of therapist experience, although the means suggest that longer survival was linked with more experienced therapists. This possibility is endorsed by the fact that three therapy cases in Group 1 were still alive at the end of the observation period after 94 months. These patients were given total survival scores of 94, even though the true mean was somewhat greater. In contrast, the procedures applied to patients in Group 4 apparently had a deleterious effect on total survival time and the interval before occurrence of distant metastases.

A number of psychosocial variables were associated with the improvement in prognosis in Creative Novation Therapy, as was found in the first study. Factors such as change in pathogenic social interactions, the will to live and increase in emotional expression were all associated with outcome. Further insight into the process of therapy was gained by carrying out a multiple regression with survival time as the dependent variable and therapy/no therapy and initial measurement of psychosocial variables as independent factors. The 13 pairs in Group 1 were included in this analysis. The initial measurement of psychosocial variables was taken after the therapist had outlined the proposed procedures to all patients. Half of them had subsequently been told that it would not be possible to make therapy available to them. In the multiple regression, the therapy/no therapy factor was insignificant ($F = 0.6$), while the variable "I pray for improvement" was highly significant (standardized partiallized regression coefficient $= 0.78$). Two other factors, the "wish to die" and hysterical "cry for help" behaviour were also significant determinants of survival time (regression coefficients $= 0.25$ and -0.33 respectively). Similar patterns were observed when outcome was recorded in terms of the interval before the occurrence of distant metastases, rather than total survival time. Once again, the therapy/no therapy variable was not significant, while the other three factors continued to play an important part.

These data suggest that the positive effects of Creative Novation Therapy in Group 1 were due in large part to psychosocial changes which had occurred before the treatment had really commenced. If the events later in therapy had had any effect on the course of disease, this would have been expressed in differences between therapy and no therapy conditions. It is possible that the initial presentation of the therapy gives patients new hope, replacing the state of hopelessness and depression which characterizes these people.

CONCLUSIONS

The studies described in this chapter indicate that psychotherapy may improve the chances of survival for extended periods in patients found to have cancer. The most effective intervention is Creative Novation Therapy, particularly when in the hands of its originator. The effects of treatment by Grossarth-Maticek may be partially ascribed to his personal impact, but is also a product of his extensive experience with this procedure. Much of the beneficial effect of the therapy may be due to the replacement of hopelessness by new optimism in the initial phases of the intervention. The results produced by other psychotherapies in the second study were less good than those found in Experiment 1. Possibly this was due to specific differences in procedure, or to the differing patient groups. We would argue that procedures which uncover psychological problems without offering immediate behavioural and cognitive alternatives may have a serious negative effect on patients with malignancies.

Psychotherapy interacted synergistically with chemotherapy in the experiment on patients with breast cancer. In the second experiment, all patients were receiving radiotherapy, so this interaction could not be analysed. The results, however, suggest that psychotherapy should not be seen as an alternative to conventional treatments, but as a supplementary procedure. The impact of psychotherapy on its own (Table 2) was modest.

The present results suggest that psychotherapeutic interventions should be seriously considered in the management of patients with cancer. Such methods may not only assist patients in their adjustment to their disease and its effect on their lives, but may also improve prognosis. However, the evaluation of psychotherapy can only be undertaken in a multi-disciplinary fashion, with careful assessment of medical, immunological and clinical as well as psychosocial aspects.

REFERENCES

Bahnson, C. B. (1976). Characteristics of a psychotherapeutic treatment program for cancer. Paper presented at the 3rd International Symposium on Detection and Prevention of Cancer, New York.

Bastiaans, J. (1967). Der Beitrag der Psychoanalyse zur psychosomatischen Medizin. In "Die Psychologie des 20 Jahrhunderts" (D. Eicke, ed.), pp. 960–995. Kindler-Verlag, Zurich.

Bastiaans, J. (1974). Neue psychodynamische und psychobiologische Aspekte der Hysterie. *Praxis Psychother.* **50,** 159–167.

Derogatis, L. R., Abeloff, M. D. and Melisaratos, M. (1979). Psychological coping mechanisms and survival time in metastatic breast cancer. *J. Am. Med. Ass.* **242,** 1504–1508.

Fox, B. H. (1981). Behavioral issues in cancer. In "Perspectives on Behavioral Medicine" (S. M. Weiss, J. A. Herd, and B. H. Fox, eds), pp. 101–134. Academic Press, Orlando, New York and London.

Greer, S. and Morris, T. (1979). Psychological attributes of women who develop breast cancer: a controlled study. *J. Psychosom. Res.* **19,** 147–153.

Greer, S., Morris, T. and Pettingale, K. W. (1979). Psychological response to breast cancer: effect on outcome. *Lancet* **ii,** 785–787.

Grossarth-Maticek, R. (1980). Psychosocial predictors of cancer and internal diseases. An overview. *Psychother. Psychosom.* **33,** 122–128.

Grossarth-Maticek, R., Kanazir, D. T., Schmidt, P. and Vetter, H. (1982). Psychosomatic factors in the process of cancerogenesis. *Psychother. Psychosom.* **38,** 284–302.

Grossarth-Maticek, R., Kanazir, D. T., Schmidt, P. and Vetter, H. (1983a). Psychosocial factors involved in the process of cancerogenesis. Preliminary results of the Yugoslav Prospective Study. *Psychother. Psychosom.,* **40,** 191–210.

Grossarth-Maticek, R., Bastiaans, J., Schmidt, P. and Vetter, H. (1983b). Psychosomatic factors in the process of cancerogenesis: The Heidelberg Prospective Study. VII World Congress of the International College of Psychosomatic Medicine, Hamburg.

Grossarth-Maticek, R., Schmidt, P. and Vetter, H. (1983c). "Psychotherapy and Radiotherapy in Cancer Patients." Heidelberg.

Holland, J. C. and Rowland, J. H. (1981). Psychiatric, social and behavioral interventions in the treatment of cancer: an historical overview. In "Perspectives on Behavioral Medicine" (S. M. Weiss, J. A. Herd and B. H. Fox, eds), pp. 235–260. Academic Press, Orlando, New York and London.

Izsak, F. C., Engel, J. and Medalie, J. H. (1973). Comprehensive rehabilitation of the patient with cancer. J. Chron. Dis. 26, 363–374.

LeShan, L. and LeShan, E. (1971). Psychotherapy and the patient with a limited life span. Psychiatry 24, 318–326.

Meyerowitz, B. E. (1980). Psychosocial correlates of breast cancer and its treatment. Psychol. Bull. 87, 108–131.

Morrison, F. R. and Paffenbarger, R. A. (1981). Epidemiological aspects of biobehavior in the aetiology of cancer: a critical review. In "Perspectives on Behavioral Medicine" (S. M. Weiss, J. A. Herd and B. H. Fox, eds). pp. 135–162. Academic Press, Orlando, New York and London.

Pettingale, K. W., Greer, S. and Tee, D. H. (1977). Serum IgA and emotional expression in breast cancer patients. J. Psychosom. Res 31, 395–399.

Simonton, O. C., Matthews-Simonton, S. and Sparks, T. F. (1980). Psychological intervention in the treatment of cancer. Psychosomatics 21, 226–233.

Yalom, I. and Greaves, C. (1977). Group therapy with the terminally ill. Am. J. Psychiat. 134, 396–400.

Index